Suggestions for Addressing Clinical and Non-Clinical Issues in Palliative Care

Edited by Marco Cascella and Michael John Stones

Published in London, United Kingdom

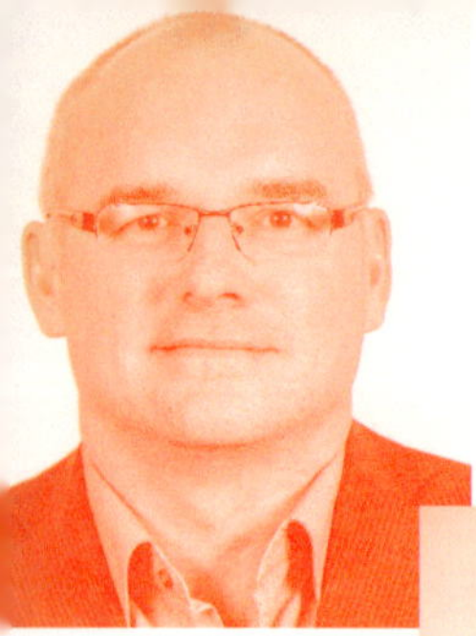
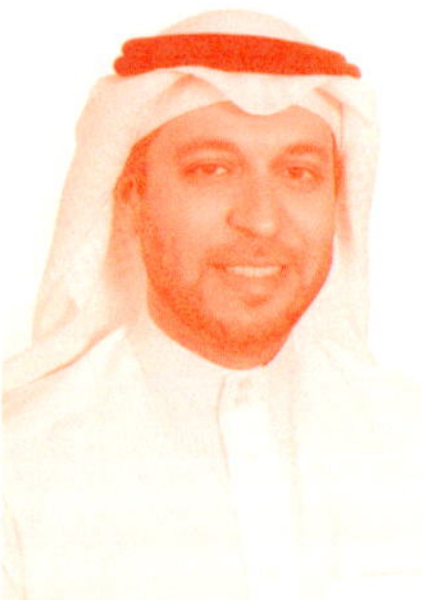
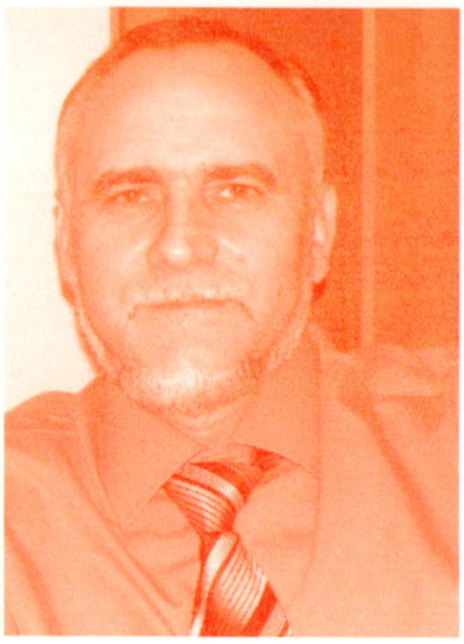
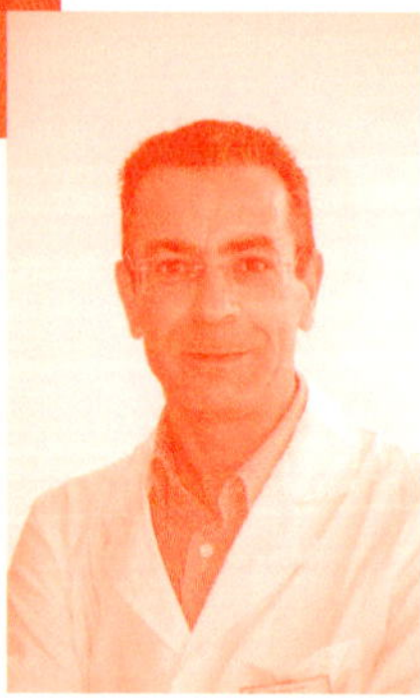
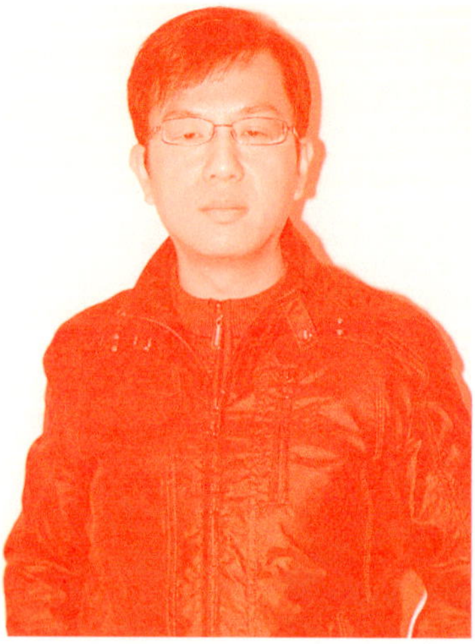
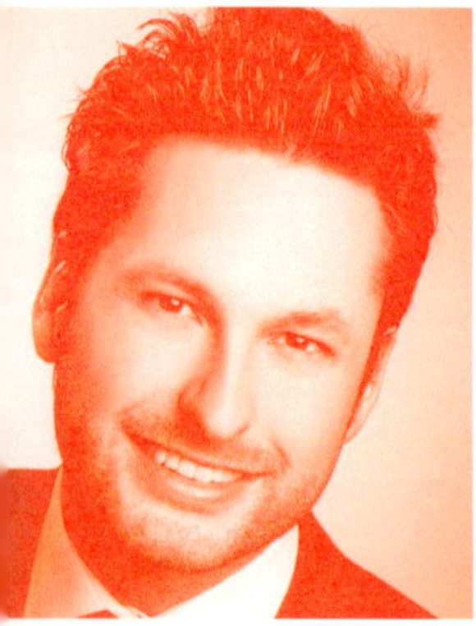
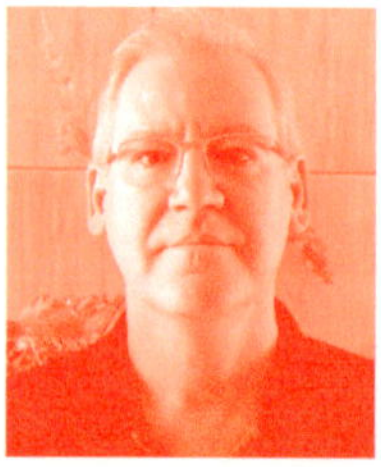

IntechOpen

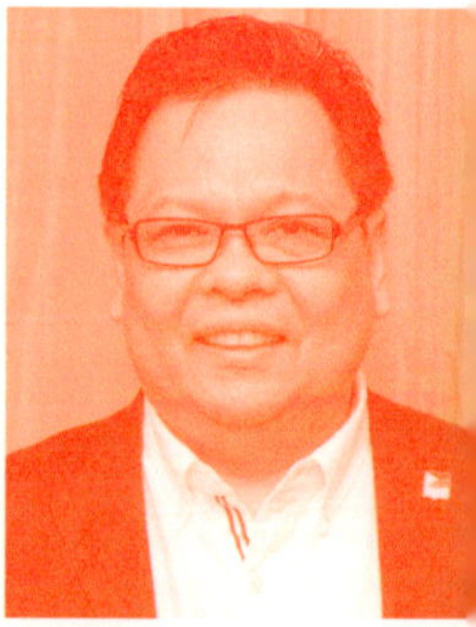
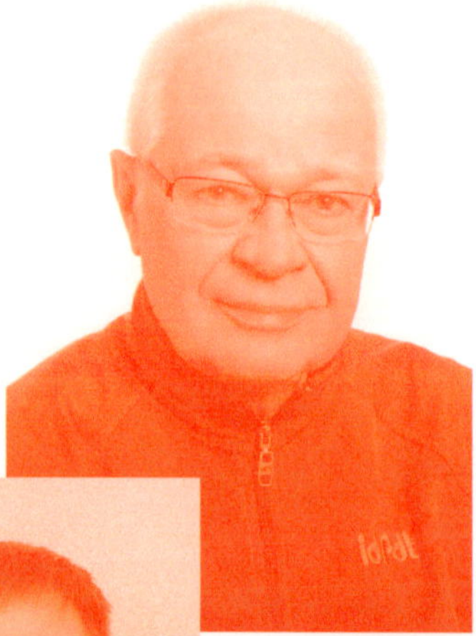
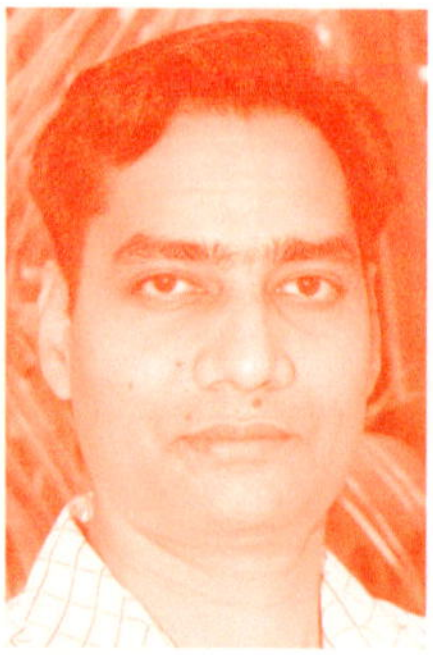
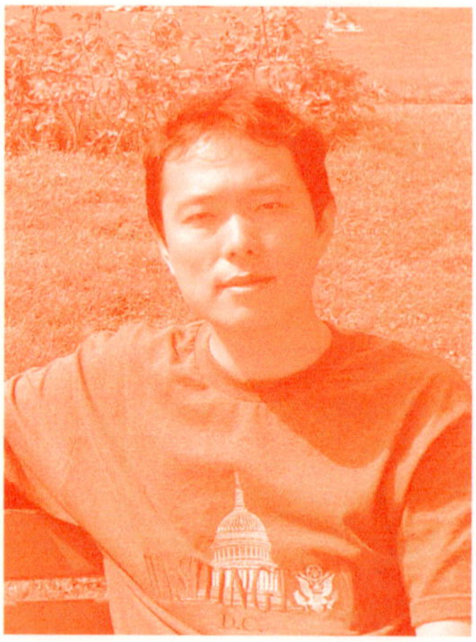
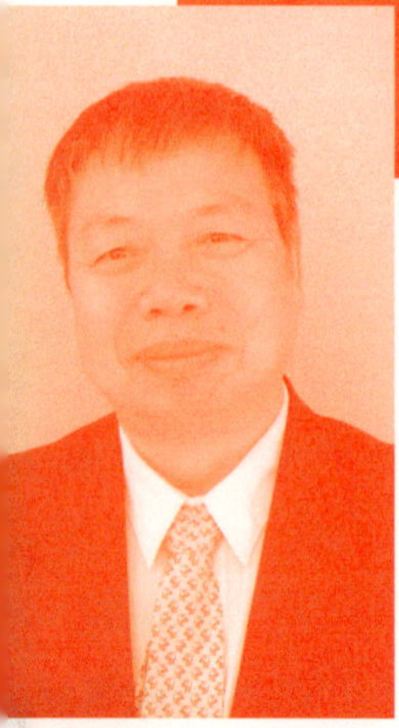
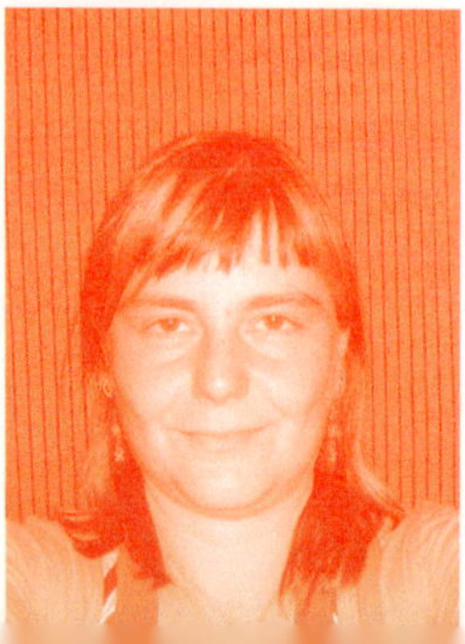

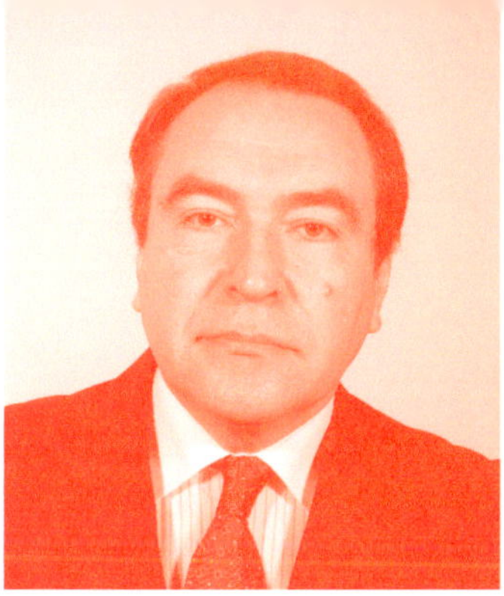

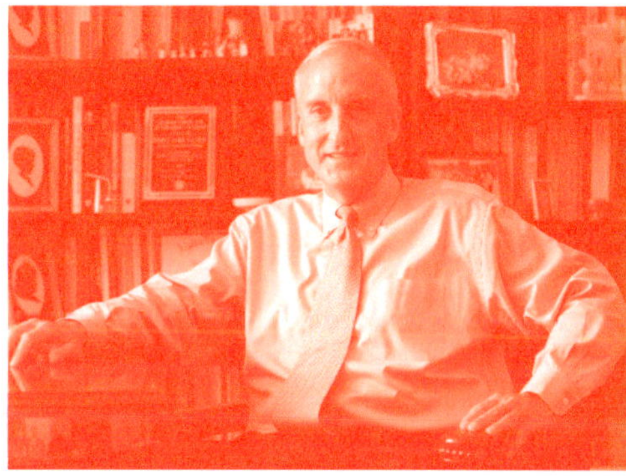

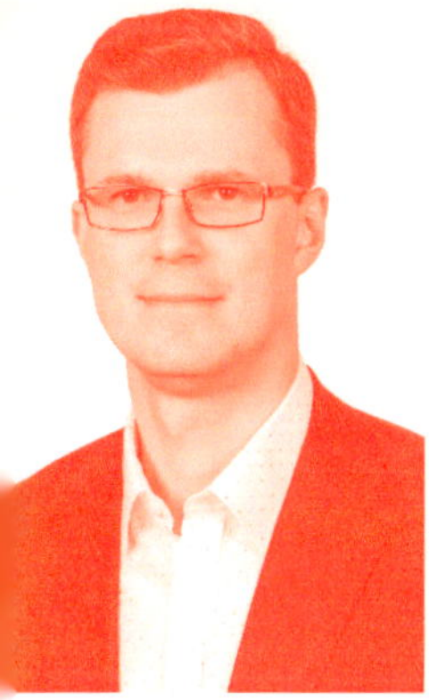

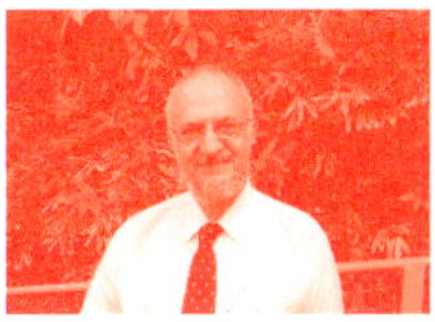

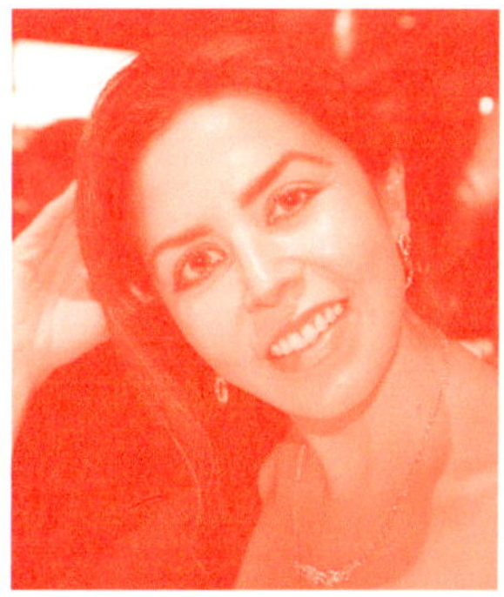

Supporting open minds since 2005

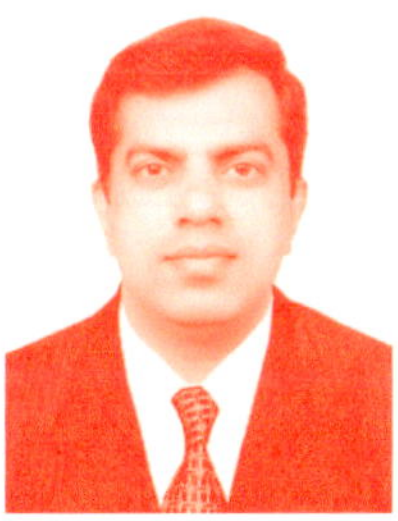

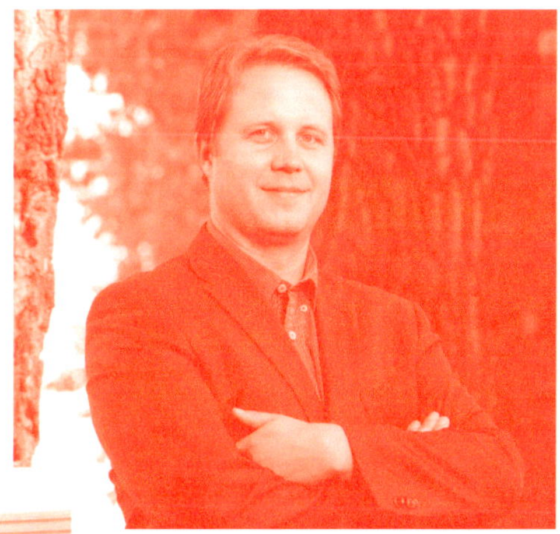

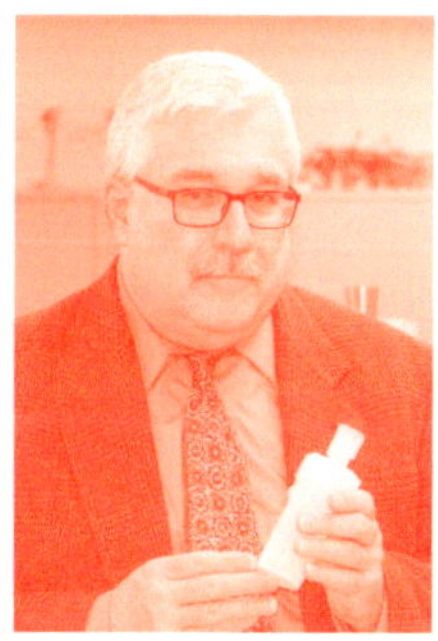

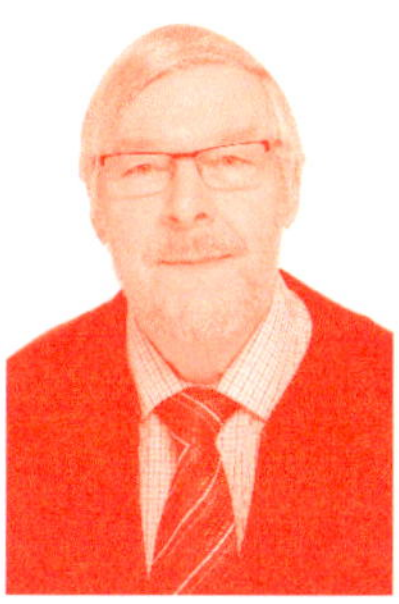

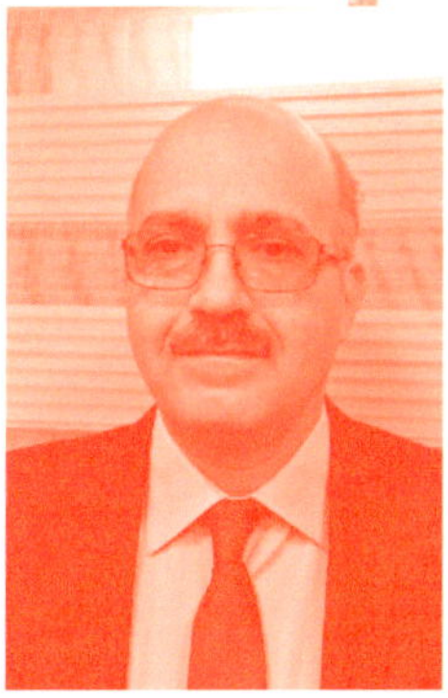

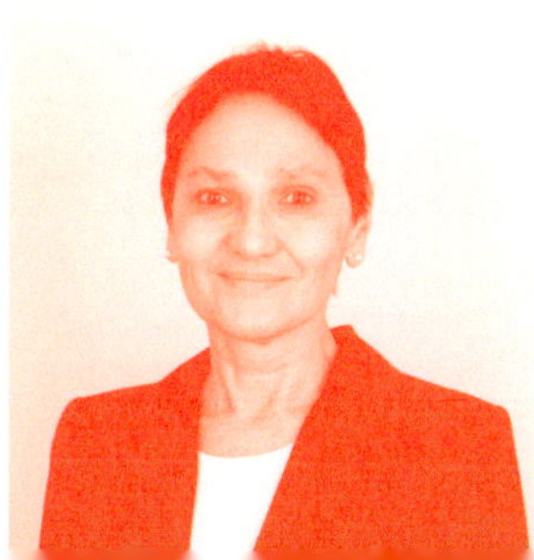

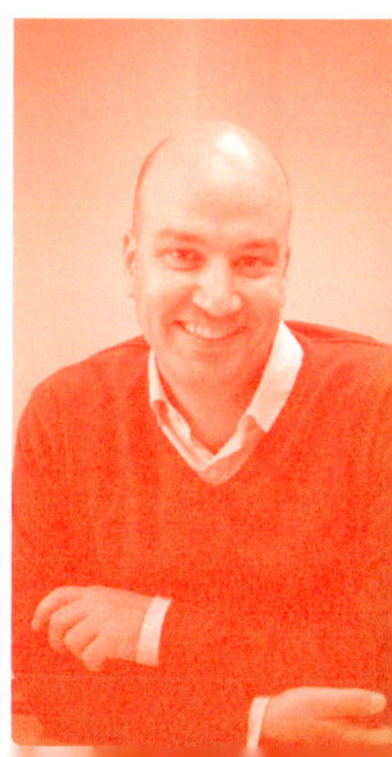

Suggestions for Addressing Clinical and Non-Clinical Issues in Palliative Care
http://dx.doi.org/10.5772/intechopen.92471
Edited by Marco Cascella and Michael John Stones

Contributors
Ekaete Francis Asuquo, Paulina Ackley Ackley Akpan-Idiok, Mira Florea, Aida Puia, Rodica Sorina Sorina Pop, Akon Ndiok, Busiswe Ncama, Emilia Oyira, Michael John Stones, Jason Randle, Peter Brink, Prasit Mahawongkajit, Farida Hanna Campbell, Monika Náležinská, Josef Chovanec, Rasheed Ofosu-Poku, Suzanne Crowe, Maeve McAllister, Roisin Ni Charra, Ann-Marie Crowe, Julie Edwards, Anshika Arora, Sonika Charak, Soumya Sharma, Manish Shandilya, Prabhu Prasad Das, Elisabetta Di Liso, María Teresa García-Baquero Merino, María Victoria Roqué Sánchez, Katherine Pettus, Kristi M. M Soileau, Chandra Mohan Srivastava, Robin Thattil, Sourav Goswami, Marija V. Sholjakova, Vesna M. Durnev, Marco Cascella, Micaela Menarguez Carreño

First published in London, United Kingdom, 2021 by IntechOpen
IntechOpen is the global imprint of INTECHOPEN LIMITED, registered in England and Wales, registration number: 11086078, 5 Princes Gate Court, London, SW7 2QJ, United Kingdom
Printed in Croatia

British Library Cataloguing-in-Publication Data
A catalogue record for this book is available from the British Library

Additional hard and PDF copies can be obtained from orders@intechopen.com

Suggestions for Addressing Clinical and Non-Clinical Issues in Palliative Care
Edited by Marco Cascella and Michael John Stones
p. cm.
Print ISBN 978-1-83969-152-2
Online ISBN 978-1-83969-153-9
eBook (PDF) ISBN 978-1-83969-154-6

For EU product safety concerns:
IN TECH d.o.o., Prolaz Marije Krucifikse Kozulić 3, 51000 Rijeka, Croatia, info@intechopen.com or visit our website at intechopen.com.

Meet the editors

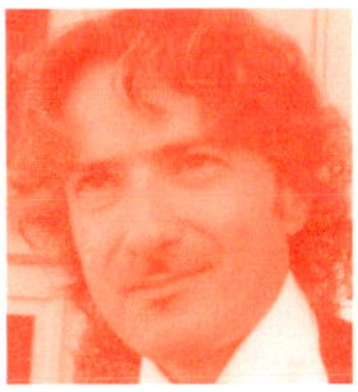

Marco Cascella, MD, works in the Department of Supportive Care at the Istituto Nazionale Tumori, Fondazione "G. Pascale" – IRCCS, Naples, Italy, where he has responsibility for research in anesthesia and pain medicine. He was granted the National Scientific Habilitation (ASN) for Associate Professor of Anesthesiology and Critical Care in Italian Universities and he is annual Professor of Physiology on the Degree Course in Biomedical Laboratory Techniques at the Faculty of Medicine, University "Federico II," Naples. Dr. Cascella graduated with honors in Medicine and Surgery in 1997 from the University "Vanvitelli" of Naples and then undertook postgraduate studies in anesthesia and intensive care, obtaining his doctorate in 2001. He acts as an editorial board member for several medical journals. He has been a speaker at numerous conferences and conventions and is the author of about 150 scientific publications, books, and book chapters in the fields of anesthesia, pathophysiology, treatment of pain, oncology, and palliative care. Dr. Cascella also heads and participates in various research projects.

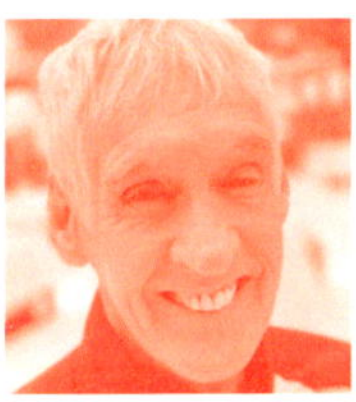

Michael John Stones is best known in academia for his contributions to gerontology. He has authored or edited 9 books, 37 book chapters, and more than 120 scientific articles, and 30 knowledge transmission articles aimed at professional or general readerships. His research interests include subjective well-being and quality of life in older people, age trends in sport and other physical performances, elder abuse, sexuality and intimacy in later life, and the use of health informatics to promote a better quality of care in long-term care settings. Applied endeavors include the development of senior resource centers in Newfoundland, assistance with the development of a resident assessment instrument for mental health used throughout Ontario, and leadership of a scientific team in Quebec that informed the provincial government about policy and practices.

Contents

Preface

Is it necessary to write an additional book on palliative care? This is the question I asked myself when IntechOpen offered me the chance to serve as editor for a book project on the topic. My main doubt was that such a vast argument must be comprehensively addressed for developing a treatise that can be useful for those who already know the subject and for students or non-healthcare providers who are approaching it [1]. Work with these features can take years to complete, and after a treatise is completed, it immediately needs updating.

The alternative is to focus the reader's attention on some aspects of the subject and to commission recognized experts to deal with the individual chapters. Although the result of this approach cannot be compared to a textbook, the editorial path is dynamic, fast, and allows the reader to extrapolate what (for example, a chapter) really interests them.

In truth, in collaboration with the publisher, we had already followed this approach in 2017. With moderate satisfaction, and according to several readers to whom I asked for an opinion, I can affirm that the book Highlights on Several Underestimated Topics in Palliative Care [2] is a decent editorial product. Other publishers have also produced multiple texts on selected issues of palliative care such as pediatric [3] and geriatric palliative care [4], symptom management [5], and ethics [6].

Data from clinical studies, evidence-based medicine investigations, and guidelines continuously enrich the wealth of knowledge in all fields of medicine and therefore also in palliative care. In addition, some topics, such as organizational and policy aspects, are very relevant in this area. On this basis, the idea was to collect updated information on selected topics in a new editorial work. In this sense, this book represents the natural complement of the previous book and the wish to publish another volume in the next 2–3 years. However, even if we started thinking of producing a book with few contributions, the enthusiasm of the authors of the chapters and the incredible commitment of the IntechOpen editorial team, led to the creation of a full-bodied volume. Given its eighteen chapters, and thanks to its systematic nature as well as to the value of the authors, it is very close to a textbook.

This book is divided into five sections.

In the first section we have an Introductory chapter.

The second deals with palliative care topics in selected clinical settings, such as palliative care of the infant and child, and in gynecological oncology. The third section focuses on the role of the caregiver. Expert readers will deepen their knowledge on this aspect of fundamental importance, while those who approach the subject will find useful information. The efforts of the authors to address this particularly sensitive subject are appreciable. Subsequently, the fourth section collects chapters on symptoms and the use/effect of drugs in these particularly vulnerable patients. Since pain is the main symptom, its careful assessment and adequate treatment are mandatory. In this context, the use of opioids represents a milestone. Nevertheless, pain is not the only symptom to address; delirium (see the introductory chapter), depression, nausea, and vomiting (especially by chemotherapy drugs) must be managed in the most appropriate way. Finally, the fifth section is dedicated to ethics, organization, and policy issues. These fascinating chapters represent the added value of this book in which I had the great honor of participating.

Marco Cascella
Department of Supportive Care,
Istituto Nazionale Tumori-IRCCS-Fondazione Pascale,
Napoli, Italy

Michael John Stones
Lakehead University,
Canada

References

[1] R. D. MacLeod, L. Van den Block. Textbook of Palliative Care. Springer. 2019

[2] M. Cascella. Highlight on several underestimated topics in palliative care. Zagreb: Intech Publisher. 2017

[3] J. Amery. A Really PRACTICAL HANDBOOK of Children's Palliative Care ICPCN. 2015

[4] S. Goldhirsch. Geriatric Palliative Care. Oxford University Press. 2014

[5] C.F.B. Regnard, D. Mervyn. A Guide to Symptom Relief in Palliative Care. Radcliffe Publishing 2010

[6] R. C. Macauley. Ethics in Palliative Care: A Complete Guidebooks. Oxford University Press. 2018

Section 1

Introduction

Chapter 1

Introductory Chapter: Delirium in Palliative Care

Marco Cascella

1. Introduction

This introductory chapter aims at presenting an overview of delirium in palliative care. In this setting, it is one of the most frequent, but often misunderstood and difficult to treat, symptoms. Moreover, this is a matter of paramount importance as delirium is associated with a heightened rate of falls, increased cognitive and functional damage, and important patient and family psychological discomfort. In these particularly vulnerable patients, distress — expressed as a feeling of fear, anguish, humiliation — can be deleterious and is ethically unacceptable. Delirium is further associated with increased healthcare costs [1].

The term delirium derives from the Latin word deliria which literally means "to come out of the trace". It refers to a serious change in the mental state that leads to confusion and reduced awareness of the environment. This change is often accompanied by perceptual symptoms, such as hallucinations, or by cognitive symptoms such as disorientation and memory loss [2]. Nevertheless, rather than a symptom, delirium is a complex neurocognitive syndrome characterized by brain dysfunction with perturbations in the degree of consciousness, attention, thinking, perception, memory, psychomotor behavior, emotional sphere, and sleep–wake rhythm [3]. These clinical features differentiate delirium from a state of agitation that can be due to other undetected symptoms or physical needs (e.g., pain or full bladder).

2. The extent of the problem

In the palliative care setting, delirium represents a frequent clinical condition. In patients with advanced cancer, for instance, research showed that its prevalence varies from 13 to 88% [4]. Despite on admission delirium prevalence ranges between 13 to 42%, the higher prevalence occurs in the last 24 to 48 hours of life (terminal delirium), when the phenomenon becomes part of the complex picture of multiorgan dysfunction [5]; in this context, delirium is particularly difficult to treat, and it is considered as the predominant symptom for starting terminal sedation [1]. Overall, the reversibility is about 30% [6] and failure to respond to treatment may become indicative of a worse prognosis already after the first week of palliative care [7].

Despite its high prevalence and clinical significance, delirium is poorly sought; of note, Rainsford et al. [8] demonstrated that the diagnosis of delirium was performed only in 30% of in-hospice patients.

3. Mechanism and causes

The genesis of delirium is multifactorial. In general, all conditions that can induce a neuroinflammatory process are potential causes of delirium. Through the action of cytokines, chemokines, tumor necrosis factor-alpha, and other inflammatory agents (e.g., interleukin (IL)-1, and IL-6), a cascade of events is activated; it culminates in endothelial and microvascular damage and alterations of the blood–brain barrier. Again, disorders of neurotransmitter pathways such as the dopamine and acetylcholine systems, involving respectively dopamine excess or acetylcholine depletion, have a key role in the pathophysiology of delirium [9]. Further, in clinically ill patients, the impairment of cerebral oxidative metabolism is another potential mechanism to be considered [10].

Although drugs such as opioids, anticholinergic drugs, steroids, chemotherapies and metabolic disorders such as metabolic encephalopathy, nutritional deficiencies, electrolyte disturbances, dehydration are the main inducers of delirium, many conditions can provoke delirium. These causes include constipation, infections, hematological changes, paraneoplastic syndromes, brain neoplasms, central nervous system (CNS) secondarisms, seizure disorders, hypoxia, hypo/hypercarbia, and environmental factors. Several acronyms are commonly used to memorize and recognize potential causes. Sometimes the cause of the delirium cannot be found (**Table 1**).

I WATCH DEATH	Infections Withdrawal Acute metabolic causes Trauma CNS pathology Hypoxia Deficiencies Endocrinopathies Acute vascular Toxins or drugs Heavy metals
DELIRIUM	**D**rugs **E**lectrolyte disturbances **L**ack of drugs withdrawals **I**nfection **R**educed sensory input **I**ntracranial infection **U**rinary/fecal retention **M**yocardial/pulmonary causes
THINK	**T**oxic Situations such as shock, dehydration, deliriogenic medications, organ failure **H**ypoxemia **I**nfections **I**mmobilization **N**on-pharmacological interventions **K** or electrolyte problems
DIMES	**D**rugs **I**nfections **M**etabolic **E**nvironmental **S**tructural

Adapted from Bush [3].

Table 1.
Acronyms used to memorize possible causes of delirium in palliative care.

4. Clinical features

According to the type of psychomotor activity, there are three subtypes of delirium:

- Hyperkinetic form. It features agitation, restlessness, with or without hallucinations.
- Hypokinetic form. It is improperly referred to as "quiet delirium" or "acute encephalopathy". This type is featured by apathy, declined responsiveness, reduced psychomotor function, withdrawn attitude, lethargy, and drowsiness.
- Mixed form. The person may exhibit a fluctuation between the hypoactive and hyperactive subtypes where there is an alternation between the hypokinetic form and the hyperkinetic form.

In palliative care, the hypoactive and mixed are the most frequent subtypes of delirium. The lack of tangible agitation and the erroneous belief that the patient is drowsy because of illness, drugs administered, or an underlying depressed habitus, make this subtype very often misunderstood. This is a serious care gap as hypoactive delirium is frequently associated with perceptual disturbances and distress [11].

5. Diagnosis

According to the recently updated guidelines of the National Institute for Health and Clinical Excellence (NICE), the assessment of delirium should be performed in all hospitalized patients who are at risk of experiencing it, including oncological and terminally ill patients (respectively up to 88% and 50% incidence) [12]. Despite this and other recommendations, the lack of a systematic assessment for delirium is a serious issue.

The Diagnostic and Statistical Manual of Mental Disorders (DSM-V, 2013) [2] defined delirium based on four criteria, namely:

- An alteration of consciousness characterized by a reduced ability to focus, maintain or shift attention.
- A cognitive change (such as memory deficit), language alteration, and the development of a perceptual disorder (such as delusion) that are not dependent on a pre-existing condition of dementia.
- A development of the disorder in a short time with daily fluctuations.
- Evidence collected from the medical history, physical examination and laboratory investigations that show that the disorder is caused by physical conditions resulting from a serious pathology, problems of alcohol abuse or drug intoxication, or withdrawal.

Of note, despite DSM-V is the gold standard for the diagnosis of delirium, it cannot be easily administered by non-psychiatrist personnel including nurses. This is a great limitation as nurses have constant contact with the patient throughout the day, and they could efficiently evaluate modifications in the patient's attention and awareness over time. Furthermore, diagnostic instruments for delirium are mostly based on the DSM-III or IV. Thus, many efforts are being made to validate updated versions or to develop new tools [13].

In addition to the DSM-V, the International Classification of Diseases (ICD) classification from the World Health Organization (WHO) is conventionally adopted. The 11th Revision (ICD-11) defined delirium as a neurocognitive disorder characterized by '*disturbed attention (i.e., reduced ability to direct, focus, sustain, and shift attention) and awareness (i.e., reduced orientation to the environment) that develops over a short period of time and tends to fluctuate during the course of a day, accompanied by other cognitive impairment such as memory deficit, disorientation, or impairment in language, visuospatial ability, or perception. Disturbance of the sleep-wake cycle (reduced arousal of acute onset or total sleep loss with reversal of the sleep-wake cycle) may also be present. The symptoms are attributable to a disorder or disease not classified under mental and behavioural disorders or to substance intoxication or withdrawal or to a medication*' [14]. Thus, this approach includes more details on non-cognitive features, and it seems to better address the problem of the diagnostic and pathophysiological difference between delirium and states of dementia.

Practically, suspicion of delirium can be induced by changes or fluctuations in usual behaviors. These fluctuations can occur in the day's course, although more severe symptoms usually manifest during the evening and the night. The diagnosis of delirium requires healthcare professionals who are trained and competent in the diagnosis of delirium. It can be made by referring to tools or simple cognitive tests, for example by having the patient recite the days of the week or the months of the year. Among the most commonly used instruments, there are the Confusion Assessment Method (CAM) [15] and the Delirium Observation Screening (DOS) scale [16]. Although the choice of tool to be used depends on the level of training of the staff, commonly used tests may require a short training period. About CAM, the training manual is available at the website of the American Geriatrics Society [17]. On the contrary, the DOS can be administered without specific training.

The CAM method was also validated in palliative care [18]. It consists of a 9-item questionnaire and a diagnostic algorithm encompassing four items/features. In particular, the features "acute onset and fluctuating course" and "inattention" are needed, along with "disorganized thinking" or "altered level of consciousness" [3]. The DOS scale is a 13-item tool. Since each item can be scored 0 or 1, the total score can range from 0 to 13 and a score of ≥3 indicates delirium. Similar to CAM, it was validated in palliative care patients [19].

Among the other tools, there is the 5-item Nursing Delirium Screening Scale (Nu-DESC) [20]. As Bush et al. [21] highlighted, it offers poor sensitivity for detection of the hypoactive form and is not validated in palliative care. Other tools are the NEECHAM Confusion Scale [22], the 13-item Delirium Rating Scale (DRS) [23] and the Memorial Delirium Assessment Scale (MDAS). This latter was also validated in palliative care [24].

6. Prevention

Prevention is based on early recognition of any precipitating causes. Pharmacological interventions, including antipsychotics, are not recommended as prophylactic strategies. For this purpose, the NICE guidelines recommend only non-pharmacological interventions [12]. Avoiding polypharmacy, in particular delirogenic drugs such as benzodiazepines, opioids, and corticosteroids is of paramount importance for delirium prevention. Moreover, in all frail patients, and even more in the presence of risk factors for delirium, multi-component preventive interventions must be implemented. These approaches are based on temporal–spatial reorientation, mobilization programs, sleep hygiene, maintenance of adequate hydration, and provision of visual and hearing aids, if used by the patient.

7. Therapy

Treatment of delirium often requires the combination of pharmacological (e.g. *major* tranquilizers) and non-pharmacological (reorientation, communication, and sleep hygiene) interventions tailored to the patient.

7.1 Causal therapy

Clinical and physical assessment including appropriate laboratory and radiological investigations can help identify the cause of the delirium. Moreover, rapid recognition and treatment of the underlying cause can often avoid resorting to more complex symptomatic pharmacological and non-pharmacological strategies. Treatment of the underlying cause may include:

- Correction of potential fluid or electrolyte disturbances
- Removal of potential pharmacological agents
- Removal of potential physical issues
- Adequate pain assessment (also looking for non-verbal signs in cognitively impaired individuals) and management [25]

For evaluating the delirogenic potential of drugs, optimizing the medication use, the DEL-FINE score can be used. Drugs (and drug withdrawal) are assigned a score ranging from "three = strong delirogenic potential" to "zero = no delirogenic potential". For instance, a score of three is assigned to amitriptyline, atropine, clomipramine, and the withdrawal of benzodiazepines, ethanol, and opioids [26].

Nevertheless, the causal treatments can often be difficult as, even when the root cause is identified, it cannot be reversible. Therefore, symptomatic treatments are often used. These treatments include pharmacological therapy and non-pharmacological strategies.

7.2 Symptomatic treatment

Drugs useful for managing delirium may include antipsychotics and in selected cases benzodiazepines including diazepam, lorazepam, and midazolam. The latter class of drug can be indicated in the case of alcohol withdrawal or epilepsy delirium. Other drugs such as α-2 receptor agonists, psychostimulants, cholinesterase inhibitors, and melatonergic drugs are also used although no recommendations have been released so far.

About antipsychotics, it was demonstrated that both conventional (e.g., haloperidol) and atypical antipsychotics including olanzapine, risperidone, quetiapine, aripiprazole are effective in the treatment of delirium. Of note, the efficacy and safety of haloperidol at low doses (up to 10 mg/day) are comparable to those of atypical antipsychotics such as risperidone, olanzapine, and quetiapine [27].

In palliative care, haloperidol is one of the most used drugs. It is commonly administrated for the treatment of delirium and for the prevention and/or treatment of nausea/vomiting (including the opioid-induced ones) [28]. Even if it represents the preferred drug in the treatment of delirium, its use is limited by concern for side effects. Usually, the onset of extrapyramidal disorders is dose-dependent and cardiotoxicity — QTc prolongation or torsades de pointes (with a QTc > 450–500 ms immediate drug withdrawal is recommended) — generally rarely occurs for low doses [29]. However, in patients under palliative care, many factors such as the severity of the underlying disease and organ damage, comorbidities, cachexia, hypoproteinemia, advanced age, and polytherapy can increase the risk of side effects. For example, haloperidol pharmacokinetics (**Table 2**) mostly depends on CYP2D6 functioning.

About doses, in mild delirium with no underlying psychiatric illness haloperidol can be used at the dose of 0.5–1 mg bid, both oral or subcutaneous (0.25–0.5 mg for elderly patients). In moderate delirium, the dose can be doubled. In severe and terminal delirium the dose is 0.5–4 mg both oral or subcutaneous (possibly repeated every 45–60 min) with a maximum of 2–20 mg/day.

Among the other antipsychotics, risperidone (0.5–4 mg/day) could be useful in patients requiring high doses of haloperidol or at high risk of developing haloperidol-induced extrapyramidal or cardiac effects. Olanzapine (2.5–10 mg/day, orally or i.m.) has an efficacy comparable to haloperidol but can induce sedation due to its antihistaminergic action; thus, it is not recommended in elderly patients with dementia or hypoactive delirium, although its use can be beneficial for the regulation of the sleep–wake rhythm [30]. Quetiapine (from 12.5–25 mg/day up to an average dose of 50–175 mg/day) has an intense antihistaminergic activity which can worsen confusion. It can also cause hypotension. Finally, the first-generation antipsychotic agent levomepromazine is also used to address intractable nausea or vomiting, and for severe delirium in the last days of life. This phenothiazine is administered orally or by subcutaneous bolus injection (10–25 mg, repeatable as required after 2 hours) or continuous subcutaneous infusion (25–100 mg/day).

It must be emphasized that the efficacy of antipsychotics and other pharmacological interventions for the treatment of delirium in palliative care is still under debate [31, 32]. The use of antipsychotics and/or other medications becomes inevitable for the management of hyperactive or mixed delirium with severe agitation and anxiety but they must be given short-term and at the lowest effective dose. Symptomatic therapy of delirium is also mandatory if it becomes a source of suffering.

T1/2	*p.o.*: after a single dose (e.g., 2–4 mg) 14.5–36.7 hrs; up to 21 days after chronic administration *i.v.*: 10.1–26.2 hrs *i.m.*: 20.7 hrs (decanoate i.m.: 21 days)
Onset of action	*p.o.*: > 1 hr. *s.c.*:10–15 min *i.v.*: seconds
Duration of action	*s.c.*: up to 24 hrs *i.v.*: 4–6 hrs
Vd	9.5–21.7 L/kg
PPB	92%
Cl	0.9–1.5 l/kg/h

Abbreviations: p.o., oral; i.m., intramuscular; s.c., subcutaneous; i.v., intravenous; Vd: Volume of distribution; PPB, Plasma protein binding; Cl, Clearance.

Table 2.
Main haloperidol pharmacokinetics.

7.3 Non-pharmacological strategies

Non-pharmacological approaches such as behavioral and educational interventions, and cognitive activities as well as methods aimed at improving sleep, vision, and hearing functioning, are useful for addressing the issue of delirium. Encouraging family visits is another effective non-pharmacological strategy to be strengthened.

Communication strategies play a role of fundamental importance. Among the many examples reported, those proposed by the Mother Élisabeth Bruyère health care organization seem to be simple and effective. According to these suggestions, it is mandatory to use a calming voice, speak slowly and in short simple sentences, present one idea at a time and if needed, repeat the sentence. It is also suggested to avoid contradicting the person, accepting his/her arguments. Finally, rapid movements or gestures that can be misinterpreted as aggressive must be avoided [33].

8. Conclusion

Although clinical experience and scientific evidence underline that delirium can lead to multiple clinical and healthcare problems and that its timely recognition and treatment can induce a remission of the clinical picture, screening of cognitive conditions and delirium remains an unmet need. As the efficacy of pharmacological treatments has not yet been proven, greater efforts must be focused on prevention and early diagnosis. In short, the strategies to be adopted for prevention are quite codified. It is crucial to recognize potential risk factors and, since according to the ICD-11, delirium is essentially featured by disturbed attention and awareness, a careful evaluation of changes in usual behaviors is mandatory. The suspicion, in turn, must direct towards the administration of validated tools. Although the effectiveness of antipsychotics and other pharmacological treatments is still questioned, the use of these drugs is especially necessary for the treatment of hyperactive or mixed delirium featuring severe agitation and self or hetero-injurious behaviors. The hypoactive subtype, although very frequent, is little recognized and requires multicomponent non-pharmacological approaches.

Author details

Marco Cascella
Department of Supportive Care, Istituto Nazionale Tumori-IRCCS-Fondazione Pascale, Napoli, Italy

*Address all correspondence to: m.cascella@istitutotumori.na.it

References

[1] Finucane AM, Lugton J, Kennedy C, et al. The experiences of caregivers of patients with delirium, and their role in its management in palliative care settings: an integrative literature review. Psychooncology 2017;26:291-300.

[2] American Psychiatric Association. (2013). Diagnostic and Statistical Manual of Mental Disorders. 5th Edn. Arlington, VA: American Psychiatric Publishing, Inc.

[3] SH Bush, S Tierney, PG Lawlor. Clinical assessment and management of delirium in the palliative care setting. Drugs. 2017;77:1623-1643.

[4] Hosie A, Davidson PM, Agar M, Sanderson CR, Phillips J. Delirium prevalence, incidence, and implications for screening in specialist palliative care inpatient settings: a systematic review. Palliat Med. 2013;27:486-498.

[5] De la Cruz M et al. The frequency, characteristics, and outcomes among cancer patients with delirium admitted to an acute palliative care unit. Oncologist. 2015; 20:1425-1431

[6] Leonard M et al. Reversibility of delirium in terminally ill patients and predicators of mortality. Palliat Med. 2008;22(7):848-854.

[7] Mercadante S, Masedu F, Balzani I, De Giovanni D, Montanari L, Pittureri C, Bertè R, Russo D, Ursini L, Marinangeli F, Aielli F. Prevalence of delirium in advanced cancer patients in home care and hospice and outcomes after 1 week of palliative care. Support Care Cancer. 2018;26(3): 913-919.

[8] Rainsford S, Rosenberg JP, Bullen T. Delirium in advanced cancer: screening for the incidence on admission to an inpatient hospice unit. J Palliat Med. 2014;17:1045-1048.

[9] Ali M, Cascella M. ICU Delirium. 2021 Jan 16. In: StatPearls [Internet]. Treasure Island (FL): StatPearls Publishing; 2021 Jan–. PMID: 32644706.

[10] Fink MP, Evans TW. Mechanisms of organ dysfunction in critical illness: report from a Round Table Conference held in Brussels. Intensive Care Med. 2002;28(3):369-375.

[11] Boettger S, Breitbart W. Phenomenology of the subtypes of delirium: phenomenological differences between hyperactive and hypoactive delirium. Palliat Support Care. 2011;9(2):129-135.

[12] National Institute for Health and Care Excellence (NICE). Delirium: prevention, diagnosis and management. Clinical guideline [CG103] Published date: 28 July 2010 Last updated: 14 March 2019. Available at: https://www.nice.org.uk/guidance/cg103. Last accessed: April 26, 2021.

[13] Adamis D, Rooney S, Meagher D, Mulligan O, McCarthy G. A comparison of delirium diagnosis in elderly medical inpatients using the CAM, DRS-R98, DSM-IV and DSM-5 criteria. Int Psychogeriatr. 2015; 27(6):883-889.

[14] World Health Organisation. ICD-11 for Mortality and Morbidity Statistics (Version : 09/2020). Delirium. Available at: https://icd.who.int/browse11/l-m/en#/http://id.who.int/icd/entity/897917531. Last accessed: April 24, 2021.

[15] Inouye SK, van Dyck CH, Alessi CA, Balkin S, Siegal AP, Horwitz RI. Clarifying confusion: the confusion assessment method. A new method for detection of delirium. Ann Intern Med. 1990;113(12):941-948.

[16] Schuurmans MJ, Shortridge-Baggett LM, Duursma SA. The Delirium

Observation Screening Scale: a screening instrument for delirium. Res Theory Nurs Pract. 2003 Spring; 17(1):31-50.

[17] American Geriatrics Society. CoCare. Hospital Elder Life Program (HELP). https://help.agscocare.org/. Last accessed: April 24, 2021.

[18] Ryan K, Leonard M, Guerin S, Donnelly S, Conroy M, Meagher D. Validation of the confusion assessment method in the palliative care setting. Palliat Med. 2009;23(1):40-45.

[19] Neefjes ECW, van der Vorst MJDL, Boddaert MSA, Verdegaal BATT, Beeker A, Teunissen SCC, Beekman ATF, Zuurmond WWA, Berkhof J, Verheul HMW. Accuracy of the Delirium Observational Screening Scale (DOS) as a screening tool for delirium in patients with advanced cancer. BMC Cancer. 2019;19(1):160. doi: 10.1186/s12885-019-5351-8.

[20] Gaudreau JD, Gagnon P, Harel F, Tremblay A, Roy MA. Fast, systematic, and continuous delirium assessment in hospitalized patients: the nursing delirium screening scale. J Pain Symptom Manage. 2005; 29(4):368-375.

[21] Bush SH, Tierney S, Lawlor PG. Clinical Assessment and Management of Delirium in the Palliative Care Setting. Drugs. 2017;77(15):1623-1643.

[22] Neelon VJ, Champagne MT, Carlson JR, Funk SG. The NEECHAM Confusion Scale: construction, validation, and clinical testing. Nurs Res. 1996; 45(6):324-330.

[23] Trzepacz PT, Baker RW, Greenhouse J. A symptom rating scale for delirium. Psychiatry Res. 1988; 23(1):89-97.

[24] Lawlor PG, Nekolaichuk C, Gagnon B, Mancini IL, Pereira JL, Bruera ED. Clinical utility, factor analysis, and further validation of the memorial delirium assessment scale in patients with advanced cancer: assessing delirium in advanced cancer. Cancer. 2000;88:2859-2867.

[25] Cuomo A, Crispo A, Truini A, Natoli S, Zanetti O, Barone P, Cascella M. Toward more focused multimodal and multidisciplinary approaches for pain management in Parkinson's disease. J Pain Res. 2019 Jul 22;12:2201-2209. doi: 10.2147/JPR.S209616.

[26] Böhmdorfer B, Rohleder S, Wawruch M, van der Cammen TJM, Frühwald T, Jagsch C, et al. DEL-FINE: ein neues Tool zur Beurteilung der delirogenen Eigenschaften relevanter Arzneimittel für die Pharmakotherapie in Europa. Z Gerontol Geriatr. 2016;49:416-422.

[27] Yoon HJ, Park KM, Choi WJ, Park JY, Kim JJ, Seok JH. Efficacy and safety of haloperidol versus atypical antipsychotic medications in the treatment of delirium. BMC Psychiatry 2013;13:240-251.

[28] Masman AD. Medication use in end-of-life care in a palliative care center. Int J Clin Pharm. 2015;37:767-775.

[29] Cascella M, Fiore M, Leone S, Carbone D, Di Napoli R. Current controversies and future perspectives on treatment of intensive care unit delirium in adults. World J Crit Care Med. 2019;8(3):18-27.

[30] Grover S, Kumar V, Chakrabarti S. Comparative efficacy study of haloperidol, olanzapine and risperidone in delirium. J Psychosom Res 2011; 71:277-281.

[31] Schrijver EJM, de Graaf K, de Vries OJ, Maier AB, Nanayakkara PWB. Efficacy and safety of haloperidol for in-hospital delirium prevention and

treatment: a systematic review of current evidence. Eur J Intern Med Elsevier Bv. 2016;27:14-23.

[32] Al-Qadheeb NS, Balk EM, Fraser GL, Skrobik Y, Riker RR, Kress JP, et al. Randomized ICU trials do not demonstrate an association between interventions that reduce delirium duration and short-term mortality. Crit Care Med. 2014;42:1442-1454.

[33] Bruyere. Delirium. Information for Palliative Care patients and their families. Available at: https://www.bruyere.org/en/about-bruyere. Last accessed: May 31, 2021

Section 2

Palliative Care in Selected Clinical Settings

Chapter 2

Palliative Care of the Infant and Child in the Paediatric Intensive Care Unit

Maeve McAllister, Ann-Marie Crowe, Roisin Ni Charra, Julie Edwards and Suzanne Crowe

Abstract

In this chapter we discuss the delivery of palliative care in the paediatric intensive care unit environment. Illustrated by challenging cases, we describe the role of intensive care in symptom management for the child with terminal or life-limiting illness. We detail the importance of a multidisciplinary team and their roles in the provision of individualised care for the child and their family. The importance of family-centred care and advance care planning is expanded upon. In addition, we explore end of life issues that are particular to children in intensive care such as withdrawal of life-sustaining therapies and organ donation. Finally, we discuss how to ensure the delivery of high-quality palliative care in the paediatric intensive care environment.

Keywords: Paediatrics, PICU, Palliative Care, Family- centred, Symptom control

1. Introduction

Although modern medicine has undoubtedly improved survival among children with life- limiting disease, there remains a substantial requirement for paediatric palliative care. Approximately 21 million children per year need the input of palliative care medicine [1].

Infants, children and adolescents who may benefit from a palliative approach to their care fall into four patterns of disease progression [2, 3]:

1. Conditions for which potentially curative treatments have failed (e.g. malignancy)

2. Life- limiting conditions for which certain treatments may prolong life, but premature death still occurs (e.g. cystic fibrosis)

3. Conditions for which treatment is almost exclusively palliative but their progression may be slow and protracted (e.g. congenital cardiac defects, neurodegenerative disease)

4. Non progressive neurological conditions which result in an increased susceptibility to complications and premature death (e.g. cerebral palsy)

IntechOpen

Paediatric Intensive Care has similarly seen the mortality amongst children decrease substantially in the last two decades to less that 5% [4]. With improved survival rates, we have also noticed an increasing need for palliative care in the management of the sequelae of chronic and progressive medical illness amongst our patients.

Palliative care in the Paediatric Intensive Care Unit (PICU) may therefore be used in the following contexts [5]:

- Life-threatening illness where life- sustaining therapies have been deemed futile and must be withdrawn.
- Uncontrollable symptoms requiring advanced care which is not available or practical on the regular ward.
- Significant morbidity secondary to progressive non-malignant illness or a chronic life- limiting conditions [6].

Delivery of palliative care in PICU requires both acceptance by the child's family that their length of life will be short, and a holistic approach from a multidisciplinary team. A focus on symptom control and family-centred care at the end of a child's life may improve the experience of death for both patient and family unit [7]. We aim to facilitate a period of time for the family which will be associated with positive memories [8].

2. The role of PICU in symptom management

'Relief of pain and other symptoms' is one of the domains of high-quality palliative care in the PICU [9]. The purpose of symptom management is to maximise comfort and improve quality of life for the child in their final hours, days or months [10]. Optimal management requires an understanding of the underlying disease process and anticipation of symptoms that may arise. Symptoms are particular to each individual patient and can vary substantially [11].

Studies show that bereaved parents have rated the management of end of life symptoms poorly [12] and it is therefore important to provide individualized care which is both tailored to the patient's specific symptoms, and acceptable within the broader context of their family.

Symptom management may be provided with non-pharmacological or pharmacological means. Although a constellation of symptoms may be seen in the child receiving palliative care, here we discuss problematic symptoms that may arise in PICU.

2.1 Pain management

Pain assessment and management is fundamental to good palliative care practice. Our goal is to alleviate pain and the fear that it garners in the child and family [13].

Pain is assessed using age-appropriate tools [14], and attention is paid to the impact of pain upon the family unit [15]. We initiate pain management in a manner that is similar to that on the ward, with adherence to the WHO analgesic ladder [16] and utilisation of opioids as the cornerstone of therapy. We employ non- pharmacological measures such as physiotherapy and cognitive behavioural therapy (CBT) in conjunction with pharmacological therapies.

We are often presented with patients with recalcitrant pain where alternatives to opioid therapy are sought. These patients may have developed opioid tolerance, side effects with increased doses or may have infiltrative or neuropathic pain that is poorly responsive to opioids.

Despite the absence of convincing evidence for their efficacy [17, 18], adjuvant agents such as clonidine, ketamine and intravenous lignocaine [19, 20] may produce a significant improvement in pain.

Other specific pain therapies may also be employed for intractable pain or to mitigate against intolerable effects of analgesic agents. Peripheral nerve blocks can be used for discrete, well-defined areas of pain secondary to tumour infiltration [21] and, may encompass neurolytic methods for permanent pain relief. Spinal administration of opioids, local anaesthetics, baclofen or other adjuvants may also be used to good effect [22]. Involvement of specialties such as anaesthesiology, pain medicine and neurosurgery can support the institution of these therapies.

2.2 Psychological support

Many children, regardless of age, will experience psychological issues at the end of life. PICU staff must actively seek and attempt to address these matters as research has shown that psychological issues at the end of life are often under recognised by staff [12, 23]. A clinical psychologist should be involved and can provide evidence- based interventions for emotional or behavioural symptoms [24]. Therapeutic interventions such as cognitive behavioural therapy and relaxation strategies are used in conjunction with pharmacological treatment for relief of distressing symptoms.

Although anxiety may be present throughout a life-limiting illness, it may be particularly pronounced at the end of life. The child may express a fear of death itself, or a fear of uncontrolled pain and suffering around the time of death [25]. Parental anxiety and fear can strongly influence this. Management is dependent upon the age and understanding of the child. Guided by the parents, a degree of open communication about their condition and provision of verbal reassurance may alleviate anxiety significantly. Conservative strategies such as relaxation, meditation, or music therapy are also beneficial. This complementary therapy can play a significant role in the provision of holistic care to patients and their families. If drug therapy is deemed necessary, benzodiazepines may be useful anxiolytics.

Cerebral irritability is occasionally a feature in the paediatric patient receiving palliative care. The child may be agitated and inconsolable. Reassurance, and the creation of a peaceful environment can be complementary to pharmacologic strategies. Gabapentin has been shown to be effective in these cases [26], but may not always be practical due to its enteral route of administration. Alternative drugs which may be utilised in cases of severe distress include; levomepromazine; clonidine; chloral hydrate and lorazepam. Formulations can be made specifically by pharmacy to allow rectal or buccal administration.

2.3 Other symptoms and their management

2.3.1 Bleeding

Thrombocytopenia, coagulopathy or local tumour effects may cause bleeding in the dying child. Simple measures can be utilised in the case of haemorrhage. The child can be nursed on dark coloured bedding. Tranexamic acid- soaked gauze can be applied to bleeding mucous membranes and adrenaline- soaked gauze can be applied directly to bleeding points. Occasionally, blood transfusion may be administered. Although this could be seen as controversial in the dying patient, justification is based on whether transfusion has the potential to improve the patient's symptoms [27]. Catastrophic bleeding, as may be seen in acute pulmonary haemorrhage, can be both a distressing and terminal event. Subcutaneous or intravenous morphine and midazolam should be administered in this scenario to ensure comfort of the patient.

2.3.2 Dyspnoea and secretions

Dyspnoea refers to the subjective sensation of finding it difficult to breathe and, may be a particularly distressing symptom for the child and family. It is important to rule out treatable causes of dyspnoea in the dying child, such as pulmonary oedema, pleural effusion, anaemia and anxiety. Simple supportive measures that may improve the child's comfort include gentle suctioning, positioning and mouth care. More specific therapies such as bronchodilators and diuretics may be administered. Interdisciplinary discussion should take place regarding the relative benefits and risks of more invasive interventions such as pleural drain or blood transfusion.

Excessive secretions are common in all stages of palliative care. Gentle suctioning and positioning to allow drainage can also be helpful here. Pharmacological measures for excessive secretions include hyoscine hydrobromide or glycopyrronium bromide.

When entering the terminal phase, secretions may pool in the upper airways and cause particularly distressing sounds, also known as the 'death rattle'. When secretions are linked with dyspnoea, administration of morphine or midazolam can be considered. Dosing intervals are based upon a perceivable change in the child's dyspnoea or distress.

To illustrate the role of paediatric critical care medicine in symptom management, a series of case vignettes are provided below. Each is a challenging case where symptoms have been difficult to optimise on the regular ward, necessitating referral to the PICU team.

Case 1:

A 4-year-old with ALL who was referred from the ward team with severe chemotherapy related mucositis and painful dermatitis. His pain had been difficult to control despite using IV morphine boluses and regular clonidine. The patient was distressed and unable to take oral fluids. A ketamine infusion was commenced with a good improvement in patient comfort. This infusion was continued over a period of days until improvement was seen in his dermatological condition. The infusion was gradually weaned and discontinued, and the patient was suitable to be transferred back to the oncology ward.

Case 2:

A 2-year-old with a terminal pelvic malignancy had invasion of her lumbosacral plexus and severe neuropathic pain. Standard palliative analgesic regimens had been unsuccessful. An intravenous infusion of lignocaine was commenced with some improvement in her symptoms. An intrathecal catheter was sited, and infusion of opioids with local anaesthetic provided her with greatly improved pain relief in her final days.

Case 3:

A neonate with central respiratory depression, seizures and limb contractures was admitted to PICU for non-invasive ventilation. A palliative care referral was made, and gabapentin was commenced for central irritability. He was subsequently discharged to the ward.

3. Communication

Communication plays a key role in the delivery of high-quality end of life care in PICU [28, 29]. In this highly technical environment, the discussion of diagnoses, interventions and prognoses must be delivered using language that the patient and family will easily understand.

When the clinical trajectory shifts and the goals of care are realigned to focus upon comfort measures, this can be a particularly stressful and disorientating time for the family. High-quality communication during this time can reduce the risk of stress-related disorders in the bereaved family [30].

As discussion shifts from procedure-oriented conversations to planning the initiation of palliative care, the PICU clinician may be out of their comfort zone [31]. Research shows that clinicians prefer to discuss technical medical issues rather than emotional issues pertaining to quality of life [32]. It is, however, important for us to recognize that by building an empathic relationship based on information sharing, we foster a supportive relationship with the family [33].

Family conferences are an essential communication platform when a child is undergoing palliative care in the PICU [34]. Members of the team and the family have the opportunity to discuss goals of care in the context of the patient's clinical condition and the family values. A trusting relationship can be built with the family and this can facilitate the transition from critical care provision to the delivery of palliative care.

Although clinicians attribute considerable importance to family conferences [35], communication with the family in PICU most frequently occurs at the bedside [33]. Regardless of location, every interaction with the family is an opportunity to build trust and understanding. The team may consider appointment of one reliable point of contact, such as a specialist nurse for the family. This will facilitate relationship building with the family and provide for consistency in communications [36].

The PICU team must be cognisant of the following barriers to effective communication that can exist: delivery of inconsistent messages regarding the care plan; time constraints; the stressful environment; and a deficit of communication training [37].

Communication strategies that have been shown to be improve the end of life experience for families in PICU include: participation of the family in decision-making; limiting the use of medical terminology; displaying honesty when a child has a poor prognosis and compassionately sharing family grief [38].

4. Family-centred care

The delivery of palliative care to a child in PICU often represents a shift away from technical critical care interventions and cure-focused management. Emotional support and quality of life become key priorities, in addition to a focus upon family- centred care.

End of life decision-making for a child is a complex and emotional process and encouragement of a family-centred approach has been shown to result in greater family satisfaction [39]. Information sharing with the family and their participation in the decision-making process are both important.

The medical team should pay close attention to the information needs and preferences of patients and their families [40], particularly when providing technical information within the often stressful PICU environment. Difficult conversations may take place during a challenging and exhausting time for the family, and professionals should provide measured and consistent communication.

Key to collaborative decision-making is a steadfast and trusted relationship between the family and those involved in the child's care. It is important to recognize that not all families will want to lead the decision-making process, particularly regarding end of life care [7]. We see a spectrum of preferred decision- making roles with some families expressing a preference for delegation of decisions to clinicians, and others wanting a more prominent role in the process [41].

Family-centred care should also focus on maintaining the dignity of the family throughout the child's PICU stay. The physical and cultural environment in PICU exerts a contextual influence on the delivery of care [42] and, even simple institutional efforts can have a profound impact on the family. Forgoing visiting restrictions to allow parental presence at the bedside, provision of family accommodation and simple measures such as covering the cost of car parking and meals will support the family during this difficult time.

5. Advance care planning

Children and their families should be provided with support in developing an Advance Care Plan (ACP) which is reflective of their wishes concerning management of their illness and end of life care. An ACP will allow families and care providers to plan for the management of both reversible deteriorations in health and irreversible changes at the end of life. This individualised approach to care has the potential to improve patient quality of life and satisfaction [43].

The ACP should be documented in the patient's medical record where it can be shared amongst all caregivers. The family and medical team may wish to update the ACP to reflect redirection of care and reprioritisation of treatment goals as the child's illness progresses.

Ideally the ACP will be in place before the child is referred to PICU, but this is not always feasible, particularly in the case of an acute deterioration. PICU medical staff should be aware of any ACP that is in place and, if there is none, provide honest and clear communication to families regarding the perceived benefits, risks and invasiveness of critical care interventions [23]. This discussion can be particularly distressing for the family and all members of the multidisciplinary team will be invaluable in providing them with support in their decision-making.

In certain circumstances, a child may have an antenatal diagnosis of a life-limiting condition and ACPs are devised with the parents in antenatal period.

6. Re-direction of care on PICU and withdrawal of life-sustaining therapies

The re-direction of therapeutic goals in PICU requires careful planning, knowledgeable staff and high-quality communication. Following the decision to prioritise the patient's comfort, certain invasive therapeutic measures are electively ceased. Staff must anticipate symptoms or problems that may arise during this period and support the family in this stressful time.

6.1 Withdrawal of ventilatory support

The initiation of invasive ventilation is prompted by severe physiological derangement or the inability of the patient to protect the airway. Mechanical ventilation may be provided via an endotracheal tube or tracheostomy and is typically anticipated to be a temporising measure until clinical stability is restored. In cases where it has been decided that invasive ventilation is no longer in the child's best interest, the process of withdrawal of ventilatory support commences.

PICU staff must be familiar with the appropriate incorporation of extubation into the end of life care. Post-extubation symptoms such as dyspnoea, secretion retention and agitation must be anticipated and managed appropriately [44]. Not every extubation will be a terminal event and staff should anticipate that the child may survive for a period of hours or days following the withdrawal of ventilatory support [44].

There should be clear communication with the family around this time. It is essential to explain the practicalities of tracheal extubation, the anticipated patient response to extubation and to decide upon a plan for symptom management in the period following extubation.

On occasion, PICU may facilitate the withdrawal of ventilatory support outside of the intensive care unit. The provision of choice in location of end of life care is increasingly advocated [45] and the child or family may express a wish to die on a ward, in hospice or at home [46, 47]. Meticulous interdisciplinary planning is required if an out-of-hospital setting is chosen [48]. The practicalities of transferring a dying child, with the potential for terminal physiological instability during transfer, must be communicated to both family and caregivers.

In some cases of life-limiting illness, we have performed tracheostomy in intubated patients to facilitate discharge to the ward or home [49].

6.2 Withdrawal of extracorporeal life support

Extracorporeal life support (ECLS), or extracorporeal membrane oxygenation (ECMO), provides mechanical circulatory support to children with cardiac or respiratory failure refractory to maximal conventional medical therapy. Although ECMO outcomes have improved [50], a number of patients will have persistent cardiac or respiratory dysfunction and cannot be successfully liberated from ECLS. Withdrawal of ECLS will be a palliative measure in these cases.

Withdrawal from this highly technical life-sustaining therapy requires collaboration with our surgical colleagues who may facilitate' bridging' or separation from the ECMO circuit, or surgical removal of ECMO cannulae.

Patients who have had ECLS for a period of time may have received prolonged high dose benzodiazepine and opioid infusions [51]. Issues such as tolerance and dependence should be anticipated as the patient may survive for a period of time after ECMO decannulation.

6.3 Transition to the ward or home

Some patients may be able to transition to the ward or to their home for their final days. This period of transition should be managed with care due to the potential for creation of additional distress for the family. The family may be concerned that the patient will not get sufficient attention on the ward and can be upset at the realisation that discharge from PICU is a definite move away from active medical treatment.

The palliative care team should be involved in this process and can provide continuity of care for the patient on the ward or, refer to community- based services. Ideally, they will already have been involved in the care of the patient and attended family conferences during the patient's stay in the PICU.

Discharge should be planned and occur in daytime hours as much as is feasible. All members of the multidisciplinary team should be aware of the planned discharge and give advice with regards to ongoing care.

7. Special considerations in paediatric palliative care

Certain aspects of palliative care management of the child differ from that of the adult. Home care is generally preferred by the child and family [3, 52]. Research suggests that parents of children who die at home have less adverse psychological effects following the death of their child than those whose children die in the hospital setting [53]. The European Association of Palliative Care provides expected standards for paediatric palliative care and advocates for the provision of palliative care within the chosen setting of the child and family [54].

Whilst family are usually involved in the palliative care of every patient, the family unit is particularly central to paediatric palliative care. Parental presence is more frequent and their dual role as direct caregivers and legal guardians can contribute to more complex and emotionally fraught end of life decisions.

Consideration must also be given to siblings of the child who is receiving palliative care. The loss of a sibling can be devastating, and so too can the course of their sibling's illness and the series of events that has led to the decision to pursue palliative care. Feelings of isolation and distress can be compounded by an emotionally distracted and sometimes physically absent parent. Unresolved, these feelings may manifest as emotional or behavioural disturbances, disengagement from school, or psychosomatic complaints [55].

The lasting after-effect of the death of a child can be devastating and life-changing for both parents and siblings. A robust bereavement care plan is important in the context as a form of preventative heath intervention.

8. Bereavement support

A family's experience of the death of a child in PICU can have significant and long- lasting impacts on their bereavement journey [56]. Attention to supportive bereavement practices within an institution is critical to assuage lasting, pathological ill effects.

Bereaved parents have recommended many low-cost resources that can support other families going through the same process [57]. These include simple interventions such as provision of a private room, creation of photographic mementos, and direct assistance to parents after the death of the child.

It is impossible to standardise bereavement aftercare as every family will have an individual response. It should be routine practice to offer information and services. The family should be provided with written information regarding the practical aspects of the mortuary or post-mortem examination process, if applicable. Information regarding counselling or bereavement support groups should also be provided.

In our institution, we routinely have a meeting with bereaved families in the months following their child's death. This provides an opportunity for the family to ask lingering questions and for healthcare professionals to offer further bereavement support or identify the requirement for specific psychological support.

9. Organ donation

Organ donation may be considered if criteria are met and if the family wishes for this. Donation may occur after brainstem death or in certain cases after death has been confirmed using circulatory criteria.

Donation can be a difficult subject to discuss with the family and, family refusal, or reluctance of practitioners to broach the topic, can be barriers to organ donation in children. Prior studies have shown that families who did not consent to donation did so due to: religious or cultural beliefs; believing that the child had suffered enough; or feeling that the donation process was too lengthy [58]. It is important to remember the sensitive nature of these concerns when discussing organ donation with the family and to provide them with support during the decision- making process [59].

The donation process requires a significant work from the PICU team. They must engage with local or national organ donation coordinators and facilitate relevant investigations. The benefits of organ donation include improved quality of life for the recipient and potential beneficial effects on the bereavement process of the parents [60].

10. The multidisciplinary team

Palliative care in PICU is delivered by a multidisciplinary team in an effort to provide a holistic approach to address the needs of the child and their family. In addition to PICU medical and nursing staff, the team ideally includes the following staff members:

- *Physiotherapy*:
  The physiotherapist facilitates interventions such as therapeutic massage, passive movements and positioning. They provide education for the family and carers regarding patient transfers and respiratory care.

- *Psychology*:
  A clinical psychologist can assess and assist in the management of emotional or behavioural disturbances in the child.

- *Complementary therapist*:
  Therapies such as, aromatherapy, massage, music and reflexology may improve the patient's quality of life or psychological wellbeing [61].

- *Pastoral care*:
  Involvement of the local pastoral care team can provide spiritual and religious support for family and staff caring for a child with life-limiting or terminal illness. Some families may wish to have their own faith leader present on PICU.

- *Social workers*:
  Medical social workers are key support for the parents. They will assist the family with planning, finances and minimising the impact on the patient's siblings. Some parents have difficulty accepting the need for palliative care for their child [36] and social work can refer them for specific psychological or bereavement support.

As aforementioned, routine meetings between the family and the interdisciplinary team should provide the family with consistent communication about the child's clinical condition and agree upon treatment goals. All team members are provided with an opportunity to discuss the patient and support the medical team and family with difficult decision-making.

11. Audit, quality assurance and follow-up

A focus on audit and quality improvement is key to the delivery of high-quality palliative care in PICU. There are many evidence-based guidelines [62] which specify standards for provision of a comprehensive paediatric palliative care service. Undertaking audit against such guidelines is essential to gauge whether care is adequate and also provides the impetus to develop local quality improvement plans.

Another simple means of assessing a unit's performance is to conduct surveys amongst both the PICU staff and parents. This will identify areas that need to be improved upon and inform local research.

It is important that the institution recognises the need to educate care providers regarding palliative care practices. Education may take place in the form of multidisciplinary teaching sessions, provision of online resources or provision of funding for staff to gain additional qualifications such as a diploma or masters in palliative care.

Development of an integrated care pathway for palliative care in PICU will provide guidance for staff. All members of the multidisciplinary team should have input in the creation of such a document. It should function as a guide in the delivery of palliative care but recognise the importance of individual patient needs.

As aforementioned, in our institution we meet with bereaved parents in the months following a child's death. We also have an ethical duty to support our staff who can be left with a profound emotional impact from caring for a dying child. A helpful means of debriefing is the 'Schwartz Round', where the multidisciplinary team can discuss the emotional impact of their work [63]. This enables staff to support each other and can strengthen relationships within the team.

12. Conclusions

Palliative care in PICU can be a complex process. Paediatric patients may require palliative care for a variety of reasons and interventions should be tailored to each specific patient. The goals of care are to enhance quality of life and relieve suffering of patients and their families.

Ideally the patient, family and multidisciplinary team will form a shared plan to guide their palliative care journey. Regular family conferences should take place to continue this collaborative process and build relationships between the family and caregivers.

Processes such as redirection of care, withdrawal of life-sustaining therapies and organ donation should be approached by the team with sensitivity and compassion.

As not all children will have an advance care plan, the PICU team need to be equipped to deliver end of life care and guidance should be in place to facilitate this. Regular audit of outcomes should guide quality improvement in palliative care practices in the PICU.

Acknowledgements

No external funds were sought or obtained for the preparation of this manuscript.

Conflict of interest

The authors declare no conflict of interest.

Abbreviations

PICU	Paediatric Intensive Care Unit
CBT	Cognitive Behavioural Therapy
ACP	Advance Care Plan
ECLS	Extra Corporeal Life Support
ECMO	Extra Corporeal Membrane Oxygenation

Author details

Maeve McAllister, Ann-Marie Crowe, Roisin Ni Charra, Julie Edwards and Suzanne Crowe*
Department of Paediatric Intensive Care Medicine, Paediatric Intensive Care Unit, Children's Health Ireland at Crumlin, Dublin, Ireland

*Address all correspondence to: suzanne.crowe@olchc.ie

References

[1] Connor SR, Downing J, Marston J. Estimating the Global Need for Palliative Care for Children: A Cross-sectional Analysis. J Pain Symptom Manage. 2017;53(2):171-7.

[2] Goldman A. ABC of palliative care. Special problems of children. BMJ. 1998;316(7124):49-52.

[3] Hynson JL, Sawyer SM. Paediatric palliative care: distinctive needs and emerging issues. J Paediatr Child Health. 2001;37(4):323-5.

[4] Paediatric Intensive Care Audit Network (PICANet). Paediatric intensive care audit network annual report (2019) 2019 [Available from: https://www.picanet.org.uk/wp-content/uploads/sites/25/2019/12/PICANet-2019-Annual-Report-Summary_v1.0.pdf.

[5] Sprung CL, Truog RD, Curtis JR, Joynt GM, Baras M, Michalsen A, et al. Seeking worldwide professional consensus on the principles of end-of-life care for the critically ill. The Consensus for Worldwide End-of-Life Practice for Patients in Intensive Care Units (WELPICUS) study. Am J Respir Crit Care Med. 2014;190(8):855-66.

[6] Fraser LK, Miller M, Hain R, Norman P, Aldridge J, McKinney PA, et al. Rising national prevalence of life-limiting conditions in children in England. Pediatrics. 2012;129(4):e923-9.

[7] Doorenbos A, Lindhorst T, Starks H, Aisenberg E, Curtis JR, Hays R. Palliative care in the pediatric ICU: challenges and opportunities for family-centered practice. J Soc Work End Life Palliat Care. 2012;8(4):297-315.

[8] Michelson KN, Steinhorn DM. Pediatric End-of-Life Issues and Palliative Care. Clin Pediatr Emerg Med. 2007;8(3):212-9.

[9] American Academy of Pediatrics. Committee on Bioethics and Committee on Hospital Care. Palliative care for children. Pediatrics. 2000;106(2 Pt 1):351-7.

[10] Kittelson SM, Elie MC, Pennypacker L. Palliative Care Symptom Management. Crit Care Nurs Clin North Am. 2015;27(3):315-39.

[11] Malcolm C, Hain R, Gibson F, Adams S, Anderson G, Forbat L. Challenging symptoms in children with rare life-limiting conditions: findings from a prospective diary and interview study with families. Acta Paediatr. 2012;101(9):985-92.

[12] Contro NA, Larson J, Scofield S, Sourkes B, Cohen HJ. Hospital staff and family perspectives regarding quality of pediatric palliative care. Pediatrics. 2004;114(5):1248-52.

[13] Bates AT, Kearney JA. Understanding death with limited experience in life: dying children's and adolescents' understanding of their own terminal illness and death. Curr Opin Support Palliat Care. 2015;9(1):40-5.

[14] Cohen LL, Lemanek K, Blount RL, Dahlquist LM, Lim CS, Palermo TM, et al. Evidence-based assessment of pediatric pain. J Pediatr Psychol. 2008;33(9):939-55; discussion 56-7.

[15] Wachholtz AB, Fitch CE, Makowski S, Tjia J. A Comprehensive Approach to the Patient at End of Life: Assessment of Multidimensional Suffering. South Med J. 2016;109(4):200-6.

[16] World Health O. Persisting pain in children package: WHO guidelines on the pharmacological treatment of persisting pain in children with medical illnesses. Geneva: World Health Organization; 2012.

[17] van den Beuken-van Everdingen MH, de Graeff A, Jongen JL, Dijkstra D, Mostovaya I, Vissers KC, et al. Pharmacological Treatment of Pain in Cancer Patients: The Role of Adjuvant Analgesics, a Systematic Review. Pain Pract. 2017;17(3):409-19.

[18] Tagami K, Matsuoka H, Ariyoshi K, Oyamada S, Hiratsuka Y, Kizawa Y, et al. The current clinical use of adjuvant analgesics for refractory cancer pain in Japan: a nationwide cross-sectional survey. Jpn J Clin Oncol. 2020;50(12):1434-41.

[19] Massey GV, Pedigo S, Dunn NL, Grossman NJ, Russell EC. Continuous lidocaine infusion for the relief of refractory malignant pain in a terminally ill pediatric cancer patient. J Pediatr Hematol Oncol. 2002;24(7):566-8.

[20] Berde C, Koka A, Donado-Rincon C. Lidocaine Infusions and Other Options for Opioid-Resistant Pain Due to Pediatric Advanced Cancer. Pediatr Blood Cancer. 2016;63(7):1141-3.

[21] Anghelescu DL, Faughnan LG, Baker JN, Yang J, Kane JR. Use of epidural and peripheral nerve blocks at the end of life in children and young adults with cancer: the collaboration between a pain service and a palliative care service. Paediatr Anaesth. 2010;20(12):1070-7.

[22] Rork JF, Berde CB, Goldstein RD. Regional anesthesia approaches to pain management in pediatric palliative care: a review of current knowledge. J Pain Symptom Manage. 2013;46(6):859-73.

[23] Mitchell S, Dale J. Advance Care Planning in palliative care: a qualitative investigation into the perspective of Paediatric Intensive Care Unit staff. Palliat Med. 2015;29(4):371-9.

[24] Edlynn E, Kaur H. The Role of Psychology in Pediatric Palliative Care. J Palliat Med. 2016;19(7):760-2.

[25] McGrath PJ, Beyer J, Cleeland C, Eland J, McGrath PA, Portenoy R. American Academy of Pediatrics Report of the Subcommittee on Assessment and Methodologic Issues in the Management of Pain in Childhood Cancer. Pediatrics. 1990;86(5 Pt 2):814-7.

[26] Hauer JM, Wical BS, Charnas L. Gabapentin successfully manages chronic unexplained irritability in children with severe neurologic impairment. Pediatrics. 2007;119(2):e519-22.

[27] Pardo-González CA, Linares A, Torres M. Transfusion therapy evidence-based recommendations for the pediatric cancer patient. Colombian Journal of Anesthesiology. 2016;44(2):151-60.

[28] Meyer EC, Ritholz MD, Burns JP, Truog RD. Improving the quality of end-of-life care in the pediatric intensive care unit: parents' priorities and recommendations. Pediatrics. 2006;117(3):649-57.

[29] Meert KL, Eggly S, Pollack M, Anand KJ, Zimmerman J, Carcillo J, et al. Parents' perspectives on physician-parent communication near the time of a child's death in the pediatric intensive care unit. Pediatr Crit Care Med. 2008;9(1):2-7.

[30] Youngblut JM, Brooten D, Cantwell GP, del Moral T, Totapally B. Parent health and functioning 13 months after infant or child NICU/PICU death. Pediatrics. 2013;132(5):e1295-301.

[31] Fine E, Reid MC, Shengelia R, Adelman RD. Directly observed patient-physician discussions in palliative and end-of-life care: a systematic review of the literature. J Palliat Med. 2010;13(5):595-603.

[32] Stapleton RD, Engelberg RA, Wenrich MD, Goss CH, Curtis JR. Clinician statements and family

satisfaction with family conferences in the intensive care unit. Crit Care Med. 2006;34(6):1679-85.

[33] Lewis-Newby M, Sellers DE, Meyer EC, Solomon MZ, Zurakowski D, Truog RD. Location of Clinician-Family Communication at the End of Life in the Pediatric Intensive Care Unit and Clinician Perception of Communication Quality. J Palliat Med. 2020;23(8):1052-9.

[34] Michelson KN, Clayman ML, Haber-Barker N, Ryan C, Rychlik K, Emanuel L, et al. The use of family conferences in the pediatric intensive care unit. J Palliat Med. 2013;16(12): 1595-601.

[35] Michelson KN, Emanuel L, Carter A, Brinkman P, Clayman ML, Frader J. Pediatric intensive care unit family conferences: one mode of communication for discussing end-of-life care decisions. Pediatr Crit Care Med. 2011;12(6):e336-43.

[36] Verberne LM, Schouten-van Meeteren AY, Bosman DK, Colenbrander DA, Jagt CT, Grootenhuis MA, et al. Parental experiences with a paediatric palliative care team: A qualitative study. Palliat Med. 2017;31(10):956-63.

[37] Hallman ML, Bellury LM. Communication in Pediatric Critical Care Units: A Review of the Literature. Crit Care Nurse. 2020;40(2):e1-e15.

[38] Butler AE, Hall H, Willetts G, Copnell B. Family Experience and PICU Death: A Meta-Synthesis. Pediatrics. 2015;136(4):e961-73.

[39] White DB, Braddock CH, 3rd, Bereknyei S, Curtis JR. Toward shared decision making at the end of life in intensive care units: opportunities for improvement. Arch Intern Med. 2007;167(5):461-7.

[40] Mitchell S, Spry JL, Hill E, Coad J, Dale J, Plunkett A. Parental experiences of end of life care decision-making for children with life-limiting conditions in the paediatric intensive care unit: a qualitative interview study. BMJ Open. 2019;9(5):e028548.

[41] Heyland DK, Cook DJ, Rocker GM, Dodek PM, Kutsogiannis DJ, Peters S, et al. Decision-making in the ICU: perspectives of the substitute decision-maker. Intensive Care Med. 2003;29(1):75-82.

[42] Hill C, Knafl KA, Docherty S, Santacroce SJ. Parent perceptions of the impact of the Paediatric Intensive Care environment on delivery of family-centred care. Intensive Crit Care Nurs. 2019;50:88-94.

[43] Rosen DA, Budwany RR. Pediatric Advance Care Plan. When Cure Is Not an Option. Crit Care Med. 2019; 47(1):140-1.

[44] Laddie J, Craig F, Brierley J, Kelly P, Bluebond-Langner M. Withdrawal of ventilatory support outside the intensive care unit: guidance for practice. Arch Dis Child. 2014;99(9):812-6.

[45] Meert KL, Sarnaik AP. Choosing between death at home or in the hospital: respecting the principle of autonomy. Pediatr Crit Care Med. 2010;11(3):438-9.

[46] Needle JS. Home extubation by a pediatric critical care team: providing a compassionate death outside the pediatric intensive care unit. Pediatr Crit Care Med. 2010;11(3):401-3.

[47] Zwerdling T, Hamann KC, Kon AA. Home pediatric compassionate extubation: bridging intensive and palliative care. Am J Hosp Palliat Care. 2006;23(3):224-8.

[48] Postier A, Catrine K, Remke S. Interdisciplinary Pediatric Palliative

Care Team Involvement in Compassionate Extubation at Home: From Shared Decision-Making to Bereavement. Children (Basel). 2018;5(3).

[49] Marshall V, Holt F, Crowe S. Tracheostomy as a Comfort Measure in Children With Life-Limiting Conditions. J Palliat Care. 2017; 32(3-4):89-91.

[50] Dohain AM, Abdelmohsen G, Elassal AA, ElMahrouk AF, Al-Radi OO. Factors affecting the outcome of extracorporeal membrane oxygenation following paediatric cardiac surgery. Cardiol Young. 2019;29(12):1501-9.

[51] Anton-Martin P, Modem V, Taylor D, Potter D, Darnell-Bowens C. A retrospective study of sedation and analgesic requirements of pediatric patients on extracorporeal membrane oxygenation (ECMO) from a single-center experience. Perfusion. 2017;32(3):183-91.

[52] Goldman A, Beardsmore S, Hunt J. Palliative care for children with cancer--home, hospital, or hospice? Arch Dis Child. 1990;65(6):641-3.

[53] Goodenough B, Drew D, Higgins S, Trethewie S. Bereavement outcomes for parents who lose a child to cancer: are place of death and sex of parent associated with differences in psychological functioning? Psychooncology. 2004;13(11):779-91.

[54] Craig F, Abu-Saad Huijer H, Benini F, Kuttner L, Wood C, Feraris PC, et al. [IMPaCCT: standards of paediatric palliative care]. Schmerz. 2008;22(4):401-8.

[55] Pettle Michael SA, Lansdown RG. Adjustment to the death of a sibling. Arch Dis Child. 1986;61(3):278-83.

[56] van der Geest IM, Darlington AS, Streng IC, Michiels EM, Pieters R, van den Heuvel-Eibrink MM. Parents' experiences of pediatric palliative care and the impact on long-term parental grief. J Pain Symptom Manage. 2014;47(6):1043-53.

[57] Butler AE, Copnell B, Hall H. When a Child Dies in the PICU: Practice Recommendations From a Qualitative Study of Bereaved Parents. Pediatr Crit Care Med. 2019;20(9):e447-e51.

[58] Hawkins KC, Scales A, Murphy P, Madden S, Brierley J. Current status of paediatric and neonatal organ donation in the UK. Arch Dis Child. 2018; 103(3):210-5.

[59] Bellali T, Papazoglou I, Papadatou D. Empirically based recommendations to support parents facing the dilemma of paediatric cadaver organ donation. Intensive Crit Care Nurs. 2007;23(4): 216-25.

[60] Merchant SJ, Yoshida EM, Lee TK, Richardson P, Karlsbjerg KM, Cheung E. Exploring the psychological effects of deceased organ donation on the families of the organ donors. Clin Transplant. 2008;22(3):341-7.

[61] Armstrong M, Flemming K, Kupeli N, Stone P, Wilkinson S, Candy B. Aromatherapy, massage and reflexology: A systematic review and thematic synthesis of the perspectives from people with palliative care needs. Palliat Med. 2019;33(7):757-69.

[62] Aidoo E, Rajapakse D. End of life care for infants, children and young people with life-limiting conditions: planning and management: the NICE guideline 2016. Arch Dis Child Educ Pract Ed. 2018;103(6):296-9.

[63] Lown BA, Manning CF. The Schwartz Center Rounds: evaluation of an interdisciplinary approach to enhancing patient-centered communication, teamwork, and provider support. Acad Med. 2010;85(6):1073-81.

Chapter 3

Home Based Palliative Care

Sourav Goswami

Abstract

Palliative care aims at improving the quality of life of a patient who is suffering from a chronic serious ailment like that of advanced cancer. Nobody wants to be away from his/her own family, especially when it's known, he has limited days to live in this world. A patient gets the best treatment when it's given in his own home and that too by his close ones. When palliative care is provided at the patient's home, it provides a sense of safety, privacy, confidentiality and peace of mind for the patient. Specialist home-based palliative care improves symptom control, health-related communication and psychosocial support. It helps in better preparing the patient and the family members to accept death. It is provided by a team of trained members which includes doctor, nurse, social worker, volunteers, physiotherapist etc. They pay regular visits at the home of the patient and provide necessary health care to the patient. Considering the increasing cost of treatment of chronic illnesses, it's sometimes hard on the part of the family to continue treatment in a hospital or hospice. It's especially true in scenarios where population are not protected financially, in countries like India. The family members also play a vital role in home-based palliative care. They get trained from the team to learn the basics of palliation. Home based palliative care needs to be integrated into regular home health care services.

Keywords: palliative care, home based, quality of life, Home PAL

1. Introduction

In today's world, non-communicable diseases like cancer, dementia, renal failure etc. are increasing in leaps and bounds. They need long term care for their chronic condition [1]. It has been estimated that around 1.5 billion people experience chronic pain round the world, and an estimated 61 million people endure unrelieved serious health-related suffering globally [1–3]. Many of them result in increasing morbidity making patients critically ill. Death is inevitable, but, today's era is giving more importance to the quality of life lived than its longevity [4]. Here comes the role of palliative care, which helps improve the quality of one's life especially in his last days and tries to decrease the burden of the disease. World Health Organization (WHO) has defined Palliative care as an approach that improves the quality of life of patients and their families experiencing problems related to life-threatening disease [5]. It is provided through the prevention, assessment and treatment of pain and other physical, psychosocial and spiritual problems.

In general, palliative care mostly functions in hospitals where the patient is admitted or may be in day care basis, where the patient needs to pay a visit to the hospital on regular basis for some procedures or sessions that help in alleviating their pain and other symptoms. Palliative care should be an admixture with the curative form of treatment which should begin from the early part of patient management. The patient, especially in his end stage of life, is happy to be with his near and dear ones, in his known home environment. This has built up the foundation of the concept of Home based palliative care (Home PAL) [6].

2. Understanding 'Home based palliative care' (Home PAL)

Home PAL is a form of palliative care that provides all the basic needs (physical, psychological, and moral) to the patient who is suffering from a chronic debilitating disease like advanced cancer, lung, renal, cardiac disease or may be dementia [7], in their homes or in a homely environment. The Home Pal is provided by a trained multidisciplinary team of doctors, nurses, social workers, physiotherapists, volunteers and others as per the need of the disease progression. The care provided by the team is at par with the standard palliative care practiced in the hospitals, institutions or hospices [8].

Teams of doctors, nurses, social workers and chaplains travel primarily to patients' homes and also to the rehabilitation centres and help in long term care of the patients, who are suffering from terminal illnesses.

3. Importance of home PAL

3.1 For the patient

The general principles of Palliative care [9] hold good in case of Home PAL as well, which can be briefly narrated as follows:

- Controlling the distressing symptoms of illness, like pain relief, etc.
- Independence.
- Intends neither to hasten nor postpone death. Rather it provides emotional, spiritual and cultural wellbeing to the patent.
- Planning for the future.
- Preparing oneself for the inevitable – death. Affirms life and regards dying as a normal process
- Will enhance quality of life, and may also positively influence the course of illness
- Caring for their family and carers.

But, to achieve those stated above, the patient should be at his peace of mind. Peace of mind comes, when he dwells in a peaceful environment which he is accustomed with since long – his own home. No one wants to die alone. Everybody wants to have his near and dear ones by his side when he is in his death bed [10].

The patient gains more confidence, when he is getting his treatment in his homely environment, where the family members are taking an active part in the process of the therapy.

3.2 For the caregiver

A person suffering from any chronic critical illness is in a debilitated state. He is not in a position to take care of himself. There comes the role of family members who come forward to take care of their loved one. Informal care by family members is unique in developing countries like India when compared with the developed world where care giving is usually in the form of paid formal care. But, this transition from being a close relative to a caregiver occurs so quickly that many a times they are not prepared for it. While providing care for their ill loved one, who is in his death bed, caregivers often neglect their own needs. This neglect, over time, comes as a heavy toll on the overall well-being of a caregiver and they feel stressed – physically, emotionally and financially [11].

That is the reason why quality of life of patient's families has been included the in the WHO's definition of Palliative care. The family members are at ease, when the patient receives treatment at home. It saves their time and money in traveling to the hospital. They can continue their regular chores and at the same time they can also learn and get trained from the expert team of Home PAL, few of the basic measures of providing palliative care like giving the proper medicine at proper time, providing physical and psychological support when needed. This helps in building confidence among the family caregivers [12]. They feel happy when their work (in the form of patient's care taking) gets recognized and they feel that their minor help is making a major impact in the quality life of the patient.

The home-based care services ensure continuity of care for patients and empower the caregiver in the family by teaching them simple and cost effective methods of patient care.

4. Things to be done to set up Home PAL

Home PAL service can be set up in a quite simple manner. The following are a gist of activities to be performed to set up the home based palliative care [13].

Like any program to be launched, we need to conduct a need base evaluation for the home based palliative care. It will help us to identify the beneficiaries, their requirements and to check if we have enough logistics to support the program. Logistics will be in term of man, material, money and time.

Once the team or the institute is satisfied with the basic evaluation, competent authorities need to be involved, informed and necessary permissions need to be taken. There is a need for setting up a formal office for the Home PAL.

Now, the action plan needs to be framed, scanned, verified and edited. This includes the resource based evaluation and what all services should be included in the charter needs to be finalized.

The Home PAL team needs to be trained efficiently in palliative care. It would be best if a trained nurse and a trained doctor can be included in the team, to begin with. If not, the dedicated team needs to get trained from a dedicated training center of palliative care.

The goal of home based palliative care is to involve community volunteers in the team. So, the community volunteers needs to be identified and proper training needs to be undertaken. The resource based evaluation, as described earlier should include the financial requirement for purchasing the necessary supplies, transportation costs and salary of the Home PAL team.

In Home PAL, the team needs to travel to the homes of the patients, which will be away from the mother institute or hospital. So, the primary care team or health workers, both government and private, need to be contacted and should be included in the community based Home PAL team. It will help in emergency care and support to the ailing patient, in times, when the Home PAL team will not be available. Also, it will help in quicker diagnosis of any emergency and better management including referral to higher centers.

IEC (Information Education Communication) and BCC (Behavior Change Communication) has a great role to play in the success of the Home PAL program. It calls for involving the public health personals, both government and private, who work with the community of that locality. The media needs to be involved as well, for better propagation of the news and information of the Home PAL. Home PAL calls for a wider support and participation from the whole community including the villagers, students, political leaders and governmental staff, for the program to succeed in achieving what it aims to do.

5. Components of Home PAL

To carry out Home PAL, we need to have a dedicated team, trained in palliative care. The patient's need to be identified beforehand. The local volunteers needs to be recruited. They are the contact persons, who would inform the households regarding the date and time of visit of the Home PAL team. Many a times, a member of the Home PAL team may directly contact a family member of the patient and inform him of their time of visit. So, the house hold should possess a mobile or a telephone for easier contact. The home environment should be a safe and accessible place for the team to store drugs and equipment, as well as to talk to the patients and family members to plan for their treatment. The dedicated space in the house for storing medicines should be a safe one outside the reach of children and the patient. They should also carry a basic set of medicines in their home care kit, including morphine to refill the stores at home. Documentation should be properly done. Home PAL forms should be prepared. It will help in proper documentation and recording of the patient details. It should include the consent form, that needs to be read and explained to the caregivers and their signature needs to be taken. The forms should also record the medicines prescribed to the patients with detailed dosage and schedule. A separate 'morphine register' should be maintained to have a note of the correct number of morphine tablets dispatched to the patients. It should be compliant with the local laws and regulations.

Importantly, in order to implement home PAL; the health care team, the patient and the family must agree that the patient can be adequately managed at home, and the treatment plan should be approved by all the stakeholders.

Now, let us come to each of the components in details.

5.1 The Home PAL team

A full-time nurse and a part-time doctor are the minimum requirements for a home-care team, although this depends on the regulatory and health system norms in the country. A multidisciplinary team of nurses, doctors, psychologists/counselors, social workers and trained volunteers or community health workers is ideal [6].

5.2 Requirements

The requirements are tabulated in **Table 1**, under the headings of basic infrastructure, personnel, home care kit and finance [6].

5.3 Home care kit

The Home PAL team should carry with them a basic home care kit, which includes some basic medical instruments, medicines for managing acute as well as chronic complains, dressing materials and nutritious supply [13, 14]. They are mentioned in details in **Table 2**.

Basic Infrastructure	Central meeting point
	Storage facilities (including for controlled drugs)
	Transport of team and home care kit
	Method of communication (telephone, mobile, etc)
Personnel	Doctors
	Nurses
	Volunteers etc.
Home care kit	Medication (including morphine)
	Equipment
	Documentation
Finance	Salaries for team members
	Transportation/vehicle hire
	Rental for room/storage facility
	Communication and printing
	Medication and equipment costs

Table 1.
Requirement for Home PAL set up.

Medical equipment and supplies	Stethoscope
	Sphygmomanometer
	Thermometer
	Tongue depressor
	Forceps
Supporting equipment	Alternating air mattress
	Aspirator
	Nebulizer
	Wheel chairs
	Walking aids
Tools	Dressing materials
	Cotton
	Scissors
	Gauze
	Gloves
	Plaster
	Transfusion materials
	IV infusion sets
	Cannula and butterfly needle
	Injector and needle
	Aspirator probes
	Urinary catheters
	Bladder
	Feeding tubes

Medicines	
Pain management	Paracetamol
	Ibuprofen
	Diclofenac
	Codeine
	Tramadol
	Morphine
	Gabapentin
Gastrointestinal symptom management	Metoclopramide
	Domperidone
	Dexamethasone
	Bisacodil
	Loperamide
	Oral rehydration salts
	Ranitidine
Psychological symptom management	Diazepam
	Haloperidol
	Amitriptyline
Antibiotics and antifungals	Ciprofloxacin
	Metronidazole
	Oxacillin
	Fluconazole
Wound therapy	Betadine solution and ointment
	Metronidazole gel
	Hydrogen peroxide
Nutritional supplements	High protein and calorie food supplements
	Iron, vitamin and mineral supplements

Table 2.
Home care kit.

	Basic	Mid level	Advanced
Doctors	Foundation courses (3–10 days)	Resident course (6 weeks)	Fellowship/Post graduate qualification in palliative care (1–3 years)
Nurses	Foundation courses (3–10 days)	Resident course (6 weeks)	Certificate course (4 months), fellowship (1 year)
Community health workers	3–6 hours to supplement prior training	Basic course (3 months/400 hours)	Advanced communication skills/ lymphedema management
Volunteers	Introductory course (3 hours)	16 hours theory + 4 clinical sessions,	Advanced communication skills and train-the-trainer course

Note: Minimum requirements for home-care team depend greatly on the format of the health system. There are countries where nurses play a larger role, and others where home care is conducted more by doctors.

Table 3.
Training requirements for the Home PAL team.

5.4 Trainings

The suggested minimum training for various members [6] of the home-care team is described in **Table 3**.

6. Role of telemedicine in Home PAL

Telemedicine, which literally means 'healing at a distance', is the practice of consultation, care, diagnosis and interaction between the physician and the patients, who are located remotely via different technologies which involves video conferencing [15]. The world has evidenced the grievousness of covid crisis, where it's either risk taking to visit a hospital or it's difficult to arrange transportation every time due to the occasional curfews and lock downs. In such a scenario, the use of technology in the form of telemedicine is surely appealing to be used for palliation as well in the home set ups. It is evidence based that telemedicine has been used to be a success in different parts of the world, especially in the European countries [16]. Telemedicine while used for palliative care has proven to improve the symptoms, quality of life and care for the patient and also results in better satisfaction to the patient and the caregiver. It also saves the doctor's time. But the most important hurdle of using telemedicine round the globe is the technology related complications. To describe briefly, most of the patients eligible for palliative care are elderly, many of them are not techno friendly. There lacks proper connectivity of internet and electricity in most of the developing nations including India, which is a must for a successful telemedicine set up [17, 18]. Though in urban areas, things could be manageable, but the scenario is just the reverse in rural set up. Moreover, there always remains a difference between the in person care and the tele care provided by the councilor or the Home PAL team, when the patient is in his last days of life. Once these challenges are taken care of, there are prospective avenues to incorporate telemedicine in the regular Home PAL services.

7. Benefits

i. Patients are more comfortable in their own home than in a hospital set up [19].

ii. In Home PAL, family members are directly involved in the process of palliative care. So, patient has an easy access to care.

iii. It provides training and support to family members to help them develop as caregivers.

iv. The home PAL team is able to facilitate quick referral to additional services.

v. Privacy and confidentiality is maintained when the care is being carried out in the home of the patient.

vi. It helps to increase community awareness of palliative care. Local resources and support networks can be mobilized and training can be provided by community health workers to others in the local area [5].

vii. Saves traveling cost and time for the patient and his family.

viii. Considering the increasing cost of treatment of chronic illnesses, it's sometimes hard on the part of the family to continue treatment in a hospital or hospice. It's especially true in scenarios where population are not protected financially, in countries like India.

8. Limitations

i. One of the limitations is to convince the patients and their families to call the care team when they experience a health crisis, for which, the Home PAL team need to build trust and rapport with the patients and their families [20].

ii. Family members may not be prepared to bring the patient to hospital in times of urgency. So, Home PAL team needs to develop preparedness among the family members to shift the patient to health care facility whenever required, which calls for advanced arrangement of money, transportation and people who will be accompanying them to hospital. Scenarios can get worse in current pandemic situations of Covid.

iii. The providers of the home PAL needs to be very sincere in paying the home visits in order to avoid care fragmentation and should never fail in their routine.

9. Best practice – example from Kerala, India

Kerala is pioneer in community-based palliative care through a socially innovative approach called the Neighborhood Network in Palliative Care in an attempt to develop a free of charge, sustainable, community led service capable of offering comprehensive long-term care and palliative care. The network aims to empower local communities to look after their chronically ill and dying patients. Funds for running the programme are raised locally by volunteers [21].

The programme was first pilot studied in 1996 in Malappuram, located in the northern district of Kerala, the state with the highest literacy rate in India. It was run by community based organizations. It was first started for cancer patients. The program was gradually expanded to include other patients who required long-term care and support such as stroke, alzheimer's disease, paraplegia and psychiatric conditions. Volunteers from the community were selected and were trained to identify the psycho-social needs of people with chronic disease in their area in order to intervene effectively with active support from a team of trained health care personnel [21, 22]. The nurses who were trained in palliative care played a vital role in this. They regularly visited the home of the patients who were enrolled in the program and provide nursing care and support at home, which included wound dressing, catheterisation, nasogastric tube insertion, and counseling. The doctors were called only for selected patients where the patient needed a physician's consultation, which was chartered by the palliative care nurse. The community volunteers also played an important role. Trained by the palliative team with the first-hand knowledge of basic nursing and palliative care, they helped patients and their families financially and emotionally. The model was a successful one. It inspired the state of Kerala to implement a palliative care policy to ensure universal coverage of palliative care services in all its local administrative units, making it the first state in Asia to develop such a policy. Home based care was considered as the corner stone of palliative care services in the policy implemented [23]. The Neighborhood Network in Palliative Care in Kerala is the best example of a community-based palliative care for low-resource countries in the world.

10. Conclusion

Considering the increasing number of critically ill patients who are in need of palliative care for long, it is high time to focus towards implementing home based palliative care measures that will help patient maintain their quality of life. It should be emphasized to include palliative care, especially home based palliative care in the primary care, community and home based health care services. Gradually, it is necessary to create and implement National health policies that integrate Home PAL services into regular home health care services.

Author details

Sourav Goswami
Associate Medical Manager, Covance, Pune, India

*Address all correspondence to: drsouravagt@gmail.com

References

[1] Knaul FM, Farmer PE, Krakauer EL, et al. Lancet Commission on Palliative Care and Pain Relief Study Group. Alleviating the access abyss in palliative care and pain relief—an imperative of universal health coverage: The Lancet Commission report. Lancet. 2017 Oct 11.

[2] Nahin RL. Estimates of pain prevalence and severity in adults: United States, 2012. J Pain. 2015 Aug;16(8):769-80.

[3] Rosenquist RW, Souzdalnitski D, Urman RD, editors. Chronic pain management for the hospitalized patient. New York, NY: Oxford University Press; 2016.

[4] Brown GC. Living too long: the current focus of medical research on increasing the quantity, rather than the quality, of life is damaging our health and harming the economy. EMBO Rep. 2015 Feb;16(2):137-41.

[5] World Health Organisation. Planning and implementing palliative care services: a guide for programme managers. Switzerland. 2018.

[6] Meier DE, McCormick E. Benefits, services, and models of subspecialty palliative care. UpToDate; 2015.

[7] Ibrahim JE, Anderson LJ, MacPhail A, Lovell JJ, Davis MC, Winbolt M. Chronic disease self-management support for persons with dementia, in a clinical setting. J Multidiscip Healthc 2017;10:49-58.

[8] Kahveci K, Koç O, Aksakal H. Home-based Palliative Care. Bezmialem Science 2020;8(1):73-80.

[9] O'Neill B, Fallon M. ABC of palliative care: Principles of palliative care and pain control BMJ 1997; 315 :801

[10] Guy M, Stern TA. The desire for death in the setting of terminal illness: a case discussion. Prim Care Companion J Clin Psychiatry. 2006;8(5):299-305.

[11] Goswami S, Gupta SS, Raut A. Understanding the psychosocial impact of oral cancer on the family caregivers and their coping up mechanism: A qualitative study in Rural wardha, Central india. Indian J Palliat Care 2019;25:421-7.

[12] Clemmer SJ, Ward-Griffin C, Forbes D. Family members providing home-based palliative care to older adults: the enactment of multiple roles. Can J Aging. 2008 Fall;27(3):267-83.

[13] Nordly M, Vadstrup ES, Sjogren P, Kurita GP. Home-based specialized palliative care in patients with advanced cancer: A systematic review. Palliat Support Care 2016;14:713-24

[14] Yeager A, LaVigne AW, Rajvanshi A, Mahato B, Mohan R, Sharma R, et al. CanSupport: a model for home-based palliative care delivery in India. Ann Palliat Med 2016;5:166-71.

[15] WHO. Telemedicine: opportunities and developments in Member States: report on the second global survey on eHealth 2009. Global Observatory for eHealth Series, 2. 2010. Available: https://www.who.int/goe/publications/goe_telemedicine_2010.pdf. Last assessed on: 31st May 2021.

[16] Hancock, S., Preston, N., Jones, H. *et al.* Telehealth in palliative care is being described but not evaluated: a systematic review. *BMC Palliat Care* **18,** 114 (2019).

[17] Worster B, Swartz K. Telemedicine and Palliative Care: an Increasing Role in Supportive Oncology. Curr Oncol Rep. 2017 Jun;19(6):37.

[18] Chellaiyan VG, Nirupama AY, Taneja N. Telemedicine in India: Where do we stand? J Family Med Prim Care. 2019 Jun;8(6):1872-1876. doi: 10.4103/jfmpc.jfmpc_264_19. PMID: 31334148; PMCID: PMC6618173.

[19] Dhiliwal SR, Muckaden M. Impact of specialist home-based palliative care services in a tertiary oncology set up: a prospective non-randomized observational study. Indian J Palliat Care. 2015 Jan-Apr;21(1):28-34.

[20] Heydari, H., Hojjat-Assari, S., Almasian, M. et al. Exploring health care providers' perceptions about home-based palliative care in terminally ill cancer patients. BMC Palliat Care. 2019. 18, 66.

[21] Philip, R.R., Philip, S., Tripathy, J.P. *et al.* Twenty years of home-based palliative care in Malappuram, Kerala, India: a descriptive study of patients and their care-givers. *BMC Palliat Care* **17,** 26 (2018).

[22] Kumar S, Numpeli M. Neighborhood network in palliative care. Indian J Palliat Care. 2005;11:6-9.

[23] Paleri AK. Showing the way forward: pain and palliative care policy of the government of Kerala. Indian J Palliat Care. 2008;14:51-4.

Chapter 4

Palliative Care in Gynaecological Oncology

Monika Náležinská and Josef Chovanec

Abstract

Palliative care in gynaecologic oncology focuses on specific and severe symptoms resulting from affected abdominal and pelvic organs and feminine genitals. These symptoms are mainly connected to advanced gynaecologic malignancies. Patients with locally advanced or recurrent gynaecologic cancers may present with various symptoms. Among those we discuss vaginal bleeding, vaginal discharge and fistulas. Vice versa non-malignant diseases and non-pelvic site diseases such as inflammations, overdose of anticoagulants, wounds or pressure ulcers may have similar clinical manifestation. Some symptoms may result from aggressive cancer treatment (oncological surgery, radiotherapy) with curative intent. Some symptoms get worse on account of the postmenopausal status (natural or artificial following any type of ovarian failure). For advanced gynae-oncological diseases it has been in practise, that the best palliative care is offered and practised simultaneously with curative treatment. The problematics of gynaecologic symptoms in palliative care represents delicate and intimate sphere and it may disturb patient's autonomy and dignity. The mission of physicians, nurses and caregivers is to consider treatment options thoroughly in context of patient's quality of life, prognosis and life conditions to fulfil the ideals of the best symptomatic and supportive care.

Keywords: gynaecologic malignancies, vaginal bleeding, fistula, vaginal packing, embolisation

1. Introduction

Our contribution to the open access book of palliative care focuses on specific and severe symptoms resulting from affected abdominal and pelvic organs and feminine genitals. These symptoms are mainly connected to advanced gynaecologic malignancies. Patients with locally advanced or recurrent gynaecologic cancers may present with various symptoms. Among those we discuss vaginal bleeding, vaginal discharge and fistulas. Problematics of pain control, oedema and ascites, nausea and vomiting, shortness of breath and malignant bowel obstruction is common to most incurable advanced diseases and these are not connected to pelvic diseases only, see specific chapters. Vice versa non-malignant diseases and non-pelvic site diseases such as inflammations, overdose of anticoagulants, wounds or pressure ulcers may have similar clinical manifestation. Some symptoms may result from aggressive cancer treatment (oncological surgery, radiotherapy) with curative intent. Some symptoms get worse on account of the postmenopausal status (natural or artificial following any type of ovarian failure). For advanced gynae-oncological diseases it has been in practise, that the best palliative care is offered and practised simultaneously with curative treatment. Optimum palliative care can only be provided by a team that may include a gynaecologic oncologist, a radiation oncologist, an interventional radiologist, a palliative care physician, nurse and a social worker to address the various problems faced by these patients [1, 2]. All described clinical situations can be well solved in hospices as well as at patient's home with the guidance of experienced mobile palliative care teams. Except for malignant bowel obstruction and severe genital bleeding, which both present extreme mental and physical load for the caregivers who witness it and it can be traumatizing experience for unprepared family members and healthcare providers.

2. Genital bleeding

Vaginal bleeding or discharge is the most common presenting symptom of advanced or recurrent gynaecologic malignancy. Patients may initially ignore bleeding if it is minimal and potentially attributable to menses. However, direct invasion of blood vessels by tumour may come to cause massive bleeding. If it is beneficial for the patient, the source of the bleeding should be determined and solved according to the possibilities (see **Table 1**). By that we mean no painful and stressing diagnostic procedures with preterminal and terminal patients. Initial management of pathologic vaginal bleeding requires a proper gynaecologic examination and considerations of placement of tight vaginal packing with haemodynamic support [1, 2]. The packing should be left in place for 24–48 hours maximum and then it must be extracted or replaced. Tight packing requires insertion of urinary catheter, because of urethral obstruction caused by packing. Prolonged packing in risky for severe inflammatory complications and fistula formation.

The aspect to consider is quality of life (relief of symptoms of anaemia versus reasonable and ethical protraction of suffering in conditions of incurable terminal status). Severe unaffected haemorrhage as the final event is really traumatizing for witnessing family members [1]. It should be well communicated in advance and if family members or caregivers do not feel comfortable with this situation, then it is better to evaluate the option of hospitalization in hospice.

In case of clinical status unresponsive to aggressive intervention, in exhausted terminal patients with severe uncontrollable vaginal haemorrhage, palliative sedation is an ethically and morally appropriate option [3].

In all other cases that are not regarded as terminal phase of incurable disease, it is useful to try to affect blood loss. Mucosal haemorrhage usually does not have any haemodynamic impact and it is rather an annoying symptom. Often it becomes a side effect of anticoagulation as a prevention of thromboembolic event in advanced oncologic disease. In that case it should be balanced which situation is more comfortable for the patient (mucosal bleeding or risk of thromboembolism). The same type of mucosal bleeding is typical for radiotherapeutic toxicity (early and late onset effect) especially in combination with postmenopausal atrophy of the affected tissues. Also, any type of inflammation of atrophic mucosa may lead to mucosal haemorrhage. Frequent showering, rinsing or irrigating with disinfectant solutions (betadine solution of maximum 10% concentration, chlorhexidine solution in commercially available remedies) is useful for both cases of mucosal bleeding, as well as trophy supporting creams (containing vitamin E). We highly recommend patient, family members and caregivers to pay attention to the best possible hygiene and skincare of genitals and frequent replacement of incontinence aids (pads, panties, diapers).

Source of haemorrhage	Possible etiology	Options for treatment
Vulvar bleeding	Inflammation in the conditions of atrophic skin and mucosa. Pressure ulcers Malignant and non - malignant tumours	Antibiotic/antimycotic ointment, frequent showering. For bleeding ulcers topical adrenalin, Monsel solution, and pressure bandage. Palliative radiotherapy in malignant affections
Vaginal bleeding	Vaginal, cervical and uterine malignant tumours of primary and secondary origin. Fistulas vesico- and recto/ entero-vaginal. Overdosing of anticoagulants. Atrophic mucosa in combination with inflammation or post - radiotherapeutic status.	First aid method – vaginal packing. For cervical and pelvic tumours interventional radiology – based embolization. Evaluation of anticoagulant therapy, adjustments of the dosage in the case of palliative approach. External radiotherapy (brachy–/external)
Urethral bleeding	Urinary inflammation Fistulas Bladder infiltration Post- radiotherapeutic atrophic mucosa Overdosing of anticoagulants	Antibiotics and anti-inflammatory drugs External palliative radiotherapy in bladder infilration Urinary catheters and antifibrinolytic drugs (tranexamic acid) intravenously or orally in case of radiotherapy-related bleeding. Percutaneous nephrostomy tubes bilaterally in fistulas Suprapubic catheter in urethral damage (surgical, tumorous)
Anal bleeding	Haemorrhoidal affections with combination of inflammatory complications. Malignant tumours of gastrointestinal and of metastatic origin. Fistulas Overdosing of anticoagulants Atrophy Radiotherapy related mucosal affections	For external annal affections of different origin: topical adrenalin, Monsel solution and packing. Anti-inflammatory suppositories and ointments. Pelvic external palliative radiotherapy for tumours in pelvis Anticoagulant drugs administered orally or intravenously

Table 1.
Sources of bleeding, possible origin and treatment options.

Bleeding from tumour surfaces or as a consequence of direct invasion of blood vessels usually represents a stressful situation. It may lead to hypotension, tachycardia, shortness of breath and disorders of consciousness. If it is in the patient's interest, and it does not interfere with quality - of life approach, it is possible to try to affect this type of bleeding by interventional radiology- based embolization (occlusion of the vessels that are supplying the anatomic sites of uncontrolled bleeding - internal iliac arteries via femoral artery) [1, 2, 4]. In theory, the same procedure can be managed by open surgery or laparoscopically by ligation of internal iliac arteries. Profit of such a risky step is questionable (aspects of the surgery - wounds, additional blood loss, anaesthesia). The effect of internal iliac obstruction comes almost immediately, in hours and days we can observe decrease in blood loss.

Other option how to reduce vessel bleeding is palliative radiotherapy (external beam radiation therapy -EBRT and/or in combination with brachytherapy). The effect of irradiation evolves in days and week. A summary of literature suggests that the most commonly described fractionation scheme for these patients is 10Gy repeated at one-month intervals to a total of 30Gy as clinical circumstances dictate and tolerance of the dosing allows. Patients who receive all 3 fractions have superior outcomes compared to those who do not, though those with the longest survival often face a recurrence of their local symptoms and an increased incidence of severe toxicity. It is therefore prudent to consider a lower dose-per-fraction for patients who may survive 10 to 12 months, or longer [2].

The duration of the effect of both mentioned procedures (interventional radiologist occlusion and palliative radiotherapy) depends on many factors (the progression rate of oncologic disease, coexistence of other comorbidities and the overall clinical status of the frail palliative patient).

If symptomatic anaemia occurs, it is a matter of discussion whether the treatment with blood transfusion is convenient. The benefits and disadvantages must be thoroughly evaluated, including economic aspects and availability of blood derivatives. Blood transfusion is questionable in the situation where severe bleeding occurs with incurable progressive disease. According to the World Health Organisation (WHO) defines palliative care as a care that affirms life and regards dying as a natural process and intends neither to hasten nor postpone death. It also emphasizes impeccable assessment as essential for effective management [5].

Regardless of the context of the patient's prognosis, quality of life and living conditions we always recommend: liquids orally or parenterally, parenteral antifibrinolytic medication if available, oxygen therapy, anxiolytic medication, morphine in the case of shortness of breath, and all other care known as the best symptomatic and supportive.

3. Fistulas

By the term fistula we mean pathologic communication between neighbouring organs, that does not normally (in conditions of healthy organism) exist. In patients with advanced progressive oncological diseases of pelvis, in patients after radical surgery +/– radiotherapy we often see vesico-vaginal and/or recto(entero-)vaginal fistulas as a consequence of super – radical curative approach. The presence of fistula leads to vaginal discharge, bleeding and develops to absolute urine and /or faecal incontinence. This problem has many aspects (physical, psychological, social, ethical), it has an overlap to the patient integrity and autonomy, especially concerning women, mothers – the pillars of the families. This situation requires a delicate approach of the family members and caregivers. For treatment options see **Table 2**.

Because of all the above-mentioned overlaps of this upsetting symptom, the surgical intervention comes always first. Surgical approach in not recommended only if the patient's condition is poor and would not have any contributions to the quality of life by means of harm and stress It makes sense to solve fistulas and prevent

Type of fistula	Patient capable of surgical intervention	Patient uncapable of surgical intervention
Vesico - vaginal	Abdominal/vaginal approach and reconstructive surgery	Bilateral nephrostomy Urinary catheter, suprapubic catheter – partial relief Continuous use of incontinence aids (pads, panties, diapers)
Recto - vaginal	colostomy	Incontinent aids
Entero - vaginal	Enterostomy (small bowel)	Incontinent aids

Table 2.
Types of fistulas and treatment options in palliative patients.

absolute incontinence even with immobile patients in otherwise good condition and low comorbidities.

In situations where fistulas cannot be bypassed, we stress again to focus on the hygiene and skincare (frequent change of incontinence pads, panties and diapers), showering genitals, disinfectant solutions (diluted betadine solution) rinsing and irrigating. Additionally, we recommend protective nutritive creams to prevent inflammation and pressure ulcers. Even when enterostomy or colostomy was constructed, some discharge from anus and/or vagina can appear, then the above mentioned also applies. The problem of the acidic intestinal content is, that it gets painful in contact with vaginal mucosa in contrast to urine, that is weakly acidic or neutral and usually does not cause any pain. Thus, with faecal incontinence good pain relief is required. If the construction of stomy is not possible and we deal with the situation of a terminal patient with poor prognosis the restriction in alimentation (feeding and eating) comes in question. Vice versa in case of a patient incapable of surgical procedure but not in preterminal nor terminal status, parenteral nutrition should be considered. Otherwise, parenteral nutrition precedes surgical treatment at least for several days for the purpose to reduce the bowel content.

As for the comfort of the patient and the caregivers we recommend air washers, aroma diffusers, fanning or other air fresheners.

4. Vaginal discharge

Most of the causes of vaginal discharge in palliative patients were discussed in previous paragraphs. Evaluation of new discharge is always warning as it may stand for fungal or bacterial infection, which can be treated in the same way as in common gynaecology practise with local disinfectants, antibiotics and antimycotics, together with good hygiene and probiotic supplementation to reinstall the normal

Type of discharge	Etiology	Treatment options
Inflammatory - purulent	Vulvar, vaginal, urinary infection Tumour growth	Disinfectant solutions (10% betadine solution, chlorohexidine solution et.)
Mycotic	Dysmicrobia of genitalia In diabetic and immobile patients	Antimycotics – suppositories, ointments, creams together with probiotics and frequent hygiene by showering and rinsing (including above mentioned disinfectants)
Watery - clear	Urinary infection Urine incontinence Vesico-vaginal fistula Ascites leak Lymph leak	Antibiotics in infection Urinary catheters, suprapubic catheters, surgical approach Paracentesis for ascites derivation Hygiene and skincare
With blood content	Severe inflammation Atrophic mucosa Post radiotherapy Fistulas Tumour growth	Disinfectants, nutritive and protective creams Surgery in fistulas if possible Antifibrinolytics in medication Vaginal packing in tumour bleeding
With faecal content	Fistulas Faecal incontinence	Surgical approach and/or best hygiene and skincare

Table 3.
Types of vaginal discharge, etiology and treatment options in palliative patients.

microbial environment of vagina [1]. In those cases where the discharge represents disease progression (in addition with bleeding and fistulas), a plan for hygiene and for treatment options has to be collaboratively developed (considering surgery procedures, conservative approach, pain relief etc.). See **Table 3**.

5. Conclusion

The problematics of gynaecologic symptoms in palliative care that we discussed represents delicate and intimate sphere and it may disturb patient's autonomy and dignity. The mission of physicians, nurses and caregivers is to consider treatment options thoroughly in context of patient's quality of life, prognosis and life conditions to fulfil the ideals of the best symptomatic and supportive care.

Acknowledgements

The chapter Palliative care in gynaecologic oncology was supported by the grant of the Ministry of Health of the Czech Republic (MHCZ-DRO, MMCI, 00209805).

Conflict of interest

The author has no conflicts of interest.

Dedication

This publication was supported by Ministry of Health of the Czech Republic, MH CZ – DRO (MMCI, 00209805).

Author details

Monika Náležinská[1,2]* and Josef Chovanec[1,2]

1 Department of Surgical Oncology, Division of Gynecologic Oncology, Masaryk Memorial Cancer Institute, Brno, Czech Republic

2 Department of Surgical Oncology, Faculty of Medicine, Masaryk University, Brno, Czech Republic

*Address all correspondence to: monika.nalezinska@mou.cz

References

[1] Kibel SM, Cain JM. Palliative care in gynecological cancer. Int J Gynecol Obstet 2015; 131: S167-S171.

[2] Lutz S, Chow E, Hosin P. Radiation Oncology in Palliative Cancer care. 1.st edition. John Wiley & Sons, Ltd. 2013.

[3] Berger AM, Shuster JL Jr., Von Roenn JH et al. Principles and Practise of Palliative Care and Supportive Oncology. 4.th edition. Lippincot Williams & Wilkins, a Woters Kluwer business. 2013.

[4] Ramondetta I. What is the appropriate approach to treating women with incurable cervical cancer? J Natl Compr Canc Netw 2013;11(3): 348-355.

[5] World Health Organization. WHO definition of palliative care. Available online. www.who.int/cancer/palliative/definition/en.

Chapter 5

Introducer Percutaneous Endoscopic Gastrostomy in Palliative Care of Patients with Esophageal Cancer

Prasit Mahawongkajit

Abstract

In the treatment of esophageal cancer and palliative care, nutritional status plays an important role in the patients' tolerance of treatment, affects the quality of life, and outcomes. Alimentation in such patients can be achieved by enteral or parenteral nutrition but the enteral route is the preferring option. Pre-pyloric feeding is easier and may result in greater nutritional benefits than post-pyloric feeding. Gastrostomy is the conventional option for intra-gastric feeding, hydration, and drug administration. Percutaneous endoscopic gastrostomy (PEG) is a minimally invasive procedure and is currently the procedure of choice. Two PEG techniques are clinically used worldwide: pull and push or introducer method. The pull-type technique is the most commonly used method, but the concerning point is that the implantation of esophageal cancer cells into the gastrostomy stroma. The introducer method is a safe alternative and effective technique for enteral feeding to the stomach with the avoidance of cancer cells seeding.

Keywords: enteral nutrition, palliative care, percutaneous endoscopic gastrostomy, introducer PEG, esophageal cancer, dysphagia, cancer cells seeding

1. Introduction

In 2018, global cancer statistics reported that the incidence of esophageal cancer and mortality were 572,000 new cases and 509,000 deaths, ranking seventh and sixth of all cause cancer morbidity and mortality, Thus, esophageal cancer is a significant global health problem [1]. Most cases present late with advanced disease, especially in the developing countries [1]. Local tumor growth leads to esophageal lumen narrowing and dysphagia and results in increasing difficulty with eating solid food, weight loss and worsening nutritional status. Improving nutritional status is a key factor in determining patient's ability to perform activities of daily living, tolerability of multimodal anticancer treatment, long-term outcomes, and quality of life [2–6].

Percutaneous endoscopic gastrostomy (PEG) is a safe and effective minimally invasive option [7, 8]. Two primary PEG techniques are used worldwide: the pull and push/introducer methods [9, 10]. The pull technique was introduced first and more widely used but cancer seeding through the gastrostomy stroma is a rare but

 IntechOpen

concern disadvantage [11–15]. Refining the pull technique led to the development of the push or introducer technique to avoid tumor seeding to the stroma [9, 16–18].

2. History and concept of the development of the introducer percutaneous endoscopic gastrostomy

Alimentation for esophageal cancer patients can be provided via the enteral or parenteral routes [2, 19, 20]; the enteral route is preferred because it utilizes the gastrointestinal tract and avoids the complications of parenteral nutrition [21, 22]. Placing the feeding tube distally to the location of the cancer is the strategy. Enteral nutrition can be provided by pre-pyloric or post-pyloric feeding (**Table 1**). Intragastric feeding is easier and might provide greater physiologic benefits than the small bowel [23, 24]. The technical approaches of pre-pyloric nutrition include a nasogastric tube (NGT), surgical gastrostomy, and PEG.

NGT is a classic approach for the patient with swallowing difficulties [25]. For early esophageal cancer, when patients may have mild dysphagia and limited luminal obstruction, a NGT should be able to pass easily. However, with advanced disease, the passing of a NGT requires endoscopic or fluoroscopic guidance to confirm the correct position of NGT before start the feeding process [8].

A surgical gastrostomy may be performed by an open approach whereby the feeding tube is placed in the stomach via an upper midline incision. This approach is associated with potential complications such as wound infection [26–29] and respiratory compromise [27, 30–33]. The laparoscopic gastrostomy was developed to minimize the risks of the open technique but it requires substantial training, a skillful surgeon, and experience [34, 35].

PEG was first performed in 1979, using the pull-type technique [36]. This approach was associated with fewer procedural complications than surgical gastrostomy [37–40]. The pull method involves inserting a string into the intragastric space through the abdominal wall. The forceps from an endoscopy grasps the string and pulls it up to the oral cavity. A feeding tube is then passed over the guide string and pushed back down the esophagus, stomach, and then out through the abdominal wall. The pull-type technique is the most commonly used method in clinical

Enteral nutrition methods	Pre-pyloric feeding	Post-pyloric feeding	Risk of cancer seeding
Nasogastric tube (NGT)	+	—	—
Nasojejunal tube (NJT)	—	+	—
Surgical approach			
Gastrostomy	+	—	—
Jejunostomy	—	+	—
Percutaneous endoscopic gastrostomy (PEG)			
Pull technique	+	—	+
Push or Introducer technique	+	—	—
Percutaneous endoscopic transgastric jejunostomy (PEG-J)	—	+	—

+ yes; – no.

Table 1.
Methods for enteral nutrition in esophageal cancer patients.

practice. However, a rare complication is the implantation of esophageal cancer cells into the gastrostomy stroma [11, 12].

The push or introducer method is an alternative PEG technique that avoids seeding cancer cells seeding by direct inoculation during the procedure [13–15, 17, 18]. The push technique involves inserting a guidewire into the stomach through the abdominal wall and then passing the feeding tube over the wire to rest in the stomach [41, 42]. In the Russell technique, once the guidewire is in the intragastric space, a dilator with a sheath is passed over the wire. After removing the dilator and guidewire, the feeding tube is inserted into the sheath, and the sheath is then peeled off [43]. The push method is associated with fewer complications than the pull method [10, 16, 41, 42].

Both PEG methods are also associated with better short-term outcomes over surgical gastrostomy in terms of shorter operative duration, less post-operative pain, and shorter hospitalization [17, 18].

3. Introducer percutaneous endoscopic gastrostomy in palliative care

In palliative care, advanced esophageal cancer patients have suffered from many symptoms such as pain, dysphagia, malnutrition, and psychological problems that depend on the tumor location with staging and the cancer current treatments [44]. Nutritional support is one of the critical roles for symptom management, especially for dysphagia and malnutrition. Also, nausea and vomiting might be the other symptom caused by chemotherapy, radiation, medication, and psychiatric issues that affected the patients' nutritional status [44, 45].

Enteral nutrition is a suitable option for managing these conditions for improving nutritional status, increasing tolerating for chemoradiation therapy, and enhancing the patients' quality of life. The preference for enteral nutrition of advanced esophageal cancer should be safe, minimally invasive with the ability to help in nutritional status. The introducer PEG is a practical choice for advanced esophageal cancer patients who had been included in palliative care [46–48].

4. Indications and contraindications

Clinical assessment to create accurate clinical staging is a crucial step for guiding the optimal management of esophageal cancer patients. Endoscopic resection is an option for the treatment of early esophageal cancer. Tri-modality therapy is an alternative for patients who have more advanced local disease and for patients with metastases group, palliative and supportive care are indicated to improve quality of life [49–51].

Esophageal cancer is often cause anorexia and dysphagia that lead to decreased oral intake and poor nutritional status, dehydration, imbalance of blood chemistry, and malnutrition. Assessing patient's performance status is a crucial for drawing up the treatment plan, irrespective of stage of the disease. Nutrition support is a key element and is indicated in patients whose nutritional status is compromised who cannot be adequately supported by eating and drinking normally. Enteral feeding is the route of first choice and preserves intestinal integrity, has a low risk of complications, and is more cost effective than the parenteral route [2, 52, 53].

NGT is a common practice for enteral nutrition. Passing a nasojejunal tube (NJT) is another enteral nutrition technique but this is technically more challenging [54]. Both NGT and NJT are intended for short-term nutritional support, usually up to four weeks [8, 9], and both require that the esophageal lumen is patent enough to accept the tubes.

Indications
For esophageal cancer Enteral nutrition support with pre-pyloric feeding Minimize the risk of cancer seeding from PEG procedure Apply for gastric decompression
Contraindications
Patient factor Unstable vital signs Sepsis Uncorrected coagulopathy Gastric outlet obstruction or intestinal obstruction **Endoscopic factor** Viscus perforation Gastric pathology Severe abdominal wall infection (especially at the site for the feeding tube) Massive ascites Pregnancy Caustic esophageal or gastric injuries Previous intra-abdominal surgery

Table 2.
Indications and contraindications.

Although surgery plays a long history of enteral nutrition, the various procedures have developed to reduce complications, pain, and additional cosmetic results. Pull-type or introducer PEG is a favored method for a minimally invasive procedure, avoiding the risk of cancer seeding compared to surgical gastrostomy [17, 18]. In addition to patients with esophageal cancer, the introducer PEG could also use in patients who indicated enteral nutrition support with pre-pyloric feeding, demand for long-term enteral feeding, the patients with head and neck cancer that could diminish the risk of cancer seeding from PEG procedure, and apply for gastric decompression [9, 25, 55, 56].

The contraindications for a PEG include: patients with unstable vital signs, sepsis, uncorrected coagulopathy, gastric outlet obstruction or intestinal obstruction as well as patients who have endoscopic contraindications such as a viscus perforation, gastric pathology or severe abdominal wall infection especially at the site for the feeding tube, massive ascites, pregnancy, caustic esophageal or gastric injuries, and previous gastric or intra-abdominal surgery (**Table 2**) [9, 57].

5. Principle of techniques for introducer percutaneous endoscopic gastrostomy

The introducer PEG is performed with the patient in the supine position under local anesthesia, intravenous sedation, or general anesthesia. EGD is necessary for visualization of the stomach during the procedure. For the patients with advanced local disease and dysphagia, the standard diameter endoscope (8–12 mm) [58] might not pass through the narrowed esophageal lumen, necessitating the use of the pediatric endoscope, which has a smaller diameter (4.9–6 mm) [59].

Gastropexy is a technique that anchors the stomach wall to the abdominal wall before the feeding tube is inserted; one method is the double needle gastropexy (**Figure 1**). The double-needle gastropexy is a device with two parallel, 20-gauge needles, and a suture-holding loop. The suture-holding loop inserts through the first needle and the suture inserts through the second needle which is grasped with

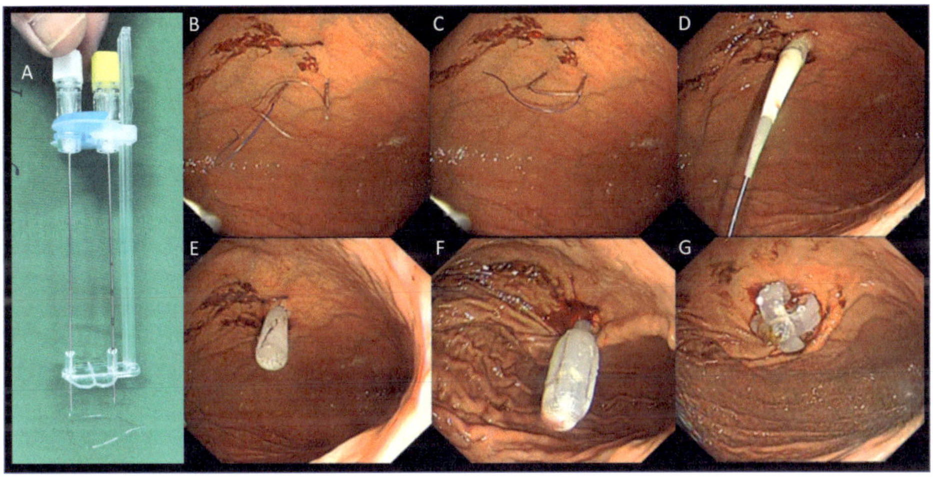

Figure 1.
Percutaneous Endoscopic Gastrostomy (PEG); Endoscopic view of introducer technique. (A) Double-needle gastropexy. (B) Puncture of the double-needle gastropexy and forming the loop to hold the suture. (C) The suture from one of the needles passes through the loop wire from the other needle and tightens the loop. The double-needle device is removed. (D) Puncture and insertion the dilating catheter over the guidewire. (E) The dilating catheter and guidewire are removed. (F) The gastrostomy tube is inserted through the sheath, and then the sheath is peeled away. (G) The bumper of a 24 Fr bumper-type gastrostomy tube (IDEAL PEG Kit; MD-43430; Akita Sumitomo Bakelite Co. Ltd., Akita, Japan).

the snare. The needles are withdrawn, and the suture is tied to the left upper quadrant of the anterior abdominal wall. A second gastropexy is performed 2–3 cm apart in the same way. The gastric wall is then punctured and the dilator inserted over the guidewire, followed by the gastrostomy tube (**Figure 1**) [16, 17].

Previous abdominal surgery of the upper abdomen is a relative contraindication because of altered intra-abdominal anatomy [9, 60]. However, there are reports that safe PEG introduction can be achieved safely with the use of transillumination (using an endoscope passed through the abdominal wall with clear endoscopic intra-gastric visualization by external palpation) [61], a plain abdominal film with air insufflation technique, and computed tomography guided PEG [62–64], and laparoscopic-assisted PEG. These techniques aim to avoid intra-abdominal organ injury [18, 65].

Although the introducer PEG is a proven effective and safe procedure, it suffers the limitation of requiring endoscopy. Passing the endoscope beyond the tumor may be difficult and there is a risk of esophageal perforation in severe esophageal luminal occlusion. In advanced cases, surgical gastrostomy and laparoscopic-assisted PEG are the alternative procedures [17, 18]. A recent study published the comparison of both techniques, and the laparoscopic-assisted PEG had advantages in the procedural duration, blood loss, postoperative pain, and hospitalization [18].

6. Complications

Although the push/introducer PEG is a minimally invasive technique that demonstrates a method in enteral nutrition [10, 17, 18, 66, 67], it is associated with several complications [9, 17, 68], including death in patients with underlying comorbidities [69].

Bleeding is the most common complication and is usually minor and manifest as oozing around the feeding tube. Apply the simple compression should stop the bleeding. If the bleeding more severe, it might be due to injury to e.g. gastric and gastroepiploic arteries. A pressure dressing is often effective but if bleeding continues, it can be treated by endoscopy, embolization, or surgery [9, 17, 57]. Selecting carefully the correct anatomical site and correcting a coagulopathy, if present, should prevent or minimize the risk of bleeding complications.

Abdominal organ injuries to the small bowel, colon, liver, and spleen may occur caused by the interposition of these organs between the gastric wall and the abdominal wall [9, 57, 70–73]. EGD should always be performed using transillumination, for clear intra-gastric visualization, and external palpation to identify and interposition of the internal organs [61]. If there is doubt, then laparoscopy can be performed to assure direct visualization of the intra-abdominal cavity [18].

Aspiration pneumonia is a severe complication and is associated with a mortality of PEG [9, 57]. Esophageal cancer patients, especially in elderly, heavy smokers with or without chronic obstructive pulmonary disease (COPD), have a higher risk of aspiration pneumonia compared to other patients and is related to residual liquid or food in the esophagus proximal to the obstruction. By technical for advanced esophageal cancer patients, the pediatric endoscope often chosen for the PEG procedure. The endoscope's small diameter is followed by the small endoscopic channel, resulting in less suction performance than the standard endoscope. Measures to reduce the risk of aspiration include the use of topical pharyngeal anesthesia rather than sedation, frequent mouth suction, and the reverse Trendelenburg position [74, 75].

The buried bumper syndrome (BBS) occurs when the internal bumper erodes into the wall of the stomach and sometimes becomes entirely buried within the gastric wall. It might cause by a disproportionate size and length of the feeding tube with the thickness of the abdominal wall. The main causative factor is excessive tightening of the external bumper, leading to increased pressure of the internal bumper on the wall of the stomach, local ischemia and gastric wall erosion (**Figure 2**). Additional risk factors include obesity, weight gain, malnutrition, corticosteroid therapy, and poor wound healing. BBS is a late complication and usually occurs > one year post PEG but it may be seen within several weeks of PEG placement. It may be asymptomatic or cause pain. Malfunction of the PEG is common, leading to leakage around the entry site, difficulty administering the feeds, fluids or drugs, infection, abscess or peritonitis [76, 77]. If BBS occurs, the tube should be removed by endoscopy, surgical intervention, or external traction, depending on the type of feeding tube and the patient's situation [9, 77, 78].

Necrotizing fasciitis is the rare and severe PEG complication and is associated with a high mortality. Local ischemia leads to bacterial infection with a mix of anaerobic and aerobic organisms from gastrointestinal tract and skin. The infection progresses rapidly along with fascial plane and causes extensive abdominal fascia necrosis [79]. Treatment includes urgent aggressive and wide surgical debridement, intravenous broad-spectrum antibiotics and close clinical monitoring in the intensive care unit [9, 80–82]. The prognosis is very poor.

Granuloma formation is a minor but common complication that results from peristomal hyper-granulation due to friction of the PEG tube and humidity due to tube leakage [83, 84]. Patients are prone to local infection and contact bleeding. Treatment includes topical antibiotics, topical steroids, electrocauterization, or cauterizing by silver nitrate. Surgical debridement may be required for sizeable peristomal granulomas [9, 83, 85].

Peristomal leakage and local infection are also minor complications that causing discomfort, pain and annoyance for patients and their families. Good peristomal hygiene and dressings combined with reducing the volume of feeds and minimizing PEG tube movements are treatment options. If these failed, removing the PEG tube and placing it in another area can be done or abandoning PEG enteral feeding for another form [9, 57, 68].

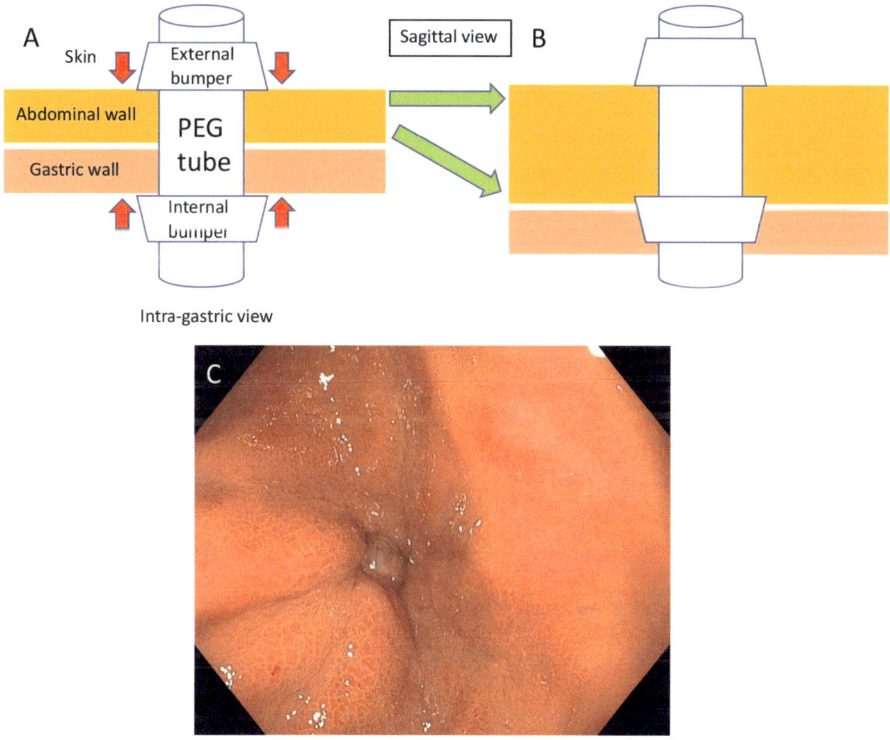

Figure 2.
Buried bumper syndrome. (A, B) The external and internal bumper held correctly in position (A) but with pressure and ischemic necrosis, the internal migrates through the gastric wall into the abdominal wall (B). (C) Endoscopic examination of a patient with the Buried Bumper syndrome.

7. Conclusion

Percutaneous endoscopic gastrostomy is a minimally invasive procedure for the patients who need enteral nutrition support, hydration, and medications. For esophageal cancer patients and palliative care, the introducer technique is the optimal technique and prevents cancer seeding from the operative procedure.

Acknowledgements

The author would like to thank Assistant Professor Jirawat Swangsri M.D., Ph.D. (Department of Surgery, Siriraj Hospital, Mahidol University) for the first case technical assistance with the introducer PEG procedure in Thammasat University Hospital.

Conflict of interest

The author declares no conflict of interest.

Notes/thanks/other declarations

Special thanks to Dr. Bob Taylor for assistance in editing the English version of this chapter.

Author details

Prasit Mahawongkajit
Department of Surgery, Faculty of Medicine, Thammasat University, Pathumthani, Thailand

*Address all correspondence to: prasit_md@yahoo.com

References

[1] Bray F, Ferlay J, Soerjomataram I, Siegel RL, Torre LA, Jemal A. Global cancer statistics 2018: GLOBOCAN estimates of incidence and mortality worldwide for 36 cancers in 185 countries. CA Cancer J Clin. 2018;68(6):394-424.

[2] Jordan T, Mastnak DM, Palamar N, Kozjek NR. Nutritional therapy for patients with esophageal cancer. Nutr Cancer. 2018;70(1):23-9.

[3] Fietkau R, Lewitzki V, Kuhnt T, et al. A disease-specific enteral nutrition formula improves nutritional status and functional performance in patients with head and neck and esophageal cancer undergoing chemoradiotherapy: results of a randomized, controlled, multicenter trial. Cancer. 2013;119(18):3343-53.

[4] Vasson MP, Talvas J, Perche O, et al. Immunonutrition improves functional capacities in head and neck and esophageal cancer patients undergoing radiochemotherapy: a randomized clinical trial. Clin Nutr. 2014;33(2):204-10.

[5] Anandavadivelan P, Lagergren P. Cachexia in patients with oesophageal cancer. Nat Rev Clin Oncol. 2016;13(3):185-98.

[6] Birnstein E, Schattner M. Nutritional support in esophagogastric cancers. Surg Oncol Clin N Am. 2017;26(2):325-33.

[7] Holmes S. Enteral feeding and percutaneous endoscopic gastrostomy. Nurs Stand. 2004;18(20):41-3.

[8] Nunes G, Fonseca J, Barata AT, Dinis-Ribeiro M, Pimentel-Nunes P. Nutritional Support of Cancer Patients without Oral Feeding: How to Select the Most Effective Technique? GE Port J Gastroenterol. 2020;27(3):172-84.

[9] Rahnemai-Azar AA, Rahnemaiazar AA, Naghshizadian R, Kurtz A, Farkas DT. Percutaneous endoscopic gastrostomy: indications, technique, complications and management. World J Gastroenterol. 2014;20(24):7739-51.

[10] Tucker AT, Gourin CG, Ghegan MD, Porubsky ES, Martindale RG, Terris DJ. 'Push' versus 'pull' percutaneous endoscopic gastrostomy tube placement in patients with advanced head and neck cancer. Laryngoscope. 2003;113(11):1898-902.

[11] Cappell MS. Risk factors and risk reduction of malignant seeding of the percutaneous endoscopic gastrostomy track from pharyngoesophageal malignancy: a review of all 44 known reported cases. Am J Gastroenterol. 2007;102(6):1307-11.

[12] Sousa AL, Sousa D, Velasco F, Açucena F, Lopes A, Guerreiro H. Rare complication of percutaneous endoscopic gastrostomy: ostomy metastasis of esophageal carcinoma. World J Gastrointest Oncol. 2013;5(11):204-6.

[13] Sinapi I, Navez B, Hamoir M. Seeding of the percutaneous endoscopic gastrostomy site from head and neck carcinoma: case report and review of the literature. Head Neck. 2013;35(7):E209-12.

[14] Köhler G, Kalcher V, Koch OO, Luketina RR, Emmanuel K, Spaun G. Comparison of 231 patients receiving either "pull- through" or "push" percutaneous endoscopic gastrostomy. Surg Endosc. 2015;29(1):170-5.

[15] Adelson RT, Ducic Y. Metastatic head and neck carcinoma to a percutaneous endoscopic gastrostomy site. Head Neck. 2005;27(4):339-43.

[16] Okumura N, Tsuji N, Ozaki N, Matsumoto N, Takaba T, Kawasaki M, et al. Percutaneous endoscopic gastrostomy with Funada-style gastropexy greatly reduces the risk of peristomal infection. Gastroenterol Rep (Oxf). 2015;3(1):69-74.

[17] Mahawongkajit P, Techagumpuch A, Limpavitayaporn P, et al. Comparison of Introducer Percutaneous Endoscopic Gastrostomy with Open Gastrostomy in Advanced Esophageal Cancer Patients. Dysphagia. 2020;35(1):117-20.

[18] Mahawongkajit P, Techagumpuch A. Gastrostomy in Patients With Previous Abdominal Surgery: A Comparative Study Between the Laparoscopy-Assisted Introducer Percutaneous Endoscopic Gastrostomy Versus Open Gastrostomy in Advanced Esophageal Cancer. Dysphagia. 2020 Apr 9. doi: 10.1007/s00455-020-10110-5.

[19] Reim D, Friess H. Feeding Challenges in Patients with Esophageal and Gastroesophageal Cancers. Gastrointest Tumors. 2016;2(4):166-77.

[20] Chen F, Fang J, Wang H, et al. Effects of nutritional support on short-term clinical outcomes and immune response in unresectable locally advanced oesophageal squamous cell carcinoma. Eur J Cancer Care (Engl). 2018;27(2):e12818.

[21] Modi RM, Mikhail S, Ciombor K, et al. Outcomes of nutritional interventions to treat dysphagia in esophageal cancer: a population-based study. Dis Esophagus. 2017;30(11):1-8.

[22] Furuta M, Yokota T, Tsushima T, et al. Comparison of enteral nutrition with total parenteral nutrition for patients with locally advanced unresectable esophageal cancer harboring dysphagia in definitive chemoradiotherapy. Jpn J Clin Oncol. 2019;49(10):910-8.

[23] Jabbar A, McClave SA. Pre-pyloric versus post-pyloric feeding. Clin Nutr. 2005;24(5):719-26.

[24] Marik PE, Zaloga GP. Gastric versus post-pyloric feeding: a systematic review. Crit Care. 2003;7(3):R46-51.

[25] Gomes CA Jr, Andriolo RB, Bennett C, et al. Percutaneous endoscopic gastrostomy versus nasogastric tube feeding for adults with swallowing disturbances. Cochrane Database Syst Rev. 2015 May 22;2015(5):CD008096.

[26] Patel SV, Paskar DD, Nelson RL, Vedula SS, Steele SR. Closure methods for laparotomy incisions for preventing incisional hernias and other wound complications. Cochrane Database Syst Rev. 2017;11:CD005661.

[27] Stone HH, Hoefling SJ, Strom PR, Dunlop WE, Fabian TC. Abdominal incisions: transverse vs vertical placement and continuous vs interrupted closure. South Med J. 1983;76(9):1106-8.

[28] Gheorghe A, Calvert M, Pinkney TD, et al; West Midlands Research Collaborative; ROSSINI Trial Management Group. Systematic review of the clinical effectiveness of wound-edge protection devices in reducing surgical site infection in patients undergoing open abdominal surgery. Ann Surg. 2012;255(6):1017-29.

[29] Bosanquet DC, Ansell J, Abdelrahman T, et al. Systematic Review and Meta-Regression of Factors Affecting Midline Incisional Hernia Rates: Analysis of 14,618 Patients. PLoS One. 2015;10(9):e0138745.

[30] Grantcharov TP, Rosenberg J. Vertical compared with transverse incisions in abdominal surgery. Eur J Surg. 2001;167(4):260-7.

[31] Brown SR, Goodfellow PB. Transverse verses midline incisions for

abdominal surgery. Cochrane Database Syst Rev. 205;19(4):CD005199.

[32] Elman A, Langonnet F, Dixsaut G, et al. Respiratory function is impaired less by transverse than by median vertical supraumbilical incisions. Intensive Care Med. 1981;7(5):235-9.

[33] Mimica Z1, Pogorelić Z, Perko Z, Srsen D, Stipić R, Dujmović D. Effect of surgical incision on pain and respiratory function after abdominal surgery: a randomized clinical trial. Hepatogastroenterology. 2007;54(80):2216-20.

[34] Mizrahi I, Garg M, Divino CM, Nguyen S. Comparison of laparoscopic versus open approach to gastrostomy tubes. JSLS. 2014;18(1):28-33.

[35] Bankhead RR, Fisher CA, Rolandelli RH. Gastrostomy tube placement outcomes: comparison of surgical, endoscopic, and laparoscopic methods. Nutr Clin Pract. 2005;20(6):607-12.

[36] Gauderer MW, Ponsky JL, Izant RJ Jr. Gastrostomy without laparotomy: a percutaneous endoscopic technique. J Pediatr Surg. 1980;15:872-5.

[37] Schneider AS, Schettler A, Markowski A, et al; Conference presentation: 36th ESPEN Congress in Leipzig, Germany on August 31st - September 3rd , 2013. Complication and mortality rate after percutaneous endoscopic gastrostomy are low and indication-dependent. Scand J Gastroenterol. 2014;49(7):891-8.

[38] Ljungdahl M, Sundbom M. Complication rate lower after percutaneous endoscopic gastrostomy than after surgical gastrostomy: a prospective, randomized trial. Surg Endosc. 2006;20(8):1248-51.

[39] Rahnemai-Azar AA, Rahnemaiazar AA, Naghshizadian R, Kurtz A1, Farkas DT. Percutaneous endoscopic gastrostomy: indications, technique, complications and management. World J Gastroenterol. 2014;20(24):7739-51.

[40] Payne KM, King TM, Eisenach JB. The technique of percutaneous endoscopic gastrostomy. A safe and cost-effective alternative to operative gastrostomy. J Crit Illn. 1991;6(6):611-9.

[41] Hogan RB, DeMarco DC, Hamilton JK, Walker CO, Polter DE. Percutaneous endoscopic gastrostomy—to push or pull. A prospective randomized trial. Gastrointest Endosc. 1986; 32(4):253-8.

[42] Kozarek RA, Ball TJ, Ryan JA Jr. When push comes to shove: a comparison between two methods of percutaneous endoscopic gastrostomy. Am J Gastroenterol. 1986; 81(8):642-6.

[43] Russell TR, Brotman M, Norris F. Percutaneous gastrostomy. A new simplified and cost-effective technique. Am J Surg. 1984; 148(1):132-7.

[44] Guyer DL, Almhanna K, McKee KY. Palliative care for patients with esophageal cancer: a narrative review. Ann Transl Med. 2020;8(17):1103.

[45] Merchant SJ, Kong W, Brundage M, Booth CM. Symptom Evolution in Patients with Esophageal and Gastric Cancer Receiving Palliative Chemotherapy: A Population-Based Study. Ann Surg Oncol. 2020 Nov 2. doi: 10.1245/s10434-020-09289-6.

[46] Kusakabe A, Sato A, Sugiura R, Koide T, Inamori M. The role of percutaneous endoscopic gastrostomy(PEG)in palliative care. Gan To Kagaku Ryoho. 2011;38 Suppl 1:85-6.

[47] Yagishita A, Kakushima N, Tanaka M, et al. Percutaneous endoscopic

gastrostomy using the direct method for aerodigestive cancer patients. Eur J Gastroenterol Hepatol. 2012;24(1):77-81.

[48] Ogino H, Akiho H. Usefulness of percutaneous endoscopic gastrostomy for supportive therapy of advanced aerodigestive cancer. World J Gastrointest Pathophysiol. 2013;4(4):119-25.

[49] National Comprehensive Cancer Network. NCCN clinical practice guidelines in oncology: Esophageal and Esophagogastric junction Cancers, version 2[Internet]. Fort Washington, PA: National Comprehensive Cancer Network; 2020. https://www.nccn.org/ professionals/physician_gls/PDF/esophageal.pdf Accessed 5 July 2020.

[50] Kitagawa Y, Uno T, Oyama T, et al. Esophageal cancer practice guidelines 2017 edited by the Japan Esophageal Society: part 1. Esophagus. 2019;16(1):1-24.

[51] Kitagawa Y, Uno T, Oyama T, et al. Esophageal cancer practice guidelines 2017 edited by the Japan Esophageal Society: part 2. Esophagus. 2019;16(1):25-43.

[52] Schattner M. Enteral nutritional support of the patient with cancer: route and role. J Clin Gastroenterol. 2003;36(4):297-302.

[53] Birnstein E, Schattner M. Nutritional Support in Esophagogastric Cancers. Surg Oncol Clin N Am. 2017;26(2):325-33.

[54] Montejo JC, Grau T, Acosta J, et al. Multicenter, prospective, randomized, single-blind study comparing the efficacy and gastrointestinal complications of early jejunal feeding with early gastric feeding in critically ill patients. Crit Care Med. 2002;30(4):796-800.

[55] Prabhakaran S, Doraiswamy VA, Nagaraja V, et al. Nasoenteric tube complications. Scand J Surg. 2012;42(1):132-8.

[56] Lucendo AJ, Friginal-Ruiz AB. Percutaneous endoscopic gastrostomy: An update on its indications, management, complications, and care. Rev Esp Enferm Dig. 2014;106(8):529-39.

[57] Hucl T, Spicak J. Complications of percutaneous endoscopic gastrostomy. Best Pract Res Clin Gastroenterol. 2016;30(5):769-81.

[58] Aydinli M, Koruk I, Dag MS, Savas MC, Kadayifci A. Ultrathin endoscopy for gastrointestinal strictures. Dig Endosc. 2012; 24(3):150-3.

[59] ASGE Technology Committee, Barth BA, Banerjee S, et al. Equipment for pediatric endoscopy. Gastrointest Endosc. 2012;76(1):8-17.

[60] Eleftheriadis E, Kotzampassi K. Percutaneous endoscopic gastrostomy after abdominal surgery. Surg Endosc. 2001;15(2):213-6.

[61] Chang WK, Yu CY, Chao YC. Positioning a safe gastric puncture point before percutaneous endoscopic gastrostomy. Int J Clin Pract. 2007;61:1121-5.

[62] Chang WK, Hsieh TY. Safety of percutaneous endoscopic gastrostomy in high-risk patients. J Gastroenterol Hepatol. 2013;28(Suppl 4):118-22.

[63] Vogt W, Messmann H, Lock G, et al. CT-guided PEG in patients with unsuccessful endoscopic transillumination. Gastrointest Endosc. 1996;43(2 Pt 1):138-40.

[64] Thornton FJ, Varghese JC, Haslam PJ, et al. Percutaneous gastrostomy in patients who fail or are unsuitable for

endoscopic gastrostomy. Cardiovasc Intervent Radiol. 2000;23:279-84.

[65] Thaker AM, Sedarat A. Laparoscopic-assisted percutaneous endoscopic gastrostomy. Curr Gastroenterol Rep. 2016;18(9):46.

[66] Giordano-Nappi JH, Maluf-Filho F, Ishioka S, et al. A new large-caliber trocar for percutaneous endoscopic gastrostomy by the introducer technique in head and neck cancer patients. Endoscopy. 2011;43(9):752-8.

[67] Foster JM, Filocamo P, Nava H, et al. The introducer technique is the optimal method for placing percutaneous endoscopic gastrostomy tubes in head and neck cancer patients. Surg Endosc. 2007;21(6):897-901.

[68] Yuruker S, Koca B, Karabicak I, Kuru B, Ozen N. Percutaneous Endoscopic Gastrostomy: Technical Problems, Complications, and Management. Indian J Surg. 2015;77(Suppl3):1159-64.

[69] Zopf Y, Maiss J, Konturek P, Rabe C, Hahn EG, Schwab D. Predictive factors of mortality after PEG insertion: guidance for clinical practice. JPEN J Parenter Enteral Nutr. 2011; 35(1):50-5.

[70] Guloglu R, Taviloglu K, Alimoglu O. Colon injury following percutaneous endoscopic gastrostomy tube insertion. J Laparoendosc Adv Surg Tech A. 2003; 13(1):69-72.

[71] Karhadkar AS, Schwartz HJ, Dutta SK. Jejunocutaneous fistula manifesting as chronic diarrhea after PEG tube replacement. J Clin Gastroenterol. 2006; 40(6):560-1.

[72] Chaer RA, Rekkas D, Trevino J, Brown R, Espat J. Intrahepatic placement of a PEG tube. Gastrointest Endosc. 2003; 57(6):763-5.

[73] Lau G, Lai SH. Fatal retroperitoneal haemorrhage: an unusual complication of percutaneous endoscopic gastrostomy. Forensic Sci Int. 2001; 116(1):69-75.

[74] Li Bassi G, Marti JD, Saucedo L, et al. Gravity predominates over ventilatory pattern in the prevention of ventilator-associated pneumonia. Crit Care Med. 2014;42(9):e620-7.

[75] Li Bassi G, Torres A. Ventilator-associated pneumonia: role of positioning. Curr Opin Crit Care. 2011;17(1):57-63.

[76] Geer W, Jeanmonod R. Early presentation of buried bumper syndrome. West J Emerg Med. 2013;14(5):421-3.

[77] Klein S, Heare BR, Soloway RD. The "buried bumper syndrome": a complication of percutaneous endoscopic gastrostomy. Am J Gastroenterol. 1990;85(4):448-51.

[78] Ma MM, Semlacher EA, Fedorak RN, et al. The buried gastrostomy bumper syndrome: prevention and endoscopic approaches to removal. Gastrointest Endosc. 1995;41(5):505-8.

[79] Chung RS, Schertzer M. Pathogenesis of complications of percutaneous endoscopic gastrostomy. A lesson in surgical principles. Am Surg. 1990; 56(3):134-7.

[80] MacLean AA, Miller G, Bamboat ZM, Hiotis K. Abdominal wall necrotizing fasciitis from dislodged percutaneous endoscopic gastrostomy tubes: a case series. Am Surg. 2004;56(9):134-7.

[81] Haas DW, Dharmaraja P, Morrison JG, Potts JR 3rd. Necrotizing fasciitis following percutaneous endoscopic gastrostomy. Gastrointest Endosc. 1988;34(6):487-8.

[82] Evans DA, Bhandarkar DS, Taylor TV. Necrotising fasciitis--a rare complication of percutaneous endoscopic gastrostomy. Endoscopy. 1995;27(8):627.

[83] Warriner L, Spruce P. Managing overgranulation tissue around gastrostomy sites. Br J Nurs. 2012;21(5):S14-6.

[84] Borkowski S. G tube care: managing hypergranulation tissue. Nursing. 2005;35(8):24.

[85] Schrag SP, Sharma R, Jaik NP, et al. Complications related to percutaneous endoscopic gastrostomy (PEG) tubes. A comprehensive clinical review. J Gastrointestin Liver Dis. 2007;16(4):407-18.

Chapter 6

Why Are We Missing the Teeth? Addressing Oral Care Neglect in the Palliative Patient

Kristi M. Soileau

Abstract

Palliative care is meant to comfort and console the mind, body, and spirit of the individual nearing the end of life to improve the quality of one's existence. It focuses on those with symptoms and stressors secondary to serious illnesses such as in cancer, pneumonia, Parkinson's disease, Alzheimer's, hypertension, diabetes, and microbial diseases. For several reasons, however, oral care and the consequences thereof in most cases go without notice for these patients. Further, the dentist is rarely, if ever, listed as necessary staff in hospice care programs. Because terminal patients' symptoms can include depression, pain, anxiety, loss of appetite, nausea, fatigue, among other issues, all related to speaking, chewing, and deglutition, this chapter will discuss why care of the mouth and dentition is typically lacking both in at-home and institutional environments, why such care is necessary, and best to meet the oral needs of patients in the later stages of life.

Keywords: oral care, ethics, end of life, palliative, dental/medical collaboration

1. Introduction

Properly implemented dental care is necessary not only for having a healthy, long lasting dentition, but also in maintaining overall systemic health and in promoting a sense of well-being. This is understandably true for the general populous, and is wholly acknowledged as such; yet there is an element of neglect in that sector of care dealing with the institutionalized elderly and infirmed.

Hospice and long-term care philosophy typically enshrouds palliation for the terminally ill and frail elderly, whose quality of life must include all aspects of comfort care management. Too often, however, medical and dental professionals and caregivers under their charge in both nursing homes and institutions simply do not elect to carry out oral care to any viable or reasonable extent. This may be from several reasons, such as difficulties encountered in patient compliance, issues with staff shortages, a sense of futility, and quite frequently an overall lack of education as to why regularly and properly implemented oral care for those unable to maintain adequate oral hygiene procedures without assistance must be given prioritization in the comfort care daily routine.

Having spent 25 years contracted with a nursing home in which I perform semi-annual oral evaluations on resident patients, and in visiting other such locales in the region, I have often witnessed the inadequacies common to most institutions where oral evaluation, preventive techniques, and palliative care of the mouth are sorely lacking. In an effort to improve the standards of oral management in the dependent and incapable, I would urge all medical institutions to mandate that a dentist be on staff, and that minimum standards programs be instituted as are appropriate, yet this is seldom the case. Even in a local faith-based hospice for which I am the gratis dental consultant, I am not listed as a member of the staff team, but rather as a volunteer.

There are multiple obstacles to be overcome to correct these inadequacies, but with compassion, candor, and competency these challenges are indeed surmountable.

2. Addressing oral care neglect in palliative care patients

In dental school in the eighties, I was offered one course on geriatric-centered care that required the students to spend a couple days observing at a nearby nursing facility, going from room-to-room with an instructor. There was, as is typically the case, no functioning, physical dental clinic. Some patients were seen by us at bedside, but with little overhead lighting. We held flashlights for one another. We gave up rather quickly on those who were combative to any extent. Positioning was difficult in many patients who were less limber than others. Nonetheless, it wasn't these incongruencies with which I take issue, but rather the fact that so little time was afforded to us students to learn to treat these types of patients and that we felt as though the paltry care we were able to administer was likely of little benefit.

2.1 Why oral care is vitally important in the terminal and dependent patient?

Palliative care serves essentially to inhibit an existence of pain and suffering. [1] The World Health Organization (WHO) defines palliative care as: an approach that improve the quality of life of patients and their families facing the problems associated with life-threatening illness, for the prevention of a life of suffering by means of early identification and impeccable assessment and treatment of pain and other problems, physical, psychosocial, and spiritual. [2]

Dental care is a fundamental part in management of patients with advanced disease, and oral care must become ensconced in the total care palliative philosophy to best maintain life quality. [3] Sischo and Broder describe a quality of life that focuses on oral health as it relates to functional and emotional well-being, expectations and satisfaction with general care, and an overall sense of self. [4]

To be certain, poor oral health can negatively affect nutrition, comfort, and social issues. [5–10] Jobbins found Candidiasis in 85% of patients studied, which can cause burning and dry mouth [11], such that palliative care is often required. [12–14] These burning and discomforting circumstances can also lead to anorexia, difficulty swallowing, problematic respiration, and inhibited verbal communicative ability. [15] Additionally, in patients with poor oral hygiene, the "bonding" that occurs with family and friends and even professional care givers can be impeded in instances of oral neglect due to offensive halitosis, unattractive tooth loss and rampant decay, heavy plaque and bleeding gums. [16] To avoid these circumstances, it is vital that all attempts possible be made to assure that the patient feels fresh, welcomed by others, and retains dignity as much as is possible.

Further, periodontal disease is a very common problem among the elderly, being linked to 46% of American adults between the years of 2007 and 2012. [17] This disease of the tissues that hold the teeth in place can create systemic medical conditions such as aspiration pneumonia [18] as well as heart disease, diabetes, and cancer. [19] Periodontitis results in the release of inflammatory cytokines, growth factors, prostaglandins, and enzymes [20], and results in many ramifications, ranging from a depressed mental state to renal disease. [21]

Of even greater interest due to its relevance in more recent times, perhaps, is the fact that a 2020 study out of the University of Toronto has stated that there is evidence showing that patients with periodontal disease may be much more likely to have heightened issues with COVID-19. [22] This is likely because in patients with active and untreated periodontal infection, already-circulating neutrophils are more excitable and ready to attack in a rather hyper-vigilant nature after a second infection, such as a viral load, is introduced into the body. The authors explain further that this cascade of events creates a susceptibility towards damage within one's body from these "primed" infection fighting cells to destroy affected tissues and organs more readily, leading to more negative outcomes. [22] This may explain why some have far more hasty and deleterious pulmonary and renal issues from COVID-19 as compared to those individuals who have no symptoms whatsoever.

In my experience, another very real challenge with oral issues in the elderly and infirmed relative to COVID-19 has been that governmental limitations on visits to nursing homes and other such institutions has impeded my getting in to perform my monthly preventative screenings over the course of the past year. This may be more inconsequential for the patient who is alert and communicative and can request an emergency visit from or to a dental professional; however, in those patients who are suffering from pain without giving outward signs of such may have issues that can only be discoverable via an on-site oral examination. This oversight does not bode well in cases such as these, and it puts into play a storm of conflicting ethical principles.

Further, in my recent visits to the home of one particular hospice patient whose diagnosis was terminal, I was there strictly to offer emotional support to the spouse. I would simply bring groceries whenever requested by the husband, who only asked for goods to be delivered that his wife needed for sustenance. It was obvious that he was not only depressed from his wife's condition, but also from the restrictive isolation he was going through socially from COVID restrictions. It was just the two of them-alone-except for the care extended by the hospice facility. I would imagine that this, and the fact that he was wheelchair-bound, made life exceptionally burdensome for this couple and others like them.

2.2 Why care of the mouth and dentition is typically lacking in the institutionalized infirmed

Some see this demand for more meticulous oral care as being futile.

It is not uncommon to find apathy among professionals and their staff members who view treatment at this level as being redundant, burdensome, unpleasant, and unfulfilling. [9] Others may feel that meticulous oral care may be "overdoing it" in these more intolerant and sickly cases. [23, 24] Thus, it is out of concern for the patients that they inadvertently neglect that oral component of care that they do not understand to be a necessary part of therapy. Still others do not like to have to restrain, force, or argue with many patients to clean their mouths or to remove their dentures, so the feat goes underperformed day after day. Plaque accumulations from both teeth and gingiva can get into the lungs and have been noted as the cause for the prior-mentioned aspiration pneumonia. [18]

A lack of supplies afforded to staff may also account for reasons of neglect. Are there toothbrushes, non-toxic toothpastes, denture storage cups and denture cleaning tablets available? Are there natural oils for caregivers to use for coating and soothing dry and burning oral tissues?

Some see this demand for more meticulous oral care as absorbing precious staff time.

And the institution in which I work, it seems that all employees are for the most part already so busy that I cannot see how time could be allotted to attend to patients' mouths with regularity, except to develop a very efficient method that is part of the daily protocol. Such a plan has yet to be established in the vast majority of institutions as far as I am able to tell.

For example, is there adequate lighting, and if not, can an institution afford to have one staff member hold a light while another performs hygiene ... and is this to be done daily, twice daily, or more? Should headlamps be purchased for each caregiver? Further, manipulating patients into positions that afford one better oral visibility in attempting bedside care can be physically taxing to those staff delegated to this function.

Certainly, since many auxiliary staff are not trained in dental schools, as are healthcare professionals, to become conditioned to working in another person's oral cavity, it can be daunting to some who must become so closely approximated to the mouth and have to deal with the unpleasantries of the smells and sights of plaque, halitosis, periodontal disease and the like.

Some see this demand for more meticulous oral care as reimbursing too little for the amount of time it takes to accomplish needed tasks.

In most cases, and perhaps even in most countries, the reimbursement fees for oral care whether for maintenance or restorative procedures in these aged and infirmed is little more than paltry. Typically, in the United States, Medicare and Medicaid funding for oral conditions is only available where medical illnesses are secondary to dental injury or disease, such as with an abscess that brings many to an emergency room. One problem with neglecting regular exams in the aged infirmed is that many individuals cannot describe their pain or even indicate that there is any discomfort whatsoever, and these infections may ultimately prove to be an undocumented cause of death.

For those patients who can verbally communicate that they are uncomfortable and have pain, it is imperative that the caregiver check for allergies and other medications being given to the patient that may not be compatible with a particular pain medication being considered for therapy. One also must be cognizant of the fact that pain medications may make these already frail patients more likely to fall or become disoriented and more confused than is normally the case. Further, it is certainly advisable to use the lowest dose and least number of pills possible for managing patient pain, and to avoid opioids, if at all possible, by using alternating doses of nonsteroidal inflammatory drugs with acetaminophen where tolerated. [25]

Distress experienced during injections may also be reduced by use of a controlled flow anesthesia system [26], and in some cases very loose teeth may be extractable with the use of a xylocaine viscous gel or topical anesthetic so as to avoid the stress of dental injections to accomplish the necessary treatment.

2.3 Moving forward to best meet the oral care needs of institutionalized patients requiring palliation

With so many questions, there seem to be very few answers in addressing this severe shortfall in caring for the oral soft tissues and dentition in this vulnerable population. But we must start somewhere, and that begins with shunning apathy and embracing the awareness that there is much ground to be gained if those who can make a difference will work towards eldercare dental equity. This starts most particularly with dentists, their staff, hospice and long-term care institutions, as well as their staff managers, physicians, nurses, and aides, all working in tandem

DOI: http://dx.doi.org/10.5772/intechopen.95606

for planning, implementing, and assessing dental programs within each healthcare setting.

Dentists must first evaluate the institutional setting in mind for enhancing change of oral care practices. Then, the dentist should consider those capabilities for stepping up oral care to levels that are reasonably within reach. After meeting with the staff administrator, and possibly even the medical staff as well, the two entities should then discuss how to implement the envisioned changes, taking into consideration the limitations the institution has therein.

For example, they should together decide if conditions exist for their patients to be evaluated yearly, biannually, or perhaps even monthly, which time frame will depend on the total number of individuals within the institution and the availability of staff as resources to help organize the entire patient "recall system". Thus, if the dental team can perform an oral exam or screening on 15 patients in one day, and the dentist is able to work for that entity one day a week, approximately 60 patients could be evaluated and their treatment plans customized/altered as need be each month. If, then, there are 180 patients in the facility, all could be covered within a three -month time frame, and this institution might well have each patient seen quarterly. However, were the dentist to only work once a month, then the patients within the facility may only receive an annual evaluation.

Of course, deflecting apathy starts with proper training, and this begins through advocacy education within the dental school itself. Schools are urged to develop a dental curriculum for "justice", placing a heavier emphasis on basic dental care for those with mental health and physical disabilities, geriatric dentistry, and nursing home oral health care. [27] Students should know that lower-paying positions and charitable services should be considered where need is significant, even if done on a limited basis. Rozas et al. speak of the "wide gap in knowledge regarding effective methods" specific to oral care in patients with dementia. [28] Oftentimes, a school can make a significant impact in a local healthcare community by sending its students to such sites on rotations, following proper planning and protocol education.

So that care can carry on properly once the dental staff is gone for the time being, the dentist must teach caregivers to make time for patients overall needs, as is practical within the scope of their environs. This program must have the goal of helping the staff implement a long-lasting oral maintenance program as efficiently and fiscally responsibly as is possible, customized to each individual patient's needs. Ellershaw and Ward are proponents of having in the curricula of all healthcare professionals those necessary educational objectives relating to the oral care in the dying. [29]

Some facilities may be able to set up an actual fully functional dental clinic complete with an air compressor, suction, reclining chair, overhead light, and amenities necessary to carry out cleanings and basic restorative procedures. They may be able to cleanse each patient's mouth after all meals. However, other entities may be unable to do little more than remove a patient's dentures nightly and soak them in a cleansing bath, hand a toothbrush and toothpaste to those capable of at least some semblance of self-care, and to attempt to clean the mouths of the remaining patients who are totally dependent for their personal hygiene. At least this would likely be an improvement over prior facility practices, and that is a start in the intended and right direction.

In all frankness, it is extremely rare for a nursing home, hospital or hospice to have a dedicated dental office, while it is much more common that there is absolutely no dental care afforded to patients by staff. In my experience, if a denture comes in and out easily, the cognizant patient is likely left to manage this at his or her discretion. In cases where the patient is demented, combative, or has a denture that is difficult to remove, or one that is causing sore areas, the denture is removed and put into a drawer or storage cup.

Moreover, without patients' being monitored for loose teeth, oral cancers, and large areas of decay, some teeth shop exfoliate during meal time, going without notice, while other patients experience pain that they cannot communicate vocally or otherwise. It is for patients such as these, as well as for those who still yearn for their regular oral hygiene protocol, that we owe our attention and service, compassion and soothing touch.

For those patients who can verbally communicate that they are uncomfortable and have pain, it is imperative that the caregiver check for allergies and other medications being given to the patient that may not be compatible with a particular pain medication being considered for therapy. One also must be cognizant of the fact that pain medications may make these already frail patients more likely to fall, become disoriented, or more confused than is normally the case. Further, it is certainly advisable to use the lowest dose and least number of pills possible for managing patient pain, and to avoid opioids, if at all possible, by using alternating doses of nonsteroidal inflammatory drugs with acetaminophen where tolerated. [25]

Distress experienced during injections may also be reduced by use of a controlled flow anesthesia system [26], and in some cases very loose teeth may be extractable with the use of a xylocaine viscous gel or topical anesthetic so as to avoid the stress of dental injections to accomplish the necessary treatment.

2.4 Suggested directives for oral palliative care management

In order to avoid oral discomfort in patients as much as is possible, the following protocol is recommended as a guide, especially for circumstances in which patients are unable to properly communicate. It is offered in a format that can be duplicated for institutional use.

Institutional recommendations for oral health standard of care when possible/practical per patient are:

Patient/Caregiver Concerns

Offer oral hygiene a minimum of once every 8 hours while in the acute care or long-term care or home.

- Refer patients and families to dental services for urgent follow-up treatment.
- Educate patients and families on the importance of good oral hygiene and follow-up dental services

Professional Caregiver/Registered Nurse Concerns:

- General assessment or evaluation of the oral cavity on admission performed at least daily and if possible, during every shift.
- Notify physician and dentist of any abnormalities causing distress present in the oral cavity.
- Assess what each patient can do independently.
- Observe for aspiration precautions and compliance while providing care.
- Provide oral care and dental care education to patients and families.

Institutional Concerns:

- Monitor staff performance.
- Provide or refer for access to dental services as appropriate.

2.4.1 Commonly identified problems reported by aides and family to the hospice staff

The following oral issues should be reported to the appropriate staff:

- Broken teeth
- Loose teeth
- Brown areas/dark staining/holes on or in the teeth
- Bleeding gums
- Swelling
- Sores
- Lumps
- Red or white patches
- Unusual-looking tissues of any type from any oral source
- Concerns of the patient of any type from any oral source

When appropriate, the hospice staff will consult with either the patient's dentist of record or the in-house dentist.

2.4.2 Xerostomia (dry mouth)

If the mouth is felt to be dry, one must treat the underlining cause as is appropriate. Not all xerostomia is secondary to a decrease in salivation or dehydration.

Other causes include:

- Anxiety and depression
- Hypothyroidism, autoimmune disease, and sarcoidosis
- Use of drugs, such as anti-muscarinics, opioids, diuretics
- Injury to the salivary glands or buccal mucosa
- Mouth breathing, or unhumidified oxygen
- A history of surgery, chemotherapy, or radiotherapy to the head and neck region

And most preferential means of palliation is to provide frequent fluids when one is able to drink, and if not, keep the mouth moistened.

Those at the end of life are vulnerable to all problems such as Candidiasis, no matter how well the mouth is cared for. It is important to check the mouth for any sore places or coatings that could indicate thrush and to treat expediently if causing the patient distress.

Saliva can be stimulated by sucking mints and candies, preferably those containing xylitol (cavity-fighting) sugar. Artificial salivas are available for purchase over-the-counter, but the effect is typically found to be no better than sipping fluids.

There is little evidence to support the use of mouthwashes, especially as they can be offensive towards the end of life; however, some individuals who have used those daily may wish to continue to do so.

Alternatives to mouthwashes, providing there is no painful thrush being treated in the mouth are as follows:

- Coconut oil on a toothette provides a comforting and pleasant-testing method of lubricating and alleviating dessication.

- Water makes an inexpensive and acceptable lubricant, but will not remove coatings around the mouth.

- Normal saline (1 teaspoon of salt dissolved in 500 mls of water) is also inexpensive and mildly antiseptic, but may not be acceptable if it is nauseating to the patient.

- Chlorhexidine mouthwash is an antibacterial and antifungal prescription used sometimes to help deter plaque buildup on the teeth.

- Sodium bicarbonate can help treat a dry, coated tongue for short periods of time.

- Commercially available glycerin and lemon mouthwash or oral swabs will actually increase dryness, as they draw water out of the mouth and my damage the enamel. These should be avoided.

Alternatives for dry mouth which can nicely simulate "feeding" and "bonding" between caregiver and the patient who can no longer swallow or manage liquids are to swab the mouth with toothette sponges dipped into such solutions as the patient may find pleasurable. These may include such items as semi-frozen tonic water and gin, semi-frozen fruit juices, coffees or teas, cold yogurts, and small dollops of coconut oil. Having the patient suck on ice chips or small pieces of frozen pears, peaches, or berries may also be soothing. The patient would best be sitting up for this to be attempted.

If the mouth is tender and sore, a topical teething anesthetic or an oral palliative mouthwash containing equal parts of xylocaine viscous, milk of magnesia, and Benadryl maybe used before and/or after application of foods and drinks.

2.4.3 Mucositis

This typically presents as dry, burning, and/or reddened tissues. It is by advisable to discontinue spicy, minty or cinnamon-containing foods and oral care products.

A liquid mixture for swabbing around the mouth after meals and before bedtime can be prescribed by a dental or medical professional. It consists of three equal parts of Benadryl (if tolerable), milk of magnesia, and xylocaine viscous, and can be easily compounded by any pharmacy.

A therapeutic regimen may consist of the following:

- use of a soft bristled toothbrush and non-irritating toothpaste (one without sodium laurel sulfate detergent and which does not contain spicy or irritating components).
- Replacement of toothbrushes weekly until healed.
- Rinsing with a sterile saline as needed.
- Removal of dentures except when needed for consumption of food.
- Soaking dentures twice a day in a 1:1 ratio of vinegar and water in solution.

If redness and pain are unresolved within seven days, consult a dentist; a treatment for Candidiasis (thrush) may be necessary.

2.4.4 Candidiasis

Often times, especially in those with poor diabetic control issues or in those using antibiotics, a fungal coating, typically white, can form on the tongue, throat, and other parts of the mouth. This "opportunistic" infection is called *Candida albicans*, and can cause a burning sensation within the mouth as well as at the corners of the lips; a palliative prescription can be administered for an antifungal medication by a dental or medical professional.

To treat the tissues, dentures must be removed during medication application to the oral tissues, and topical agents may be used on the dentures themselves. Sponge swabs maybe used to apply the medications for hospice patients who may be unable to rinse with liquid suspensions.

Systemic agents including ketoconazole, fluconazole, and/or amphotericin B may be required for severe or intractable cases. Candidiasis may be treated according to severity by one or more of the following medicinal agents:

- Nystatin suspension 100,000 IU (5 ml = 1tsp) four times daily for 1 to 2 weeks. The medication is to be held in the mouth for one minute, with a swish and swallow approach. An oral sponge may be employed if rinsing is not possible. This is the first choice of therapy if a patient is unable to safely hold a tablet/troche in the mouth.
- Clotrimazole troches 10 mg per troche
  This is to be used five times daily for two weeks. This is the first choice of therapy if a patient is able to hold the tablet in the mouth without risk of aspiration.
- Fluconazole tablets 100 mg. This is to be taken as two stat, then once daily for two weeks. This is preferable for moderate to severe cases or if topical treatment is impractical.
- Dentures may be soaked overnight in a few drops of Nystatin suspension mixed into a cup of cool or room temperature water.

2.4.5 Dysphagia (difficulty with swallowing)

Dysphagia is defined as difficulty in swallowing. It may be an acute or chronic condition that affects oral intake and is usually indicative of some disease process.

Because this condition is common with a patient's deconditioning near the end of life, many healthcare providers consider it relatively trivial and it is therefore unreported or underestimated. It is also frequently overlooked due to the presence of more prominent symptoms, such as pain or shortness of breath.

Difficulty swallowing liquids can indicate poor muscular control, and difficulty swallowing solids may indicate physiologic abnormality, such as a tumor. Sudden onset may be indicative of a psychogenic etiology.

Dysphasia has been detected in approximately 30% of patients with stroke, and 40 to 60% of patients with neurodegenerative disease, and in approximately 20% of patients with cancer, all of which may be treated with palliative care. It can cause or exacerbate other problems, such as weight loss, debility, and aspiration pneumonia, and in some cases it can hasten death.

Other routes of food administration (intravenous nutrition or gastrostomy feeding tubes) may be used in patients who are unable to eat. Often times, because patients may present with difficulty swallowing, the caregiver must be cautious in cleaning the mouth with use of too much liquid or lubricants such as coconut oil (which rapidly liquidates). Therefore, proceed with care when swabbing food/drinks substances during "feeding", as well as in cleaning and lubrication of the mouth.

2.4.6 Orally-related impediments to verbal communication

Please attend to this as is possible by applying lubrication consistently to the lips and oral cavity when they are dry.

(See section on Xerostomia for more in-depth discussion on methods of alleviating dry mouth.)

2.4.7 Poor Oral hygiene

Proper oral care is important, as it maintains self-esteem, comfort, a sense of well-being, and our ability to communicate, socialize, and enjoy taking in sustenance.

An additional significant problem among palliative care patients is poor oral hygiene. This is likely due to a number of factors, including the patient's cognitive and physical disabilities; a lack of optimal preventive devices and supplies; and the caregiver's inadequate knowledge, attitudes, and experience regarding provision of oral care to people other than themselves.

Finding particles of food, accumulated plaque and calculus (tartar), and mucus and saliva on the patient's teeth, palatal and buccal tissues, and dentures is common, yet is objectionable to many individuals.

Preventive care protocols should be established early and maintained throughout the palliative care process. A number of preventive protocols are appropriate for these patients:

Basic palliative oral care protocol

Keep lips moist at all times with a lip balm, coconut oil, or some such substance.

1. Keep intra-oral tissues moist at all times using saliva substitutes or coconut oil, applying with oral sponges or by the having patient rinse where possible.

2. Clean the teeth with a manual or power brush and fluoridated toothpaste (avoiding those that may be more irritating, such as mint or cinnamon-or those that tend to be dessicating, such as those with detergents like sodium laurel sulfate). Make a watery toothpaste slurry in instances where patients may risk choking on thick dentifrices. Perform this after each meal as is possible.

3. Clean between teeth with floss, and if necessary, using floss-aiding holders and devices. Brushes that fit between teeth are also available and can be very helpful. Perform this daily. Avoid use of water jet devices to clean food from between teeth.

4. Clean soft tissues of the inside of the mouth to remove adherent debris with a soft brush or oral sponge dipped in coconut oil or a saliva substitute.

5. Clean dentures (full coverage or partial) after eating with a denture brush while holding the appliance low in the sink and under a gentle stream of running cool (or slightly warm) water. They may be soaked in commercial denture cleaning solutions. Do not soak in harsh or toxic chemicals.

Poor oral hygiene can lead to aspiration pneumonia, a leading cause of death in nursing homes. It involves aspiration of bacteria from the teeth, dentures, and oral tissues into the lungs, complicated by difficulty swallowing and loss of protective reflexes such as coughing. Pneumonia presents with fever, altered mental status, and decreased oral intake. It eventually leads to fatal respiratory failure or sepsis.

Other factors leading to aspiration pneumonia are immunocompromised status; Alzheimer's; psychotropic and sedative drug administration; active periodontal disease; bedridden status; history of CVA, bulbar palsies; esophageal disease, COPD, CHF, GERD; intubator/ventilator use; aspirators; dysphasia, and other abnormalities of the protective airway mechanism; poorly fitting oral prostheses; and xerostomia.

2.4.8 Caries (tooth decay)

Caries, or cavities, are caused by an adequate cleansing of the bacteria from around and between the teeth. Hygiene must be performed properly by cleaning around and between the teeth as frequently and thoroughly as is possible after meals.

Exposed root surfaces, being softer than the enamel on the crown of the tooth, are especially susceptible to decay, and should be afforded appropriate attention.

We are seeing new trends emerge in the dental health needs of older adults as life expectancy and dentate status continue to change through the years, and we must continue meeting these challenges.

2.4.9 Periodontal disease (loss of the supportive tissues around the teeth)

Periodontal disease is a bacterial control issue in which the spaces between the teeth and gums can harbor damaging bacteria that, if not cleaned properly or frequently enough, will result in loss of bone, loosening of teeth, and life-threatening infections in the mouth and around the body.

Signs and symptoms which are indicative of periodontal disease include:

- Gums that bleed when brushed
- Gums that are red, swollen, or tender
- Gums that have receded or pulled away from the teeth
- Purulence (pus) between the gums and the teeth
- Movement or displacement of permanent teeth
- Halitosis (bad breath)

Adequately maintained oral care can alleviate this disease's progression and symptomatology.

2.4.10 Care of partial denture patients (and when is it okay not to wear the partials any longer?)

Independent mouth care for those with teeth or partial dentures:

- Dentures should be removed and soaked/brushed separately, low and over a sink or basin.
- Caregivers should wash hands and wear gloves.
- A soft toothbrush or oral sponge should be angled against the gumline, gently brushing teeth and an up-and-down motion with short strokes.
- Brush the patient's tongue.
- Apply lip moisturizer consistently as is necessary.
- Use toothpaste slurry or coconut oil for brushing, avoiding harsh or burning types of toothpastes, such as those with sodium laurel sulfate, mint, or cinnamon.

Discontinuation of denture-wearing is acceptable, if they are providing less benefit than they are creating discomfort and frustration for the patient. Usually, the hospice patient can maintain his same level of nourishment after discontinuing the use of his complete or partial dentures by changing the textures of foods eaten and by eating/being fed more slowly.

If the patient in fact is distressed while wearing his dentures, but is also having trouble functioning without them, a dental professional should examine the dentures for sore spots, poor fit, need for reline, and the like, as is possible.

2.4.11 Further Care in Cleaning the teeth: when flossing is a challenge

Daily brushing, flossing, and rinsing are three of the most important steps to having healthy teeth and gums. Yet, debilitated patients may have trouble wrapping floss around the fingers or in keeping a steady hand. They may also be intolerant to a caregiver's putting two fingers far back into the mouth.

There are a few methods that may make interdental cleaning easier. The patient or caregiver can use floss picks to clean under gums and in-between the teeth, where plaque and food work their way under the gingiva every day and can lead to gum disease.

Other options include soft picks (thin, feathery, rubber toothpicks), and various floss folders, all of which can be used with one hand by the patient. For caregivers, it is easier to reach the back of the mouth by using a long-handled floss aid, a thin instrument shaped rather like a slingshot, across which floss can be threaded.

Flossing (or the closest semblance thereof) is necessary in accessing areas under the gums where a toothbrush cannot reach. It is important to brush after meals and to floss at least before bedtime each day.

Water jet irrigation devices are not generally recommended for hospice patients.

2.4.12 Care of Full Denture Patients (and when is it okay not to wear dentures any longer?)

The use of dentures is common in the hospice population of patients. Numerous studies involving long-term care facilities show that, while many patients have dentures, a small proportion of these dentures are actually worn, because of issues with comfort and function. This proportion is likely higher in palliative care patients because of comorbidities, including xerostomia (dryness), Candidiasis, and general physiologic debilitations and losses.

Atrophy of facial muscles in stroke or advanced head and neck cancer patients can contribute to the inability for dentures to stay in properly. Looseness of the denture can also be brought about by significant weight loss or from resorption over previous years of the bony architecture underneath the denture.

Various treatments being administered for palliative care patients can exacerbate sores in the mouth, causing a patient distress while wearing the denture, even when not eating or talking with it.

Discontinuation of denture-wearing is acceptable, if the dentures are providing less benefit than they are in creating discomfort and frustration for the patient. Usually, the hospice patient can maintain his same level of nourishment after discontinuing the use of his dentures by changing the textures of foods eaten and by eating/being fed more slowly.

If the patient in fact is distressed while wearing his dentures, but is also having trouble functioning without them, a dental professional should examine the dentures for sore spots, poor fit, need for reline, and the like, as is possible.

Oral Hygiene Plan of Care for the Edentulous Patient With or Without Dentures

- Remember that dentures are not necessary for proper eating, communicating, and other such functions.

- Dentures should be labeled on the inside with the patient's name written using an indelible marker or placed within the acrylic by a professional.

- Oral care should be provided after meals and as is necessary.

- Caregivers should wash hands and wear gloves.

- Dentures should be removed and safely set aside while cleaning the teeth.

- Dentures should be brushed with a toothbrush and toothpaste low in a sink or basin.

- Clean the grooved areas of dentures with the brush.

- Use cool or slightly warm water.
- Brush the patient's tongue and wipe the oral tissues (cheeks, palate, and under the lips); coconut oil can provide a nice-tasting and lubricating medium.
- Reinsert the dentures.
- Apply lip moisturizer.

2.4.13 Care of the Oral Tissues (tongue, cheeks, inside and outside of lips, floor and roof of the mouth)

These tissues should be cleaned anytime the teeth and/or dentures are cleaned. This can be accomplished either by rinsing (where the patient is capable), or by wiping the mouth with a lubricating substance, such as a saliva substitute or coconut oil placed on either a piece of gauze or a toothette sponge.

Take care not to choke patients with hasty or over-abundant use of these substances.

3. Conclusion

Oral care is an important component of institutionalized healthcare for the dependent and terminal because:

- Palliative care and dental health go hand-in-hand.
- The demographic of older adults who are entering hospice care is growing and likely will continue to constitute an increasingly larger populous engaged with end-of-life caregiving.
- The comorbidities and physiological changes associated with these aging individuals make them more vulnerable to oral health problems.
- With aging comes the use of multiple prescriptive and over-the-counter medications, causing a potential rise in medication errors, drug interactions, and adverse drug reactions, all of which are important in oral care considerations, particularly where local anesthetics and analgesics are concerned.
- The physical, sensory, and cognitive impairments often seen in this group may create challenges both with oral health self-care as well as with patient education and communication.
- Dental conditions associated with the aging mouth can include xerostomia (dry mouth), root and coronal caries (decay), and periodontal (gum) disease.
- Oral health related quality of life is a multi-dimensional concept which considers the totality of the patient's oral health, functional well-being, emotional well-being, expectations and satisfaction with care, and sense of self.
- Patient oriented outcomes with a focus on quality of life can enhance our understanding of the relationship between oral health and general health,

while demonstrating that improving one's palliation goes beyond the caregiver's simply assisting with or treating dental maladies.

- Appropriate oral care delivered adequately and expediently, will enhance the hospice patient's quality of life through a more esthetic and comfortable experience of well-being.

- This will include one's experiencing enhanced socialization, more pleasurable eating and drinking, freedom from pain and discomfort, and an enhanced ability to communicate verbally.

- Further, this will prevent medical problems such as bacteremia, aspiration pneumonia, and poor diabetic control issues.

- It will also help to manage patient complaints such as halitosis (bad breath), speech problems, dysphasia (trouble eating), and an inability for maintaining adequate nutrition and hydration.

- It will help to manage consequences from comorbid medical conditions such as Sjogren's syndrome, arthritis, strokes, radiation, and chemotherapy.

The most generous detail about delivering -and receiving-palliative care is that it focuses a great deal on kindness, and not so much on clinical perfection. There is really no general standard of care, as each individual is unique in his or her tolerance, basic needs, and willingness to allow intervention. Responsibilities as mentioned for facilities and dental providers in serving the terminally ill can certainly appear a bit daunting, yet palliative care only requires a caregiver to offer the best therapy possible in light of any situation that may exist. It is not so linked to stipulations and mandates, but rather to heartfelt compassion and a well-intended effort to soothe and comfort a person both physically and psychosocially.

Dentistry has long been absent in the role played in delivering such care, and as such, personal dignity and the sense of well-being aided by oral maintenance are concomitantly remiss. Dentists must step up to avail to caregivers in both institutions and at home a more well-understood prescriptive program for oral care that can be implemented at the various stages of need for end-of-life patients. Further, collaborative efforts among dentists, physicians, institutions, and their respective staff members must be strengthened to assure that care of the oral cavity does not continue to go unattended.

Finally, increased awareness to address these issues must begin in dental and medical schools, as students should learn early on about elder care, volunteerism, and advocacy. Without advances in oral care management of the infirmed and terminal, the void in these patients' receiving comprehensive systemic and psychological palliation will increase as the percentage of the elderly continues to rise.

Author details

Kristi M. Soileau[1,2]

1 Private Periodontal Practice, New Orleans, LA, USA

2 Louisiana State University Health School of Dentistry, New Orleans, LA, USA

*Address all correspondence to: kmsperio@gmail.com

References

[1] Abel EK. The Inevitable Hour: A History of Caring for Dying Patients in America. Baltimore, MD: Johns Hopkins University Press; 2013:166-169

[2] World Health Organization. Palliative care for older people: better practices. 2011:1-25. http://www.euro.who.int/__data/assets/pdf_file/0017/143153/e95052.pdf. [Accessed 2018-02-28]

[3] Saini R, Marawar P, Shete S, Saini S, Mani A. Dental expression and role in palliative treatment. Indian J Palliat Care. 2009;15(1):26-29. DOI:10.4103/0973-1075.53508

[4] Sischo L, Broder HL. Oral health-related quality of life: what, why, how, and future implications. J Dent Res. 2011;90(11):1264-1270

[5] Slaughter A. Providing Dental Care for Older Adults in Long Term Care. Philadelphia, PA: University of Pennsylvania School of Medicine; 2006

[6] Chen X, Kistler CE. Oral health care for older adults with serious illness: when and how? J Am Geriatr Soc. 2015;63(2):375-378. DOI:10.1111/jgs.13240

[7] Wiseman M. The treatment of oral problems in the palliative patient. J Can Dent Assoc. 2006;72(5):453

[8] Meier DE, McCormick E, Arnold RM, Savarese DM. Benefits, Services, and Models of Subspecialty Palliative Care. 2017. https://www.uptodate.com/contents/benefits-services-and-models-of-subspecialty-palliative-care. [Accessed 2018-02-28]

[9] Miller S, Ryndes T. Quality of life at the end of life: the public health perspective. Generations. 2005;29(2):41-47

[10] CDHB Hospital Palliative Care Service. Oral Care in Patients at the End of Life. Canterbury, New Zealand; 2013. http://cdhb.palliativecare.org.nz/Oral%20Care%20in%20Patients%20at%20the%20end%20of%20life.pdf. [Accessed 2018-02-28]

[11] Jobbins J, Bagg J, Finlay IG, Addy M, Newcombe RG. Oral and dental disease in terminally ill cancer patients. Br Med J. 1992;304(6842):1612. DOI:10.1136/bmj.304.6842.1612

[12] Spolarich E. Medicines and Your Mouth [Health Resource]. 2013. https://www.toothwisdom.org/a-z/article/medicines-and-your-mouth/. [Accessed 2018-02-28]

[13] Roderick R. Reasons Why You Have Dry Mouth. 2016. https://www.toothwisdom.org/a-z/article/reasons-why-you-may-have-dry-mouth/. [Accessed 2018-02-28]

[14] Salinas T. Dry mouth treatment: tips for controlling dry mouth. Mayo Clinic. 2017. http://www.mayoclinic.org/diseases-conditions/dry-mouth/expert-answers/dry-mouth/FAQ-20058424. [Accessed 2018-02-28]

[15] Bean L. Monitoring the mouth—oral considerations for hospice patients. 2017. http://wilbeadme.com/general/monitoring-the-mouth-oral-considerations-for-hospice-patients/. [Accessed 2018-02-28]

[16] Treister N. Palliative care: overview of mouth care at the end of life. palliative care: overview of mouth care at the end of life. 2016. https://www.uptodate.com/contents/palliative-care-overview-of-mouth-care-at-the-end-of-life. [Accessed 2018-02-28]

[17] Eke PI, Dye BA, Wei L, Slade GD, Thornton-Evans GO, Borgnakke WS. Update on prevalence of periodontitis

in adults in the United States: NHANES 2009-2012. J Periodontal. 2015;86(5):611-622. DOI:10.1902/jop.2015.140520

[18] McLearan S. Guidelines for Providing Dental Services in Skilled Nursing Facilities. Center for Oral Health. 2013 http://www.centerfororalhealth.org/images/lib_PDF/Skilled_Nursing_Facility_Dental_Services_Guidelines.pdf. [Accessed 2018-02-28]

[19] Atchley M. Mouth body connection: a holistic approach to dentistry. Dental Bliss. http://dentalbliss.com/mouth-and-body-connection-a-holistic-approach-to-dentistry/. 2016. [Accessed 2018-02-28]

[20] Rajesh K, Hegde S, Kumar MS, Thomas D. Poor periodontal health: a cancer risk? J Indian Soc Periodontal. 2013;17(6):706-710. DOI:10.4103/0972- 124x.124470

[21] Goldie M. How depression threatens oral health, and other oral-systemic links. Dentistry IQ. 2016. http://www.dentistryiq.com/articles/2016/03/how-depression-threatens-oral-health-and-other-oral-systemic-links.html. [Accessed 2018-02-28]

[22] Vollick E. U of T researchers discover mechanism linking gum disease to heart disease, other conditions. 2020. https://www.utoronto.ca/news/u-t-researchers-discover-mechanism-linking-gum-disease-heart-disease-other-conditions. [Accessed 2020-11-19]

[23] Kelsch N. Hospice hygiene: oral comfort for end-of-life patients. National Magazine Dent Hyg Professionals. 2009:72-80

[24] Kennedy C, Brooks-Young P, Gray CB. Diagnosing dying: an integrative literature review. BMJ & Support Palliat Care. 2014;4(3):263-270. DOI:10.1136/bmjspcare-2013-000621

[25] Chang A, Bijur P, Esses D, Barnaby D, Baer J. Effect of a Single Dose of Oral Opioid and Nonopioid Analgesics on Acute Extremity Pain in the Emergency Department: A Randomized Clinical Trial. JAMA. 2017 Nov 7;318(17):1661-1667. DOI: 10.1001/jama.2017.16190. PMID: 29114833; PMCID: PMC5818795.

[26] Soileau, K, DeGenova, A & Yu, Q. Blood pressure monitoring following individual carpules of anesthetic utilizing computer-controlled anesthetic delivery. BDJ Open 6, 21 (2020). https://doi.org/10.1038/s41405-020-00049-y

[27] Welie JV. Justice in oral health care: the preferential option for the poor. In: Welie, JV (ed.) A Social Justice Perspective on Oral Health Care. Milwaukee, WI: Marquette University Press; 2006:127-138

[28] Rozas NS, Sadowsky JM, Jeter CB. Strategies to improve dental health in elderly patients with cognitive impairment. J Am Dent Assoc. 2017;148(4):236-245. DOI:10.1016/j.adaj.2016.12.022

[29] Ellershaw J, Ward C. Care of the dying patient: the last hours or days of life commentary: a "good death" is possible in the NHS. BMJ. 2003;326(7379):30-34. DOI:10.1136/bmj.326.7379.30

Section 3

A Focus on the Caregiver Role

Chapter 7

Caregiver Distress in Cancer

Anshika Arora

Abstract

Cancer is a chronic disease with associated physical, emotional, social, financial and spiritual problems. The primary caregiver takes care of all these cancer-related issues for the patient. In India, usually a family member or loved one is the caregiver of the patient. The caregivers themselves feel distress and many factors may be associated with their psychological well-being. Pattern of distress may vary according to phases of the disease like at diagnosis, during ongoing oncological treatment, recovery period, remission period, recurrence of cancer, during end of life care and bereavement. Identifying and understanding caregiver distress is the first step. Active listening and good communication is important to unearth the real concerns and fears in order to relieve the distress. This chapter covers components of caregiver distress, assessment, physical, psychosocial and spiritual factors associated with distress and its management. Lastly, some recent literature related to prevalence and factors associated with caregiver distress.

Keywords: caregiver distress, cancer, palliative care, psychological distress, good death

1. Introduction

The incidence and prevalence of cancer has been increasing in developing countries in the last few decades. Cancer is viewed increasingly as a chronic disease, with prolonged management and increased rates of survival, leading to long term care requirements of the patient. In developing countries like India, the primary caregiver for long-term and intensive care of a cancer patient is preferably the family member, and sometimes family member is the 'only option' available to the patient as caregiver. The caregiver is usually a close relative like parent, child, sibling, spouse or a friend. This person usually has a deep relationship with the patient and more importantly, a significant emotional co-dependence. Cancer diagnosis and treatment not only affects patients but also their family, resulting in psychological distress.

In cancer treatment, there has been a shift from in-patient care to ambulatory and out-patient care. This increases demands on the patient's caregiver towards unmet physical, psychosocial and spiritual needs of the patient. Most of the caregivers have little preparation or training to take up this role. With newer modalities of treatment, cancer patients have prolonged survival through all stages of disease, making it more of a chronic disease. These trends have definitely increased the caregiver burden. The act of caring for a sick patient is multifaceted. The caregiver needs to have dedicated time to take the patient for hospital appointments and care for disease and treatment related problems at home as well. The caregiver then may face loss of personal work due to lack of time. They may eventually develop varying degrees of emotional and psychosocial distress. There is ample literature on the palliative care needs of cancer patients. However, there is limited literature on the psychosocial needs of the relatives or caregivers of cancer patients. A significant proportion of caregivers have unmet needs for emotional support. They may have unaddressed fears regarding the patient's prognosis, disease related information and treatment details. Furthermore, caregivers of patients with advanced disease usually have distress symptoms like anxiety and depression. Caregivers face extreme demands right through the course of the cancer, survivorship and also during bereavement.

2. Components of caregiver distress

The common psychological distress problems would be- anxiety and anxiety disorders, low mood and depressive disorders and adjustment disorders (**Table 1**).

Whenever a person perceives threat, '*anxiety*' is the natural response. This response helps to enhance their actions in order to take care of the threat. When does this natural response of anxiety become a problem? Either the threat is out of person's capability to resolve, or the anxiety hampers with the person's ability to act appropriately in the situation. So, 'anxiety' may be seen as a spectrum between normal response to persistent to severe anxiety (**Figure 1**).

Some people experience anxiety in response to day to day stressors lifelong, for them anxiety due to caring for someone's cancer is just another symptom of their own chronic anxiety problem. This may be seen more as 'chronic anxiety'. On the other hand, some people may experience 'acute anxiety'. It is generally a temporary response to a particular stressor, for example, being delivered the news of metastatic and incurable cancer in the patient, or the news of recurrent cancer. In a caregiver, anxiety may be related to –

- caring for a patient with uncontrolled symptoms like, pain or dyspnoea,
- fear of unknown like, prognosis of the patient,
- anticipation of symptoms post treatment like, chemotherapy induced nausea and vomiting,
- lack of sleep, either due to distress, or caring for the patient at night continuously,
- fear of being left alone after the death of the patient, etc.

Some people may be suffering from anxiety disorders like- panic disorder, generalized anxiety disorder and mixed anxiety and depressive disorder. It is commonly seen that people with symptoms of anxiety usually have adjustment disorder or varying degrees of depression.

1	Anxiety and anxiety disorders
2	Low mood and depressive disorders
3	Adjustment disorders

Table 1.
Components of caregiver distress.

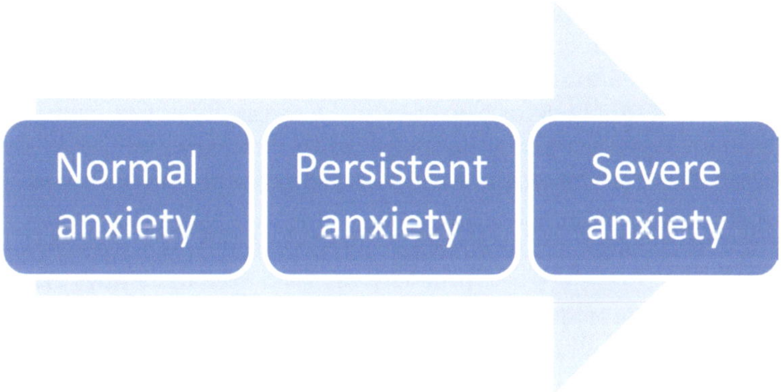

Figure 1.
This figure shows the spectrum of caregiver's response to the perceived threat posed by cancer in their loved one.

Caregivers suffer from low mood very often. '*Depression*' is a common occurrence in cancer patients, and is also common in their caregivers. There is a spectrum of mood disorders ranging from sadness to adjustment disorder to depression. Depression is not the same as feeling sad. The common features seen in depression are- inability to experience pleasure (anhedonia), helplessness, hopelessness, feelings of loss and a flattening of all feelings. They may feel irritable, worthless; there may be lack of interest in daily activities or recreational activities; suicidal ideation is important to look for. There may be physical features like lack of sleep, weight loss, fatigue, reduced energy level and lethargy. Depressive disorders are usually under diagnosed in caregivers. This results from lack of active screening, lack of focus on the caregiver, more focus on the cancer patient, social cover-up by the caregiver and other simultaneous psychiatric problems like anxiety.

There will be many people with distress, who do not fall into the diagnostic criteria for depression or anxiety if the diagnostic criteria are applied strictly. These people may have '*adjustment disorders*'. The main components of adjustment disorders are- they occur in response to a stressor, they usually last for a short duration of time (acute in nature), there will be emotional turmoil and distress and finally this results in function impairment. The diagnosis of adjustment disorder is more of a clinical judgment. The main temporality to remember is that the distress should start within 1–3 months of the stressor and be relieved within 6 months of resolution of the stressor. It is important to acknowledge adjustment disorders if distress is recognized in the caregiver, because otherwise, they may be inappropriately diagnosed to be depressed and prescribed unnecessary medications.

3. Assessment of caregiver distress

It has been seen in cancer patients, that regular and ongoing *evaluation* of psychological distress improves the management and treatment of psychiatric issues. This eventually contributes to better outcome, patient satisfaction, doctor-patient partnership, and improved overall care [1]. This is true even for caregiver distress. Regular screening and ongoing evaluation is as important aspect for good quality of life in the patients and their caregivers. Distress is defined as

"a multifactorial unpleasant emotional experience of a psychological, social or spiritual nature that interferes with coping."

There are various tools and scales to screen for distress. Definitions for specific mental disorders are provided in Psychiatric Association's *Diagnostic and Statistical*

Manual (DSM-5) [2]. A visual analog tool, the distress thermometer, is used as a self-report method to screen and measure distress. This tool has been validated against other tools used to screen for psychological distress [3]. *Distress thermometer* is an invaluable tool to screen for psychological distress. It has two components; one is a visual analogue scale ranging from 0 to 10. Zero being no distress and 10 being extreme distress. The second component asks the person to answer a series of yes or no questions pertaining to- practical problems, family problems, emotional problems, spiritual/religious problems and physical problems. This scale measures the global distress score, the list of problems are then used to identify areas that need focused care. The *Hospital Anxiety and Depression Scale* is self administered 14 question scale. This validated tool can be used to screen caregivers for anxiety and depression. A score from 0 to 21 is generated for both anxiety and depression, 0–7 indicates normal, 8–10 borderline and 11–21 abnormal score. People with abnormal score can then be reviewed in detail for anxiety and depression. Another tool useful for depression is *Beck Depression Inventory* (BDI). BDI is a self reporting, 21-item rating tool. It measures attitudes and the symptoms of depression. A shorter version with 13 items is called BDI-II. It has an internal consistency of 0.73 to 0.92. For anxiety, *Beck Anxiety Inventory* (BAI) tool can be used. It again consists of 21 items and is a self reporting rating questionnaire. Instrument *General Health Questionnaire* (GHQ-12) is a validated tool to assess the severity of any mental problem a person may have suffered from in the past few weeks. This instrument consists of 12 items, 4-point scale, with total score ranging from 0 to 36. A higher score indicates a worse mental problem. *Psycho-Oncology Screening* is a screening tool, specific for cancer. The screening is based on 5 to 10 minutes of standardized interview, which comprises of

- questions related to socio-demographic characteristics,
- questions related to medical characteristics, and
- questions on the subjective experience associated with psychological distress in the past 3 days

To assess the third point, Psycho-Oncology Screening tool uses 6 items, rated from 0 to 4. Any patient with >9 points on this rating scale is considered distressed. Another validated, self administered tool is the *Psychological Distress Inventory*, used to measure distress in cancer patients. *Mental Health Quotient* is an online assessment tool. It captures the complete mental profile of an individual, ranging from "Clinical to Thriving". Another useful tool to screen for distress and unmet needs of a person is *Needs Evaluation Questionnaire* (NEQ). It is again a self-administered tool, with 23 items with dichotomous answers. The *Kessler Psychological Distress Scale* (K 10) comprises of 10 items with scores ranging from 1 to 5 for each item (minimum possible score 10, maximum score 50). The grading is done as per following cut-offs

- 10–19 Likely to be well
- 20–24 Likely to have a mild disorder
- 25–29 Likely to have a moderate disorder
- 30–50 Likely to have a severe disorder

4. Physical factors affecting caregiver distress

Patients with advanced cancer usually have multiple physical symptoms, with varying degrees of severity. In addition to this, the symptoms burden is dynamic, i.e., ever changing in severity and pattern, as the disease profile changes. The **Table 2** shows the prevalence of common physical symptoms in an advanced cancer patient.

The caregiver of an advanced cancer has to be able to care for above symptoms. Seeing your loved one in pain or with anorexia can be a source of distress, caring for someone with dyspnea can be quite scary and cause a lot of distress in the caregiver. Due to fatigue, patients with terminal cancer are unable to carry out recreational or occupation activities and even sometimes activities of daily living. Their caregiver, usually a family member, is equally affected emotionally by the changes in life style the patient may have to make to adapt to constant fatigue. In an Indian study, the researcher asked about the most bothersome symptoms reported by parents of dying children. Pain (85%) and respiratory distress (73%) were the commonest [5]. Much of the fear is due to past experiences of uncontrolled symptoms. This eventually leads to anticipatory psychological distress in both patients and their caregivers. In India, many complex factors like cost, scarcity of medical facilities in remote areas, taboo, etc., contribute to reduced expert medical care opportunities and hospice care. Advanced cancer patients with smelly fungating wounds, oro-cutaneous malignant fistulas, large bed sores, bowel and bladder dysfunction are being managed primarily at home by caregivers. The caregivers have the added responsibility of taking over the nursing role, usually full time. This may leave little or no time for personal needs, being a source of distress. Consider a patient who has a colostomy due to malignant bowel obstruction, this patient will have body image issues. He may become socially recluse, irritable, depressed and feel overall limited by the colostomy bag. Seeing him in psychological pain, the patient's caregiver and loved ones may find it distressing. So, change in body image of a patient whether due to a stoma, or amputation, or mastectomy not only affects the psyche of the patient but their family members and caregivers.

Symptom	Frequency (%)
Pain	35–96
Anorexia	30–92
Fatigue	32–90
Delirium	6–93
Dyspnoea	10–70
Depression	3–77

Table 2.
Prevalence of common symptoms in patients with advanced cancer. [4].

5. Psychosocial factors affecting caregiver distress

Being diagnosed with cancer is a life-altering event in a patient's life. Nature of his/her response to diagnosis, treatment etc. will impact mood of the patient and quality of the social support. Managing strong emotional responses will affect patient's family and vocational exchanges. Similar points could be envisioned for the caregiver. In a country like India, the caregiver, usually a close family member is the first to receive the news of diagnosis of cancer; even before the patient. During this early period of breaking bad news and details of disease related prognosis, the caregiver goes through psychological problems like- acute stress disorder. Usually, the person may go through phases of disbelief, fear, anxiety, in-ability to sleep, blame, anger and intrusive thinking etc. Now, their lifestyle may never remain the same. They go from the routine activities to a whirlwind of hospital appointments, tests, investigations and consultation with multiple doctors. Consolidating all the information shared with them regarding the disease and treatment during these consultations and then, the mammoth responsibility of taking the right decisions can be quite daunting. The caregivers could quickly move from acute stress to more chronic post-traumatic stress disorder [6–8]. During the stage of active treatment of cancer the caregiver may experience exhaustion, helplessness and disruption of social roles. As the treatment ends and follow up period starts, there may be fears of disease recurrence, long-term treatment side effects, higher vulnerability and sudden isolation. In India, another important factor to consider is feeling of *taboo*. Generally, people fear that if the society comes to know that their family member has cancer, the family will be socially isolated, to the extent that they may be considered bad luck to be around. The constant effort to keep the secret of cancer in the family is a cause of distress. *Collusion* is another important consideration in context of India. The primary caregiver keeps the knowledge of diagnosis or the knowledge of disease prognosis to themselves. They hardly allow the medical team to disclose cancer diagnosis to the patient in order to protect their loved one from mental trauma and resulting distress. But this *conspiracy of silence* between the caregiver and the medical team is a source of constant psychological distress in the patient, as well as the caregiver. The psychodynamics of the family is any way disturbed by the diagnosis of cancer in a family member. Adding on that, the pressure of hiding diagnosis from the patient, all while struggling through diagnostic tests and treatment of cancer will generate stress and tension for the caregivers. Collusion also blocks honest discussions among the family members and preparation for parting. Caregivers may have mixed states and degrees of depression, anxiety, psychological distress; they may find it difficulty in falling asleep or staying asleep. All these affect their quality of life. Collusion, if not resolved is a source of immense distress to family members during bereavement period too.

6. Spiritual factors affecting caregiver distress

Spirituality is about valuing the non-material aspects of life, it is also concerned intimately with day to day reality. "Spirituality can be defined as *awareness of the transcendent*, the awareness of something beyond ordinary human knowledge or experience" [9]. It concerns with the whole life. The *4S model* of a human being involves- the 'soma' (physical), social, psychological dimensions; embraced and enhanced by the spiritual dimension. Relationship with the ultimate reality, meaning of life, purpose of living, deeper meaning behind experiences and harmony with other beings and the universe are some aspects spiritually is concerned with. Religion is a shared system of beliefs and certain rituals. One's spirituality may be either independent or dependent on their religious believes. Whether one calls it spirituality or soul or '*atma*' or the spirit, it is about exploring and discovering the meaning or purpose of one's identity and life.

Dealing with major life-stressors, like diagnosis and treatment of cancer, has been shown to trigger post-traumatic growth in the patients and their caregivers. There may be an altered perspective on what really matters in life, what is the meaning behind life [10]. The higher domains like life appreciation, relating to other's problems, empathy, compassion and spiritual matters are seen to be affected in patients and their families [11, 12].

The following are some of the spiritual needs of a caregiver-

- *Guilt or Shame* Person feels they are reaping the results of their past actions. They are being punished for their ill actions by suffering like this. They feel that they deserve this misery and do not deserve any better. The concept of '*karma*'.
- *Intense suffering* Receiving bad news, long periods of caring for a cancer patient can lead to isolation, loneliness and vulnerability. This intense suffering may overwhelm the caregiver into feelings of suicide.
- *Sense of –lessness* Caregivers may develop feelings of helplessness, hopelessness and meaninglessness. Some people are able to cope with this, but others may become withdrawn and depressed. They may feel - 'What's the point of going on if it's going to be like this?'
- *Breaking up with God* Some may question God and other religious authorities- "Why us, what did we do to deserve this?" and feel angry. Others may just break their ties with God and the religious believes they had been following till now. For some, their relationship with God may change- "Now I can't ask for help from God and talk to Him the same way."
- *Premature stoicism* Stoicism is defined as- "the endurance of pain or hardship without the display of feelings and without complaint." In Indian culture, the family members and loved ones feel this overpowering need to take care of their cancer patient. The caregiver often feels that he or she cannot let down their patient and thus feel they have to do it all. They also endure suffering, without complaining, as part of this duty towards the family member.
- *Nightmares* Each one of us may have had that vivid dream about falling endlessly or being stuck in a box and unable to get out, at some point of time in our lives. Cancer caregivers, if asked, share that they frequently get these nightmares.

Thus, the interplay of elements like experiences, values, beliefs, relationships, assumptions, motivation, dreams, aspirations, thoughts and emotions determines the spiritual health or *qualify of spiritual health*.

7. How can one help

Medical professionals and health team may be able to reduce caregiver distress related to cancer if it is identified early and adequate steps are taken to relieve the causes of distress. Also, they can work with caregivers to help them attain something of emotional significance from the experience of loss or suffering [13]. Cancer patient caregivers will benefit from improving their *coping skills* and learning more adaptive coping skills (**Table 3**). They need to preserve their emotional balance, sense of know-how, sustain social relationships and above all, be prepared for the uncertain future. Expression of emotions to social support system is shown to improve optimism and reduce distress in cancer patients [14–16]. Similar strategies

Improving coping skills
Learning adaptive skills Group psychotherapy
Good communication

Table 3.
Proposed interventions to relieve caregiver distress.

aimed at increasing the social support for caregiver may be desirable. *Adaptive coping*, in terms of emotion focused and problem focused, may help the caregiver to match their response to a difficult medical situation. Avoidant strategies may not be that adaptive and useful in the long run [17, 18]. The components of adaptive coping are- facing not fleeing, altering the perception, coping actively, social support and expressing emotion. The caregiver of a terminally ill cancer patient needs to be able to cope with uncertainty of eminent death. Usually they are anxious to know the 'time left with the patient'. It is good to ask the caregiver that why they wanted to know in the first place. They may express a particular concern, like, the wedding of a loved one or travel plans. This opens a forum for discussion and scope for addressing the real concerns. Acknowledging that living with this kind of uncertainty is in fact difficult for most people will help the caregiver to get some perspective. Lastly, discuss certain coping strategies like living only one day at a time, living and planning till the next event like a birthday, learning to hope for the best but be prepared for the worst.

Group psychotherapy has already been shown to be efficient in providing psychological support to cancer patients [19, 20]. The same concepts could be applied to support cancer caregivers. The components of group therapy include- social support, emotional expression, demystifying dying, living in the present and re-organizing life priorities, family support enhancement and effective communication with medical team.

Good communication skills on the part of the medical team are a starting point for identification of distress in the cancer caregivers. A good approach would be to identify not just the telltale signs and symptoms of distress (like depression), but identify all psychological issues relevant to the caregiver at that moment. The person may be in a phase of denial or anger or disbelief or sadness. Identifying these and working on the core issue may serve better to take care of psychological distress. For example, if a cancer caregiver has received news of cancer recurrence in the patient, he may be in 'denial' for some time. This is a usual response when one is unable to deal with the weight of the reality and looks for alternate explanations. The 'denial' may result in anxiety. Rather than treating the anxiety with drugs, addressing the core issue, which was 'denial' in this case, acknowledging its effect on the person and an open honest discussion may be a better path to take. In addition to verbal communication, an effective way of conveying the message is 'non-verbal cues'. These include things like eye contact, facial expression, act of sitting with the person, posture, placement of hands, pace of voice, voice pitch and touch. For effective communication 'privacy' is equally important. The person should feel safe and confident to share their emotions and thoughts. Another important aspect is not to hurry up the conversation, we have to create the illusion of 'time' and should not interrupt as far as possible. Lastly, 'avoiding medical jargon' will allow for a smoother conversation and better understanding on the part of the caregiver. Nodding from time to time, reflective questioning, picking up cues from caregiver's statements, asking and validating their feelings, picking up non-verbal cues and finally summarizing the contents of the whole conversation are part of *active listening*. Active listening will help finding out about caregiver's emotions, feelings and concerns. Asking 'open questions' is better than asking leading or closed questions if you want to understand their feelings and concerns.

Leading question- *Are not you feeling less anxious today?*

Closed question- *Do you feel anxious today?*

Open question- *How is your anxiety today?*

What worries you so?

How do you think you feel today as compared to our previous consultation?

Next important thing to remember as a medical professional is to not use 'distancing behaviors'. Non-verbal cues like facial expression, looking very busy and tone of voice; labeling a patient, e.g., 'she is cancer colon patient; lecturing, criticizing, making threats, issuing orders, addressing only the physical problems, using closed questions, inappropriate humor and normalilsing prematurely are examples of distancing behaviors.

7.1 Management of anxiety

The first step is impeccable assessment keeping the following components in mind. Firstly, look for the common features of anxiety like- vigilance, scanning, autonomic hyperactivity, increased motor tension and excessive worrying. Secondly, we need to assess the character of anxiety, whether it is acute or chronic in nature, whether it is part of a psychiatric syndrome. Thirdly, there may be some features leading to anxiety, which may be reversible. For example, the patient's symptom control could be better or the medical team could address anxiety resulting from fear of unknown prognosis by counseling the caregiver in depth regarding patient's cancer related prognosis. It is important to note here that, one needs to give ample time to listen to the caregiver, so the real reasons behind the anxiety could be explored. The main concerns and worries mentioned by the caregiver will be helpful in understanding the reasons behind anxiety. Just the act of sharing these concerns may result in decreased anxiety. Treatment approach could be pharmacological or non-pharmacological. The non-pharmacological options are- psychological counseling, progressive muscular relaxation and distraction. The main pharmacological management is use of benzodiazepines like- Lorazepam, Diazepam, Midazolam and Clonazepam. Medications should be used only for short period to break the cycle of anxiety; non-pharmacological approaches are the main stay of management.

7.2 Management of depression

As with management of anxiety, we assess for the reversible causative factors and try to eliminate these. Enough emphasis cannot be given to the fact, that spending time with the caregiver, active and patient listening is important to uncover the main concerns and fears. Addressing these fears and concerns, emotional and social support and counseling are the main stay of management. Tricyclic antidepressants may be used in a few instances.

7.3 Management of adjustment disorders

Psychotherapy is the main stay of treatment. The focus will be on spending enough time with the caregiver and listening to his/her concerns and fears. Thereafter, focus will shift to addressing these concerns, help them find solutions to problems that are reversible. There will be need to resolve conflicts. For example, there may be ongoing conflict due to collusion, the patient may not be aware of the diagnosis or the prognosis. The caregiver, the patient and the medical team are bound to face conflict at multiple points of time in the management of cancer of this patient. Addressing the issues around collusion in this case will reduce distress in the caregiver. It is important to make an effort to improve communication between patient, caregiver and the medical team. The practical family issues and social issues like taboo and isolation need to be addressed to improve distress. There are formal approaches to manage adjustment disorders like- cognitive behavior therapy and problem solving therapy.

8. A good death

Caregiver of a patient who is nearing his death may feel a heightened need for reconciliation, affirmation, forgiveness and acceptance. It is important to note that *death is the not the ultimate failure*, poor quality of death and a demoralizing death is the real failure. Patient dying in a hostile environment of ICU, away from the physical and emotional support of the loved ones, is demoralizing to the family. Collusion prevents the spiritual nourishment between patient and caregiver, leading to a poor quality of death and distress in the bereavement period. *How can one achieve a 'good death'?* Taking care of physical issues like pain and dyspnoea at end of life of the cancer patient can be of great help. Patient and caregivers should have had adequate time and support to be able to accept death as a real eventuality and say a healthy 'good bye'. They should have had time to express love for each other. There should be openness to accept failures of life, forgive others and each other, reconcile with other family members. The achievements in life as an individual and as a family unit should be reviewed and acknowledged together. Lastly, the life journey as a whole may be evaluated and discussed among the family.

9. Recent literature on cancer caregiver distress

There are studies evaluating prevalence of distress in caregivers of cancer patients and its associated factors. In a study conducted on 641 Chinese adult cancer patients and their caregivers, it was found that *one-third* caregivers had experienced anxiety and depression and with similar degree. The factors that were found to affect the anxiety and depression in patient-caregiver dyads were- marital status, age, gender, level of information about disease, type of cancer and treatment, being the spouse, duration in role as caregiver, time spent daily on care giving, pre- and post-cancer family relationship and financial burden due to cancer treatment [21]. These factors associated with the caregiver distress may affect it with varying degree of severity. A review article published in 2018 found that caregiver distress was related to psycho-physiological elements like blood pressure and poor health related behaviors. Problem focused coping reduced depression and improved adjustment in this study [22].

Caring for children with cancer also leads to caregiver distress and burden. There may be some association between the child's symptoms and caregiver's distress. At the time of diagnosis, the parent of child may feel grief and severe anxiety. A study on psychological adjustment in families of 159 children with cancer found that during the first year of diagnosis the caregivers have clinically significant distress but the children are well adjusted [23]. Caregivers of 100 acute lymphoblastic leukemia children in Hydrabad (India) were enrolled in a study, which showed, that both mothers and fathers did not experience significantly different burden, however they used different coping strategies for the distress they felt [24]. Study published in 2016 concluded that symptoms of children being treated for cancer and financial difficulty were significantly associated caregiver distress and burden [25].

In a randomized controlled trial published in Oncologist in 2017, 350 patients and their caregivers were randomized to either early integrated palliative care or regular oncological care. This intervention improved the total distress and depression scores, but no change in anxiety score were noted [26]. It has been frequently reported that psychological distress is substantially high in a nuclear family, so family based approach is needed and most effective in cancer care. The caregiver-patient dyad unit should be the focus of assessment and intervention [27]. In a study on 43 lung cancer patient and caregiver dyads, it was found that patient's Lung Cancer Symptom Scale scores correlated positively with caregiver distress and burden scores [28]. Another study on 91 lung cancer patients and caregiver dyads found that the burden, anxiety, depression, Quality of life of the caregivers was affected by the Quality of life of the patient and not their stage of disease [29].

A study aimed to assess the inter-relationship of patient and caregiver distress at the time of diagnosis of incurable cancer. They enrolled 350 patients and 275 family caregivers within 8 weeks of diagnosis of incurable cancer. They found that patients reported more depression and caregivers more anxiety [30]. The anxiety and depression were found to be interrelated in the patient and their caregiver with good correlation. A review article published in 2016 on caregivers of ovarian cancer patients found that with time the experience of the caregiver changes. During the first year of diagnosis of cancer there is minimal compromise in well being and Quality of life, however there is steady decline as the disease progresses [31]. In pediatric cancer patients health related quality of life of the children has been significantly related to the caregiver distress, with age of the child being a significant covariate [32].

There has been limited research on caregivers of head and neck cancer patients. This study interviewed 31 long term caregivers of head and neck cancer patients. Emotional distress was found related to – understanding of illness, fears, restrictions in lifestyle, change in body image, financial burden, co-morbidities and witnessing suffering [13].

A study looked at the bereavement outcome in relation to age of advanced cancer patients [33]. They interviewed caregivers of 199 advanced cancer patients at the time of diagnosis and shortly following death of the patient. They concluded that relatives of patients in middle age (40–59 years) had greater grief and related distress symptoms like depression during bereavement period. In contrast, the relatives of young-old patients (60–79 years) had greater distress during caring period and relief of distress during the bereavement period.

An Indian study [34] explored the association between distress and somatization in 100 cancer patients and their caregivers. They found that the depression and anxiety found in patient and their caregiver had significant correlation; the caregiver's distress significantly correlated with somatization in the patient. Thus, psychological evaluation and management of the caregiver distress is essential for well being of the cancer patient. A study looked at gender differences in 377 cancer caregivers in Albania and found that female caregiver had higher levels of distress and poorer quality of life as compared to male caregivers [35]. An interventional study randomized 65 patient-caregiver dyads to group intervention and 66 to usual care, the interventional group had better Spiritual well-being scores, caregiver Quality of life scores at short and long term [36].

Medical professionals and health team may be able to reduce caregiver distress related to cancer if it is identified early and adequate steps are taken to relieve the causes of distress. Also, they can work with caregivers to help them attain something of emotional significance from the experience of loss or suffering [13].

10. Conclusion

There are various factors that may affect caregiver distress. The demographic and geographic factors like distance of travel from home to the hospital, frequency of hospital visits, ease of public or private travel, financial issues, loss of work, level of education. Patient and disease factors like age, stage, prognosis, type of treatment, physical symptoms, presence of stoma or tubes, knowledge of prognosis. Caregiver factors like gender, age, relation to the patient, duration of care-giving, total time spent daily caring, etc. Various psychological and spiritual elements have to be considered as well. In the clinical setting, physicians and medical team do not monitor caregiver burden regularly. Distress in caregivers is usually under recognized, under reported and under treated. In India, first and second degree relatives are the primary source of care and support system for cancer patients, though simultaneously they experience considerable distress themselves.

Author details

Anshika Arora
Department of Surgical Oncology, CRI, HIMS, Swami Rama Himalayan University, Dehradun, India

*Address all correspondence to: anshika00mittal@gmail.com; anshikaarora@srhu.edu.in

References

[1] Holland JC, Andersen B, Breitbart WS, et al. Distress management. *J Natl Compr Cancer Netw* 2010;8:448-485.

[2] American Psychiatric Association. *Diagnostic and Statistical Manual of Mental Disorders 5th Edition*. Vol. DSM-5. Washington, DC: American Psy chiatric Association; 2013.

[3] Jacobsen PB, Donovan KA, Trask PC, et al. Screening for psy chologic distress in ambulatory cancer patients. *Cancer* 2005;103:1494-1502.

[4] Solano JP, Gomes B, Higginson IJ: A comparison of symptom prevalence in far advanced cancer, AIDS, heart disease, chronic obstructive pulmonary disease and renal disease. J Pain Symptom Manage 31:58-69, 2006.

[5] Kunal Das, Tanvi Khanna, Anshika Arora et al. Parents' acceptance and regret about end of life care for children who died due to malignancy. Supportive Care in Cancer. https://doi.org/10.1007/s00520-019-04806-0

[6] Green BL, Rowland JH, Krupnick JL, et al. Prevalence of posttraumatic stress disorder (PTSD) in women with breast cancer. *Psychometrics* 1998;32: 102-111.

[7] Koopman C, Butler LD, Classen C, et al. Traumatic stress sy mptoms among women with recently diagnosed primary breast cancer. *J Trauma Stress* 2002;15:277-287.

[8] Cordova MJ, Andry kowski MA, Kenady DE, et al. Frequency and correlates of posttraumatic stress disorder-like sy stems following treatment for cancer. *J Consult Clin Psychol* 1995;63:981-986.

[9] Mayne M (1995) *This Sunrise of Wonder*. Fount, London, p. 21.

[10] Tedeschi RG, Calhoun LG. The posttraumatic growth inventory: measuring the positive legacy of trauma. *J Traumatic Stress* 1996;9:455-471.

[11] Cordova MJ, Cunningham LL, Carlson CR, et al. Social constraints, cognitive processing, and adjustment to breast cancer. *J Consult Clin Psychol* 2001;69:706-711.

[12] Cordova MJ, Cunningham LL, Carlson CR, et al. Posttraumatic growth following breast cancer: a controlled comparison study. *Health Psychol* 2001;20:176-185.

[13] Balfe M, Maguire R, Hanly P, et. al (2016). Distress in long-term head and neck cancer carers: a qualitative study of carers' perspectives. J Clin Nurs. Aug;25(15-16):2317-27. doi: 10.1111/jocn.13242.

[14] Trunzo JJ, Pinto BM. Social support as a mediator of optimism and distress in breast cancer survivors. *J Consult Clin Psychol* 2003;71:805-811.

[15] Giese-Davis J, Koopman C, Butler L, et al. Change in emotion-regulation strategy for women with metastatic breast cancer following supportive expressive group therapy . *J Consult Clin Psychol* 2002;70:916-925.

[16] Cordova MJ, Andry kowski MM. Responses to cancer diagnosis and treatment: posttraumatic stress and posttraumatic growth. *Semin Clin Neuropsychiatr* 2003;8: 286-296.

[17] Lazarus A, Folkman S. *Stress, Appraisal, And Coping*. New York: Springer; 1984.

[18] Folkman S, Moskowitz J. Positive affect and the other side of coping. *Am Psychol* 2000;55:647-654.

[19] Yalom I. *Theory And Practice Of Group Psychotherapy*. New York: Basic Books; 1995.

[20] Spiegel D, Classen C. *Group Therapy For Cancer Patients: A Research-Based Handbook Of Psychosocial Care*. New York: Basic Books; 2000.

[21] Qiuping LI, Yi LIN, Yinghua XU and Huiya ZHOU (2018). The impact of depression and anxiety on quality of life in Chinese cancer patientfamily caregiver dyads, a cross-sectional study. Health and Quality of Life Outcomes.16:230. https://doi.org/10.1186/s12955-018-1051-3

[22] Teixeira RJ, Applebaum AJ, Bhatia S, Brandão T (2018). The impact of coping strategies of cancer caregivers on psychophysiological outcomes: an integrative review. Psychol Res Behav Manag. May 24;11:207-215. doi: 10.2147/PRBM.S164946.

[23] Katz LF, Fladeboe K, King K, et.al (2018). Trajectories of child and caregiver psychological adjustment in families of children with cancer. Health Psychol. Aug;37(8):725-735. doi: 10.1037/hea0000619.

[24] Chivukula U, Kota S, Nandinee D (2018). Burden Experience of Caregivers of Acute Lymphoblastic Leukemia: Impact of Coping and Spirituality. Indian J Palliat Care. Apr-Jun; 24(2):189-195. doi: 10.4103/IJPC.IJPC_209_17.

[25] Edmond SN, Graves PE, Whiting SE, et. al (2016). Emotional distress and burden among caregivers of children with oncological/hematological disorders. Fam Syst Health. Jun;34(2):166-71. doi: 10.1037/fsh0000181.

[26] El-Jawahri A, Greer JA, Pirl WF, et. al (2017). Effects of Early Integrated Palliative Care on Caregivers of Patients with Lung and Gastrointestinal Cancer: A Randomized Clinical Trial. Oncologist. Dec;22(12):1528-1534. doi: 10.1634/theoncologist.2017-0227.

[27] Caruso R, Nanni MG, Riba MB, et. al (2017). The burden of psychosocial morbidity related to cancer: patient and family issues. Int Rev Psychiatry. Oct;29(5):389-402. doi: 10.1080/09540261.2017.1288090.

[28] Tan JY, Molassiotis A, Lloyd-Williams M, et. al (2018). Burden, emotional distress and quality of life among informal caregivers of lung cancer patients: An exploratory study. Eur J Cancer Care (Engl). Jan;27(1). doi: 10.1111/ecc.12691.

[29] Borges EL Franceschini J, Costa LH, et. al (2017). Family caregiver burden: the burden of caring for lung cancer patients according to the cancer stage and patient quality of life. J Bras Pneumol. Jan-Feb;43(1):18-23. doi: 10.1590/S1806-37562016000000177.

[30] Jacobs JM, Shaffer KM, Nipp RD, , et. al (2017). Distress is Interdependent in Patients and Caregivers with Newly Diagnosed Incurable Cancers. Ann Behav Med. Aug;51(4):519-531. doi: 10.1007/s12160-017-9875-3.

[31] Petricone-Westwood D, Lebel S (2016). Being a caregiver to patients with ovarian cancer: A scoping review of the literature. Gynecol Oncol. Oct;143(1):184-192. doi: 10.1016/j.ygyno.2016.07.007.

[32] Pierce L, Hocking MC, Schwartz LA, et. al (2017). Caregiver distress and patient health-related quality of life: psychosocial screening during pediatric cancer treatment. Psychooncology. 2017 Oct;26(10):1555-1561. doi: 10.1002/pon.4171.

[33] Francis LE, Kypriotakis G, O'Toole EE, et. al(2016). Cancer patient age and family caregiver bereavement outcomes. Support Care Cancer.

Sep;24(9):3987-96. doi: 10.1007/s00520-016-3219-x.

[34] Padmaja G, Vanlalhruaii C, Rana S, et. al (2016). Care givers' depression, anxiety, distress, and somatization as predictors of identical symptoms in cancer patients. J Cancer Res Ther. Jan-Mar;12(1):53-7. doi: 10.4103/0973-1482.146088.

[35] Burnette D, Duci V, Dhembo E (2017). Psychological distress, social support, and quality of life among cancer caregivers in Albania. Psychooncology. Jun;26(6):779-786. doi: 10.1002/pon.4081.

[36] Lapid MI, Atherton PJ, Kung S, et. al (2016). Cancer caregiver quality of life: need for targeted intervention. Psychooncology. Dec;25(12):1400-1407. doi: 10.1002/pon.3960.

Chapter 8

The Exceptional Role of Women as Primary Caregivers for People Living with HIV/AIDS in Nigeria, West Africa

Ekaete Francis Asuquo and Paulina Ackley Akpan-Idiok

Abstract

In Africa, women play an indispensable role in family life. The normative roles of women extend from reproductive role to the raising of children and caring for sick family members. These roles are very unique and are dictated by culture, religion and beliefs. Despite these, their contributions in caregiving remain unrecognized except by the beneficiaries. Caregivers of people living with HIV/AIDS (PLWHA) experience high level of burden due to the expanded role and inadequate preparation for the caregiver's duty. A descriptive cross-sectional research design was utilized to elicit data from 260 participants in Calabar municipality, Nigeria. Caring for PLWHA is an exceptional service due to exacerbation of symptoms and co-morbidities peculiar to terminal phase of HIV. The study revealed gender inequalities in burden levels. Significant relationships ($p < 0.05$) also existed between burden of care, availability of support and duration of care during this study. Despite the perceived consequences, the family care givers were still determined to continue caregiving role. This informs the need for governmental support to ameliorate the negative consequences of caregiving by female caregivers.

Keywords: women caregivers, burden, PLWHA, Nigeria

1. Introduction

Africa is a patriarchal society with women role detected by ethno-religious ideologies, economic as well as socio-cultural factors. These factors inform assignment of resources and responsibilities which is often laden with inequities between men and women [1, 2]. However, women have proven to be the central crux that holds family together while serving as primary caregiver to children and elderly globally as well as facilitating or hindering change in family life [3]. Additionally, with the scourge of HIV in the African society, the responsibility rest on them, a situation describing AIDS as having "a woman's face" in Africa [4]. While HIV prevalence continues to soar in Africa, it is eroding the health of women directly as well as indirectly diminishing their skills and productivity which adversely affects family life [4, 5].

An average of 75.7 million (55.9 million–100 million) people have been infected with HIV with about 32.7 million (24.8 million–42.2 million) AIDS-related death recorded since the onset of HIV epidemic in 1981 [6]. Presently, UNAIDS fact sheet [6] reveal about 31.6 million–44.5 million (38.0 million) people living with HIV, with about 1.7 new infection in 2019. African disproportionately bear the burden of HIV with about 25.7 million people living with HIV and 470,000 AIDS related death in 2018. Although global effort has been directed to combat HIV impact in Africa, the continent still contributes about two thirds of global new HIV infections with about 1.1 million people infected in 2018 [7]. Nigeria remains Africa's most populous country, with about 1.9 million people living with HIV, 130000 new infection, and 53,000 AIDS-related death in 2018 [6]. The high prevalence of HIV will invariably invoke strain on family life especially when affected member returns home for succor.

The African nuclear family is a potent therapeutic force, and highly sensitive to the needs of its member, by providing physical, financial, emotional and spiritual support. Studies reveal that family remains the primary entity in caring for individuals, through which socialization, trust, loyalty and inter-family cooperation develops, and many counts on these attributes in adverse health condition [8, 9]. These attributes attracts afflicted members and act as a succor especially during terminal stage of HIV with co-morbidities [9, 10]. Caregiving although a normative role, is assumed most often by people without preparation or questioning even though it may disrupt work, family and social life of the caregivers. As the number of people living with HIV/AIDS increases, the demand for family members who assume caregiving role increases [11]. Moreover without appropriate restructuring of existing role to accommodate new caregiving roles, the increase in responsibility may constitute burden, which is detrimental to the caregiver's health as well as quality of care rendered to the care recipient [10–12].

2. Women and HIV

Women disproportionately bear the burden of HIV and this is often secondary to gender inequalities which are obvious in economic status, cultural and societal norms. Women and girls constitute more than half the population of PLWHA, accounting for 18.8 million prsons. Studies reveal that in every 4 minutes, three young women are infected with HIV with approximately 870,000 new HIV every year among women and girls [13]. Additionally among female age 15–49, AIDS-related illnesses remains the leading cause of death [14]. Although, no HIV gender disparity existed in children, gender disparities became obvious during adolescence, with girls accounting for 75 per cent (130,000) of new HIV infections among adolescents, globally in comparison to about 44,000 adolescent boys [14]. In sub-Saharan Africa, young women are two times more likely to be infected with HIV than male and they account for 59% of all new HIV infections [6]. Women also disproportionately bear the burden of HIV in Nigeria, among 1,800,000 adults with HIV, and the majority, 1,000,000 (55.56%) were women. New HIV infection among those aged 15–24 years were more (26000) among female compared to 15,000 among their male counterparts [6]. New HIV infections among young women aged 15–24 years were almost double those among young men: 26000 new infections among young women, compared to 15,000 among young men. The high prevalence among female is fueled by biological vulnerability, gender inequalities which encouraged early and forced marriage, lack of information on sexuality, lack of negotiating power as well as economic autonomy [15]. The need to bridge the gap by improving the quality of life of females by encouraging social justice with equal access to employment, education, health services and freedom from discrimination and violence had been advocated as a panacea for ending HIV epidemic by 2030 [4]. In spite of high HIV burden among women, they also bear the brunt of caring for those affected, a double jeopardy.

3. Women and caregiving

It is imperative that as humans navigate through life with changing demographics that some will have to function as caregivers. Caregiving is a role expected of family members however, the irrefutable strength of informal caregiving lies on female family caregivers, whose role are often designated by ideologies and endorsed by culture. It has been asserted that caregiving is feminized and women are socialized into nurturing roles [16]. Studies affirmed that round the world women make-up about 57 to 81% of informal care givers for family members with chronic disabilities [17–21]. Females commenced their caregiving activities at a very young age and maintain this role as they aged [22]. Most often their roles are not recognized by other family members and health care system except by the care recipient [23].

A Canadian study revealed that in every five persons there was a female family caregiver who provided 70 percent or more of required caregiving needs [24]. In the United States, about 41 million family caregivers served 34 billion hours of care to recipient with functional disabilities accounting for an estimated $470 billion of unpaid caregivers [23]. The female form (65%) majority of family caregivers and about 80% provide care to elderly relative or friend [25]. Another study revealed that 82.8% of family caregivers were females in a study with 583 family caregivers [26]. A similar report was obtained from an Australian research where 2.65 million family caregivers in 2015, were females (12.3%) and only 9.3% were males [27]. Studies in Nigeria also revealed gender difference when it comes to caregiving, where majority were female, (67.3%) and experience a higher level of burden than men [12, 28]. In France majority of caregivers were women and whenever one caregiver was needed to provide care it was most often female [29]. Additionally, daughters form three-quarters of those caring for their elderly parent, and 70% of those caring for their spouses were wives while men tend to seek professional assistance with care duties [29]. Similarly among couples, women most often shoulder caregiving role than their spouses [30]. When it comes to physical care or personal care, such as bathing or getting dressed, women are more likely (19% vs. 8%) than men to provide such care to care recipients [31]. It has been affirmed that caregiving is a traditionally driven activity earmarked for women [32].

4. Duration of care

Unlike formal caregivers, informal caregivers may not have stipulated time period for caring and are often required to perform multiple task both planned and unplanned for the day with progressive increase in activities over time which induces burden [10, 11]. A study affirmed the disparity between men and women caregiving involvement with changing demographics and suggested the need for more male involvement in order to reduce caregiving burden on women [30, 33]. The period spent providing care to a sick family member differs between men and women. The variation however exists between the types of care provided as well as duration, thereby exacerbating women perceived burden. Studies have revealed disparity in hours between men and women providing care, that women provides full time care with an average of 9 hours 45 minutes, that is, with an additional 2 hours more than men, who provide 7 hours 20 minutes of care [30, 34]. With regards to gender specific differences in providing care, women approach to caregiving is more comprehensive (more hands-on care) supporting care recipient with activities of daily living. Furthermore, women provide care for longer duration than men, with caregivers spending more than 11 hours per week [32, 35, 36]. The feminization of female role in caregiving and home centered care give a greater sense of family obligation with longer duration spent in caregiving than men [37–39]. Another report stated that duration of care increased among cultures and societies who designate caregiving as a woman's primary role [39]. Additionally, females' care giving role commenced at a younger age and persists as they grow older with an average age for female primary caregivers ranging between 30 and 55 years [22].

5. Gender and caregivers burden

African traditional gender norms feminize caregiving and exclude men and boys from caregiving. The normative women roles extend from reproductive role to nurturing infant and sick family members and remain progressive all through their lifetime [40]. However, these roles remain unrecognized except by the beneficiaries. Therefore, personal sacrifice comes with fulfillment of this role, while some female may have to leave school to provide care [41]. The added responsibility may overshadow the individual coping ability and it manifest as stress or burden. Caregiver's burden is defined as an individual response to physical, emotional, psychological, financial as well as social stressors in Ref. to caregiving experience [42]. Burden maybe objective or subjective. Objective burden refers to disruption in household routines, social relations, leisure, time, finances, work as well as physical health which is often observable [43–45]. Subjective burden refers to how the caregiver appraises the caregiving task [44]. However it has been reported that objective burden depends on subjective appraisal of the caregiving task [44]. Report reveals that caregivers of PLWHA experienced high level of burden [34]. With common sessional symptoms and exacerbation in terminal phase of HIV, many are overwhelmed with caregiving demands resulting in burden [46]. Moreover burden may be compounded with lack of support and financial constraint. Studies revealed higher level of both subjective and objective burden among females compared to males [17, 38, 47, 48] and higher level of physical and social burden [49]. But women experienced more objective burden which is often associated with physical task of caregiving [40]. Similarly, another report stated that women are directly involved in providing personal care which is more demanding and significantly contributes to burden [11, 33]. Studies in Nigeria also affirmed a significant relationship between caregiver's burden and gender with 67.5% female accounting for those with high level of caregivers' burden [10, 28]. Similarly, another study in Lagos, Nigeria also affirmed higher level of burden among female and more stressor emanating from financial, physical as well as emotional domain of burden scale.

5.1 Caregiving and support

The high prevalence of HIV in Africa and Nigeria, coupled with improvements in treatment modalities and life expectancy predict the inevitable loss of autonomy as disease trajectory progressed into AIDS. It has been noted that in spite of prophylaxis for opportunist infection and antiretroviral therapy in preventing AIDS associated illness, PLWHA will still be sick and have disability in functional ability, hence require care [50]. This terminal stage invariable signals the need for either formal or informal caregivers. Studies also revealed that HIV infected individuals return to their homes for physical and psychological support and adequate discharge preparation which incorporate health care team; and family care givers become imperative [50]. However, health care system especially in developing countries do not have the capacity to provide long-term services, they rarely involved family caregivers in the discharge planning, neither are they educated about their roles. Patients are discharged home without contact with family caregivers and most health systems lack structured and effective discharge plans [51, 52]. But effective discharge planning plays a role in continuity of care [53]. Although there are benefits associated with caregiving such as fulfilling normative role and reciprocity when the chips are down [10, 54]. Reducing the cost of institutionalization and receiving care in an environment one is familiar with as well as being in the company of loved ones improved the quality of life of the care recipient. Moreover, during caregiving bonding relationship develops between the caregiver and recipient, but the type of relationship depends on the age of caregiver and recipient [55]. It is however pertinent to note that in spite of family resiliency with care, their experience of physical and emotional strain should never be ignored [56]. Most caregivers are "hidden" patients which health care professional fail to recognize [57]. Besides, while discharging the patient they fail to think about continuity of care to full recovery, based on the implicit assumption that family members would care for them, without educational preparation on how to managed discharged patient. The assumption of caregiving role without preparation might affect the individual coping mechanism resulting in the experiencing of stress or burden. Caregiving has both positive and negative consequences although the two may exist concurrently [57]. Excessive life stressor on the other hand results in negative consequences and without adequate intervention may affect role performance [58]. This informs the need for family caregivers support. Support is conceptualized as what others do to help the individual cope [58]. This conceptualization of involving significant others in the caregivers' capability constitute the principal theme that is exemplified in this study.

The forms of support have been categorized into three namely: (a) instrumental aid (actions or resources provided to aid caregiving responsibilities), (b) socio-emotional aid (infer demonstrations of love, caring, esteem, sympathy and group belonging) and (c) informational aid (communications of information that makes life challenges easier) [59]. These forms of social support buffer the negative consequences of caregiving. Although men have jobs more than female [30], the female combine caregiving most often with productive and reproductive activities, therefore they need support for adaptation as responsibilities changes or increases, in order to ensure quality care and life of the care recipient. This study therefore seeks to assess the level of burden experienced by all caregivers of PLWHA, identify and compare the gender differences in the degree of perceived burden, ascertain the duration of care, assess the availability of support as well as the willingness of caregivers to continue caregiving in the future.

6. Materials and method

6.1 Location of the study

The study was conducted in Calabar Municipality, a local government in Cross River State (CRS) of Nigeria between June to December 2009. Cross River State is one of the 36 States of the Federal republic of Nigeria situated in the South South zone of Nigeria. Calabar Municipality has an area of 142 km^2 and a population of 179,392 by the 2006 census. Calabar Municipality otherwise called '*Efik eburutu*' has a rich cultural heritage and very hospitable. Compared with other communities in Nigeria, they operate the patriarchal system with male preference and dominance. Moreover the families take responsibilities for their sick member. CRS operate the three tier health care system which includes primary, secondary and tertiary, however the health facility is skewed to the urban area. The University of Calabar

Teaching Hospital (UCTH) is a tertiary institution and a referral center to other health care facilities. The facility offers both inpatient and outpatient services and collaborates with nongovernmental organizations (NGOs) in the treatment of PLWHA from rural/urban areas and neighboring country, Cameroun. The state is one the 12 + 1 states which contribute about 70% of HIV burden in Nigeria. UCTH is one of the centers for the management of PLWHA. The high HIV prevalence (10.4%) at the study site inform the choice of study setting [10, 60].

7. Study design and participants

The study utilized a cross-sectional descriptive research design with a convenient sampling technique. Two hundred and ninety nine (299) participants were selected for the study; however 260 completely filled their questionnaires and were aware of care recipient HIV status. Family caregivers were recruited through HIV clinic of the UCTH and Positive Development Foundation (NGO) visitation list of voluntary caregiver of PLWHA. Information letter and invitation were posted at UCTH HIV clinic and the Positive Development Foundation office where interested and willing participants were contacted by the researcher. This study is part of the research project previously published [10]. Therefore participants who met the inclusion criteria were individuals: who have been a primary caregiver for more than 1 month, have awareness of the care recipient status or have provided care for PLWHA patient with some functional abilities as a family member. Family caregivers age cuts across all age brackets, and often include children under the age of 16 [61]. The role of primary caregiver as associated with this study involved participants who provided unpaid physical support such as helping in activities of daily living, food preparation, shopping, managing scheduled medication, managing finances, overseeing medical appointment and emotional support to PLWHA. Questionnaires were coded and contact information was not included to ensure confidentiality. Ethical consent for the study was obtained from Health Research Ethics Committee of UCTH Calabar. Consent was also obtained from the Managing Director of Positive Development Foundation who helped to identify PLWHA caregivers. Informed consent was also obtained from study participants after full explanation of the aims and objectives of study. Participants were appreciated for their time.

8. Instrument and measures

Structured questionnaires were the instrument for data collection, two versions of the questionnaire was developed: the English version and the Efik version (local dialect). The Efik version was translated from English into Efik and back-translated into English by experts to prevent loss of meaning. The researcher and trained field assistants helped with data collection through face to face contact, however some questionnaires were deposited with the caregivers who filled and returned within 1 week. The structured questionnaires consisted of 41 items, 7 demographic variables, 22 from Zarit Burden Interview (ZBI) scale and 12 measuring social support. Reliability of the instruments was attained through test–retest method. The questionnaires were administered to 10 caregivers of PLWHA in Calabar South. After 2 weeks the same questionnaire was administered again to the same subjects. Their responses during the two occasions were correlated using Pearson product-moment correlation to obtain a reliability coefficient ranging from 0.85 to 0.96.

9. Demographics

Seven items make-up the demographic variables which included: participant's age, marital status, their current occupation, highest educational qualification, household income level, number of people in the household and duration of care. Duration of care was categorized into two namely: hours spent per day and years spent as a caregiver of PLWHA. Duration of care was predefined for the caregivers.

9.1 Caregivers burden

The Zarit Burden Interview (ZBI) scale is a caregiver self-report questionnaire consisting of 22 items. Each item reflected the impact that patient disabilities have in the caregiver's life. The caregiver endorsed the degree of physical, emotional and social discomfort experienced on a 5-point Likert scale ranging from never, rarely, sometimes, quite frequently, or nearly always. The 22 items validated ZBI scale had reliability coefficient ranging from 0.88 to 0.92. Scores ranged from 0 to 88 and a high score is associated with higher level of burden.

9.2 Support

The support questionnaire contained 12 items which assessed the extent of support received in the form of information, financial help, emotional support as well as physical help with caregiving activities. The instrument was pilot tested with a reliability coefficient of 0.85 to 0.96. Caregivers indicated the extent of support received on a 4-point Likert-type scale, ranging from lots of support, some support, very little support and no support.

9.3 Data analysis

Descriptive and inferential data were obtained using Statistical Package for the Social Sciences (SPSS 16.0 software) which generated the frequency and percentages of the values. Chi-square test and T-test was used for inferential statistics. The level of significance was also determined at the p value of 0.05. The ZBI scale scores ranged from 0 to 88. The scores were categorized into four namely: 0 to 20 represented little or no burden; 21 to 40, mild to moderate burden; 41 to 60, moderate to severe burden; and 61 to 88, severe burden [62]. The support instrument was grouped into two namely: availability of support for "lot of support and some support," and lack of support for "very little support and no support."

10. Results

10.1 Socio-demographic characteristics

Table 1 describes the socio-demographic variables of 260 caregivers of PLWHA who participated in the study. The majority of caregivers were females 199 (76.5%). Age ranged from 10 to 80 years, with majority between 31 and 40 years, however the females formed the majority in all age ranges. Marital status revealed majority (93/35.8%) were single females. The majority (77/29.6%) had tertiary education as the highest educational qualification and (89/34.2%) caregivers were employed, while 60 caregivers left school to care for their loved ones with majority 49 (18.8%) among the female caregivers of PLWHA (**Table 1**).

G	Age (years) Range n (%)		Marital status Type n (%)		Educational qualification Type n(%)		Occupation Type n (%)		Duration of care (hr/day) Range n (%)		Years of care Range n (%)	
F	10–20	22 (8.5)	Married	79 (30.)	Primary (Basic)	22 (8.5)	Employed	89 (34.2)	3–8	16 (6.2)	<1	67 (25.8)
	21–30	31 (11.9)	Single	93 (35.8)	Secondary (high)	31 (11.9)	Un-employed	31 (11.9)	9–12	145 (55.8)	1–2	90 (34.6)
	31–40	63 (24.2)	Divorced	10 (3.8)	Tertiary	77 (29.6)	Business/ farming	79 (30.4)	13–24	38 (14.6)	2–3	32 (12.3)
	41–50	46 (17.7)	Widowed	8 (3.1)	Never been to school	20 (7.7)	Employed	89 (34.2)	—	—	>3	10 (3.8)
	>51	37 (14.2)	Living together/ domestic partner	9 (3.5)	Left school for caregiving	49 (18.8)	Un-employed	31 (11.9)	—	—	—	—
T	**199 (76.5)**		**199 (76.5)**		**199 (76.5)**		**199 (76.5)**		**199 (76.5)**		**199 (76.5)**	
M	10–20	3 (1.2)	Married	34 (13.1)	Primary (Basic)	4 (1.5)	Employed	11 (4.2)	3–8	36 (13.8)	<1	34 (13.1)
	21–30	8 (3.1)	Single	15 (5.8)	Secondary (high)	16 (6.2)	Un-employed	29 (11.2)	9–12	17 (6.5)	1–2	19 (7.3)
	31–40	22 (8.5)	Divorced	4 (1.5)	Tertiary	28 (10.8)	Business/ farming	21 (8.1)	13–24	8 (3.1)	2–3	6 (2.3)
	41–50	15 (5.8)	Widowed	5 (1.9)	Never been to school	2 (0.8)	Employed	—	—	—	>3	2 (0.8)
	>51	13 (5.0)	Living together/ domestic partner	3 (1.2)	Left school for caregiving	11 (4.2)	Un-employed	—	—	—	—	—
T	**61 (23.5)**		**61 (23.5)**		**61 (23.5)**		**61 (23.5)**		**61 (23.5)**		**61 (23.5)**	

Note: G, gender; F, female; M, male; T, total.

Table 1.
The socio-demographic characteristics of caregiver respondents.

10.2 Gender difference in duration of care

Gender difference existed in the duration of care provided for PLWHA. The least duration 3–8 hours was spent by 36 (13.8) male caregivers while only 16 (6.2) female caregivers spent the same. 9–12 hours majority were spent by 145 (55.8) female caregivers. 13–24 hours of care was provided mostly by 38 (14.6) female caregivers. With reference to the years spent in caregiving, the majority 90 (34.6) female caregivers spent between 1 and 2 years, while the least 10 (3.8) female and 2 (0.8) male caregivers provided care to PLWHA for more than three years (**Table 1**).

Table 2 describes the household income as well the number of people in the household. The majority 130 (50%) family caregivers of PLWHA lived below a household income of US$6.00/day while only 15 (5.8%) family caregivers spent US$14.00 and above. The majority 153 (58.9%) lived in a household with about three to six members and only about 19 (7.3%) lived in small households with one to three persons (**Table 2**).

Table 3 describes gender difference in the level of burden among family caregivers of PLWHA ranging between 14 and 71 on ZBI Scale (**Table 3**); among the 49 (18.8%) caregivers that experienced no burden, the majority were females 39 (15.0) while 10 (3.9%) males. The 46 (17.7) female caregivers experienced mild to moderate while providing care. Ninety-three (35.8) caregivers experienced moderate to severe burden and the majority 69 (26.6) were females. Fifty-one (19.6%) family caregivers experienced severe level of burden in providing care to PLWHA and majority 45 (17.3) caregivers were females.

Household income level US$/Day		
Variables	**Frequency**	**Percentage (%)**
Less than US$6.00	130	50.0
US$7.00-US$8.00	59	22.7
US$9.00-US$10.00	25	9.6
US$11.00-US$12.00	18	6.9
US$13.00-US$14.00	13	5.0
US$14.00 and above	15	5.8
Number of people in the household		
1–3	19	7.3
4–6	153	58.9
7 and above	88	33.8

Table 2.
Household income and the number of people in the household.

Gender				
Level of burden	**Female (%)**	**Male (%)**	**N = 260 (%)**	**Range**
No burden	39 (15.0)	10 (3.9)	49 (18.9)	0–20
Mild to moderate	46 (17.7)	21 (8.1)	67 (25.8)	21–40
Moderate to severe	69 (26.6)	24 (9.2)	93 (35.8)	41–60
Severe burden	45 (17.3)	6 (2.3)	51 (19.6)	61–88
Total	**199 (76.5)**	**61 (23.5)**	**260 (100.0)**	**0–88**

Table 3.
The distribution of burden on Zarit burden interview (ZBI) scale.

Level of burden	Class interval (range)	Class mark (x)	F1 (female)	F2 (male)
No burden	0–20	10.0	39	10
Mild to moderate burden	21–40	30.5	46	21
Moderate to severe	41–60	50.5	69	24
Severe burden	61–88	74.5	45	6
Total	**0–88**		**199**	**61**

Note: T-test Cal. = 1.27. T-test tab. = 1.62, N = 260, $p < 0.05$.

Table 4.
The relationship between gender and caregivers burden.

Significant statistical relationship existed between gender and caregivers burden assessed with the students t test. Calculated t test value of 1.27 at $p < 0.05$, indicated a significant relationship between the levels of burden experienced by gender (**Table 4**).

11. Availability of support to caregivers

One hundred and eight (108, 41.5%) family caregivers received no form of support, while 152 (58.5%) received some form of support. The forms of support received included information on practical and coping skills 6 (0.2%), financial assistance 36 (13.9%), help with care giving 72 (27.7%), while 38 (14.6%) caregivers received emotional support. There was no difference in the types of support by gender (**Figure 1**).

In-spite of burden experienced by the majority of family caregivers, 213 (81.9%) representing 171 females and 42 males, were willing to continue with caregiving, while 47 (18.1%) caregivers (28 females and 14 males) did not feel like continuing with caregiving role (**Figure 2**).

Table 5 presents the relationship between availability of support and caregivers burden. One hundred and eight (108) caregivers received no support, 12 caregivers experienced no burden, 23 caregivers experienced mild to moderate burden, 37 caregivers experienced moderate to severe burden while 36 caregivers experienced severe burden. A chi-square value of 25.1 at $p < 0.05$, reveal a significant relationship between availability of support and caregivers burden.

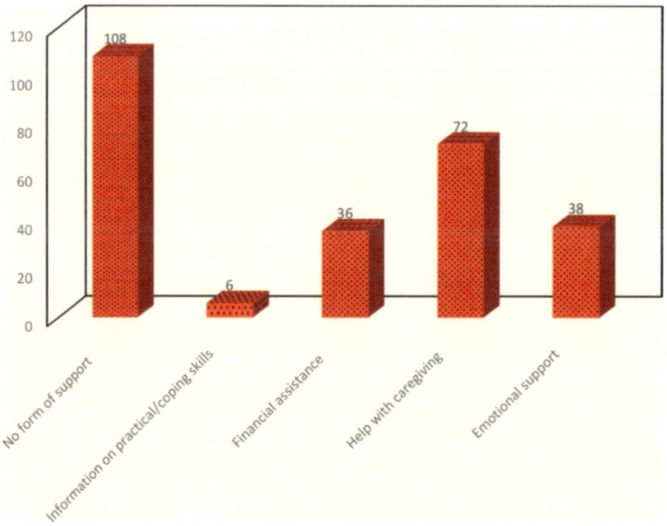

Figure 1.
Assessing the extent of support to caregivers of PLWHA in Nigeria.

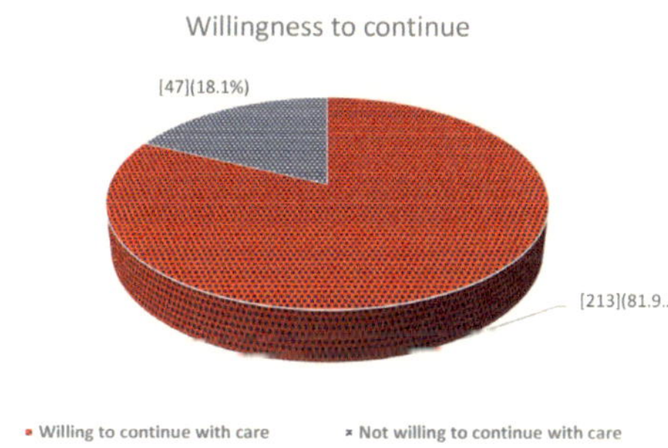

Figure 2.
The caregiver's willingness to continue in caregiving role.

Availability of support	No burden	Mild to moderate burden	Moderate to severe burden	Severe burden	Total
Received any form of support	37 (28.7)	44 (39.2)	56 (54.4)	15 (29.8)	152
Received no support	12 (20.4)	23 (27.8)	37 (38.6)	36 (21.2)	108
Total	**49**	**67**	**93**	**51**	**260**

Note: Figures in parentheses are expected frequencies. $\chi2$ Cal. = 25.1. $\chi2$ Tab. = 7.81, df = 3, N = 260, $p < 0.05$ where "$\chi2$ Cal." and "$\chi2$ Tab." Represents Chi square calculated and Chi square tabulated, respectively.

Table 5.
The relationship between availability of support and caregivers' burden.

12. The duration of care for caregivers

Fifty-two family caregivers provided 3–8 hours of care per day, however a majority of 28 caregivers experienced no burden, 10 caregivers experienced mild burden, eight caregivers experienced moderate to severe burden while six caregivers experienced severe burden. Among 162 caregivers that delivered care for 9–12 hours per day, the majority 73 caregivers experienced moderate to severe burden while 23 respondents experienced severe burden. Forty-six family caregivers provided care for 13–24 hours per day, five caregivers experienced no burden, seven caregivers perceived mild to moderate burden, while the majority 22 caregivers experienced severe burden (**Table 6**).

A chi-square value of 80.0 at $p < 0.05$ revealed a significant relationship between duration of care and caregivers burden (**Table 6**).

Duration, hours/day	No burden	Mild to moderate burden	Moderate to severe burden	Severe burden	Total
3–8	28 (9.8)	10 (13.4)	8 (18.5)	6 (10.2)	52
9–12	16 (30.5)	50 (41.8)	73 (58.0)	23 (31.8)	162
13–24	5 (8.7)	7 (11.9)	12 (16.5)	22 (9.0)	46
Total	**49**	**67**	**93**	**51,260**	**260**

Note: Figures in parentheses are expected frequencies. $\chi2$ Cal. = 80.0, χTab. = 10.65, df = 6, N = 260, $p < 0.05$.

Table 6.
The relationship between duration of care and caregivers' burden.

13. Discussion

The high disease burdens in low and middle countries outweigh the available capacity and resources of the health care system, which prevent institutionalization for full recovery. Early discharge depicts the need for family caregivers, most often female who assumes caregiving role without adequate preparation as it is obvious in this study. This finding corroborates with previous report that about four to five million people serve as caregivers with the majority being women and they provide more than 80% of the care needed by HIV individuals [63]. Even though the proportion of male involved with care giving is on the increase, specific gender differences still exist as caregiving remains the traditional role of women [32].

Caregiving though a rewarding role with intrinsic benefit is laden with burden especially while caring for PLWHA at the terminal phase. This finding is consistent with other studies which affirmed that caregiving adversely affect the physical, social and psychological wellbeing of the caregiver [10, 11, 46]. The demanding role of caregiving, which requires patience, empathy and show of affection irrespective of the physical disabilities of the care recipient, is an attribute which most women acquire from birth [64]. This commensurate the finding of this study that the burden of care in HIV/AIDS affected household rest more on women and girls than men. Similarly, previous reports identify women as the primary caregivers in most households and societies [19, 22, 65]. It is however pertinent to note that female dominance in caregiving is in consonance with the Nigerian patriarchal system which culturally relegate caregiving and domestic chores to women and girls except where there are no eligible females. This is also similar to studies which report caregiving as being culturally feminized and women are socialized into nurturing roles [16, 65]. It is obvious that the traditional gender norms emancipate men from caregiving thereby exacerbating burden of care on primary caregivers who are predominantly females.

In-spite of female dominance in caregiving this study revealed that majority of primary caregivers experienced high burden level (**Table 3**). This stipulates the degree to which caregiving to PLWHA impacts on physical health, emotional, financial and social life of the caregiver. It is obvious that the physical labor of accomplishing activities of daily living especially in the presence of functional disabilities of the care recipient invoke burden. This finding is similar to studies that asserted that caregivers experienced a high level of burden which produces detrimental effects on the carer's own health [10, 54, 66]. This study revealed that burden may also be exacerbated with the lack of resources to spend on medication and other basic household needs especially where household spend less than $6 dollars/day (**Table 1**). This is apparent because HIV disproportionately affects low and middle income countries especially in Africa, which contributes two thirds of global new HIV infections [7]. Encouraging care provision in homes is regarded as a cost-effective strategy for governments and the private sector, but little consideration is given to the physical, emotional and economic costs to households and the caregivers who take on the additional burdens, many of whom are often poor and living below US$ 1.00 to US$1.25 per day [10, 67, 68]. In sub-Saharan Africa, not only does correlation exist between poverty and HIV infection but HIV remained the exact outcome of poverty in the region with sexual trade, migration, polygamy, and teenage marriages as its predictors [69].

This study revealed a significant relationship between gender and level of burden, this obvious because women perform more hands on care than men, probably due to their cultural normative perception. This corroborates with previous report [70], which affirmed that women experienced more burden than men due to their propensity to execute more personal care tasks as primary caregivers and are less likely to obtain formal help. It is however pertinent to note that people rarely acknowledged the psychosocial and physical impacts of caregiving on women's well-being. While most female caregivers ignore their personal health concerns to consummate the challenges of caregiving, some apparently sacrifice work or school to provide care in addition to reproductive and household economic roles [41, 65, 71, 72]. The caregiver has a right to be supported, valued and compensated appropriately to ensure a high quality care [41]. Without appropriate intervention to ameliorate the impact of burden of care, it produces negative consequences which often manifest as symptoms of depression and anxiety and may subsequently induced changes that could lead to physiological ailment like hypertension, heart disease and suppressed immune responses [10, 19, 73–76]. It is therefore appropriate to recognize caregivers as potential patients and give them the necessary support as much as can be achieved when their well-being is jeopardized [72].

This study also reveals that female caregivers spend more hours and years in providing care than male counterparts. This is obvious because men are regarded as heads of family and if young, they are expected to be in school, therefore they spend less hours in caregiving. However, caregiving is regarded as unique women role; therefore, most female caregivers live with care recipients and may spend 24 hour/day providing care without any social activities or regards to personal needs. This corroborates previous reports [41, 77] that men's low contribution in caregiving is sociocultural since they are expected to provide financial support for their families. However, other studies revealed disparity in hours between men and women providing care, with women delivering more encompassing and full time care than men [23, 30, 34, 78]. A significant relationship also existed between duration of care and caregivers burden (**Table 6**). This agrees with the report that irrespective of the duration of care, caregiving depletes the personal resources of the caregivers and induced burden without appropriate coping abilities [79, 80]. Family caregivers in this study had limited support in terms of financial assistance, information on practical and coping skills, emotional support as well as help with caregiving. Most caregivers assume role without educational preparation and may not be familiar with the type and extent of care needed. It is wrong to assume that caregivers have essential knowledge and skills required to care for an ill relative without training or providing some form of support [80]. Similarly, giving caregivers information on practical and coping skills reduces caregiver's burden or their perception of caregiving as burdensome [81]. Studies affirmed the need for adequate information and proper training on practical and coping skills, to fear of HIV contagion which may induce anxiety and reduce quality of care rendered [10, 66].

Although care recipient symptoms play a critical role in accounting for levels of caregiver's depressiveness or willingness to continue in caregiving role [82]. The willingness to continue despite the high burden experienced with caregiving role, depend to a great extent on caregivers internalize coping behavior [83]. Additionally it may also be accredited to adherence to cultural norms and expectation, strong family bond, fraternal love for the sick as well as sheer need. Annotations analogous to role theory [84] asserted that caregivers strive to fulfill a normative expectation to avoid criticism by others. Similarly, role theory, affirmed that a person's behavior is indirectly or directly influenced by the social environment [85]. This normative role in Nigeria, which is backed by persistent influence of traditional norms, values and behavior, is practiced as deified and not routines [64]. However, studies recommend that, the provision of social support and counseling before the assumption of caregiving role, alleviate burden and enhance willingness to continue with role [65, 86].

It was however obvious that majority of caregivers who decline future caregiving role did not received any form of support, while spending over 9 hours per day providing care. This findings substantiate other studies which assert that increased burden with limited support validate burnout as well as physical and psychological incapacitation [12, 87]. Therefore, with the global commitment to achieve universal access to prevention, care, support and treatment for those PLWHA, there is need to reflect on what these goals might mean in terms of burden on women and girls [41].

14. Conclusion/recommendation

The high prevalence of HIV in Sub-Saharan Africa, consumer's preferences and the cost of inpatient care depicts the shift from hospital to home care and predict the need for family caregivers, who will be directly involved with the care of PLWHA at home. This shift invoke high level of burden on family caregivers who have little knowledge and skills for HIV management. Strategies for countering caregiver's burden must be identified and addressed through providing adequate support as well as seeking measures to enhance male involvement in family caregiving. This could be accomplished by creating public awareness of negative impact of caregiving as well as encouraging equal distribution of household and caregiving responsibilities. Additionally, ensuring the health care system adherence to discharge policies by providing adequate information on practical and coping skills, as well as community resources for family caregivers of PLWHA is strongly advocated. With the high prevalence of HIV, there is need for periodic counseling sessions where caregivers of PLWHA can meet with medical professionals for advice. Creating caregiver's forum would provide avenue to vent pressure and discussed problems and challenges encountered in the course of caregiving. It is pertinent for health care professionals to recognize family caregivers as potential patient and develop comprehensive assessment format which will incorporate assessment of both PLWHA and their caregivers during hospital visits. Finally there is need for promulgation of policy that recognizes and support female caregivers of PLWHA in Africa.

14.1 Limitation

This study was restricted to caregivers of PLWHA in Calabar municipality. The study did not also identify households that were predominantly male or female controlled.

Conflict of interest

"The authors declare no conflict of interest."

Author details

Ekaete Francis Asuquo* and Paulina Ackley Akpan-Idiok
Department of Nursing Sciences, Faculty of Allied Medical Sciences, University of Calabar, Calabar, Nigeria

*Address all correspondence to: ekaeteasuquo@unical.edu.ng; ekaetefasuquo@yahoo.com

References

[1] Akinola AO. Women, Culture and Africa's Land Reform Agenda Psychology. 2018. DOI: 10.3389/fpsyg.2018.02234

[2] Food and Agriculture Organization (FAO). The State of Food and Agriculture 2010-2011. Women in Agriculture: Closing the Gender Gap for Development. Rome: Food and Agriculture Organization of the United Nations; 2011

[3] Gran M. The global role of women—Caretakers, conscience, farmers, educators and entrepreneurs. Development Impact, Reaching Children's Potential. 2019. Available from: https://globalvolunteers.org/global-role-of-women/

[4] Sidibe M. Women and Girls and HIV. UNAIDS executive director. 2017. Available from: https://www.unaids.org/sites/default/files/media_asset/women_girls_hiv_en.pdf

[5] Annan K. Opinion: In Africa, AIDS Has a Woman's Face. New York Times. 2002. Available from: https://www.nytimes.com/2002/12/29/opinion/in-africa-aids-has-a-woman-s-face.html

[6] UNAIDS. Country Nigeria. 2020. Available from: https://www.unaids.org/en/regionscountries/countries/nigeria

[7] World Health Organization. HIV/AIDS: Regional Office for Africa. 2020. Available from: https://www.afro.who.int/health-topics/hivaids

[8] AARP. Caregiving in the U.S. 2009. Available from: http://www. caregiving.org/data/04finalreport.pdf

[9] Sethi B. Family as a potent therapeutic force. Indian Journal of Psychiatry. 1989;**31**(1):22

[10] Asuquo EF, Etowa J, Adejumo P. Assessing the relationship between caregivers burden and availability of support for family caregivers of HIV/AIDS patients in Calabar, south East Nigeria. World Journal of AIDS. 2013;**3**(4):335-344. DOI: 10.1236/wja.2013.34043

[11] Lee SJ, Li L, Jiraphongsa C, Rotheram-Borus MJ. Caregiver burden of family members of persons living with HIV in Thailand. International Journal of Nursing Practice. 2010;**16**(1):57-63. DOI: 10.1111/j.1440-172X.2009.01812.x

[12] Asuquo EF, Adejumo P, Etowa J, Adejumo A. Fear of HIV susceptibility influencing burden of care among nurses in south-East Nigeria. World Journal of AIDS. 2013;**3**:231-238

[13] UNAIDS. Women and Girls and HIV. 2018. Available from: https://www.unaids.org/sites/default/files/media_asset/women_girls_hiv_en.pdf

[14] UNAIDS. Women and HIV—A Spotlight on Adolescent Girls and Young Women. 2019. Available from: https://www.unaids.org/en/resources/documents/2019/women-and-hiv

[15] UNICEF. Gender and HIV/AIDS. 2020. Available from: https://data.unicef.org/topic/gender/gender-and-hiv-aids/

[16] Aronson J. Women's sense of responsibility for the care of old people: But who else is going to do it? Gender & Society. 1992;**6**:8-29

[17] del-Pino-Casado R, Frías-Osuna A, Palomino-Moral PA, Ramón Martínez-Riera J. Gender differences regarding informal caregivers of older people. Journal of Nursing Scholarship. 2012;**44**(4):349-357

[18] National Alliance for Caregiving & AARP. Caregiving in the US. 2004. Available from: http://www.caregiving.org/data/04finalreport.pdf

[19] National Alliance for Caregiving and AARP. Caregiving in the US. 2009. Available from: http://www.caregiving.org/data/FINALRegularExSum50plus.pdf

[20] Tang B, Harary E, Kurzman R, Mould-Quevedo JF, Pan S, Yang J, et al. Clinical characterization and the caregiver burden of dementia in China. Value in Health Regional Issues. 2013;**2**(1):118-126

[21] Sharma N, Chakrabarti S, Grover S. Gender differences in caregiving among family - caregivers of people with mental illnesses. World Journal of Psychiatry. 2016;**6**(1):7-17. DOI: 10.5498/wjp.v6.i1.7

[22] Forever Young Information. Survey Confirms Woman Assume Major Burden as Caregivers. 2013. Available from: http://foreveryoungnews.com/posts/2086-survey-confirms-woman-assumemajor-burden-as-caregivers

[23] Reinhard SC, Feinberg LF, Houser A, Choula R, Evans M. Valuing the Invaluable: 2019 Update Charting a Path Forward. 2019. AARP Public Policy Institute. Avaialble from: https://www.aarp.org/content/dam/aarp/ppi/2019/11/valuing-the-invaluable-2019-update-charting-a-path-forward.doi.10.26419-2Fppi.00082.001.pdf

[24] Home Care Ontario. Family Caregiving. 2015. Available from: https://www.homecareontario.ca/home-care-reports/other-home-care-publications/family-caregivingCaregiving Family Caregiver Alliance; National Center on Caregiving. https://www.caregiver.org/27-things-you-may-not-know-about-women-and-caregiving

[25] Coffey S. Twenty seven things you may not know about women and Caregiving. Family Caregiving Alliance. National Center on Caregiving; 2019. Available from: https://www.caregiver.org/27-things-you-may-not-know-about-women-and-caregiving

[26] National Alliance for Caregiving. Caregiving Costs: Declining Health in the Alzheimer's Caregiver As Dementia Increases in the Care Recipient. 2011. Available from: http://eldercareworkforce.org/caregiving-costs-declining-health-in-the-alzheimers-caregiver-as-dementia-increases-in-the-care-recipient/

[27] Australian Bureau of Statistic. 4430.0–Disability, Ageing and Carers, Australia: Summary of Findings. 2018. Available from: https://www.abs.gov.au/ausstats/abs@.nsf/mf/4430.0?OpenDocument

[28] Olagundoye O, Akhuemokhan V, Alugo M. Towards caring for caregivers: Assessing the burden of care and experience of associative stigma among caregivers of patients with 17 chronic mental illnesses at a mental health care facility in Lagos Metropolis, Nigeria. Family Medicine & Primary Care Review. 2017;**19**(2):149-155

[29] Gaymu J, Festy P, Poulain M, Beets G. Future elderly living conditions in Europe. INED, Cahier. 2008;**162**:315

[30] Bonnet C, Cambois E, Cases C, Gaymu J. Elder Care and Dependence: No Longer Just a Women's Concern? Population and Society No.83. 2011. Available from: https://www.ined.fr/fichier/s_rubrique/19151/pesa483.en.pdf

[31] Stepler R. 5 Facts about Family Caregivers. Pew Research Centre. 2015. Available from: https://www.pewresearch.org/fact-tank/2015/11/18/5-facts-about-familycaregivers/#:~:text=2Adults%20ages%2045%20to,most%20likely%20to%20be%20caregivers.&text=A%20significant%20share%20of%20adults,age%20group%20to%20be%20caregivers

[32] Scerri C. The curvy side of dementia: The impact of gender on prevalence and caregiving. Journal of

the Malta College of Pharmacy Practice. 2014, 2014;**20**:37-39

[33] Swinkels J, Tilburg TV, Verbakel E, Groenou V, Broese M. Explaining the gender gap in the caregiving burden of partner caregivers. The Journals of Gerontology Series B. 2019;**74**(2): 309-317. DOI: 10.1093/geronb/gbx036

[34] Petite S, Weber A. Les effets de l'Allocation personnalisée d'autonomie sur l'aide dispensée aux personnes âgées, DREES, Études et Résultats, 459; 2006

[35] Calasanti T, Bowen E. Spousal caregiving and crossing gender boundaries: Maintaining gendered identities. Journal of Agricultural Studies. 2006;**20**:253-263

[36] Chappell NL, Hollander M. Aging in Canada. Toronto, Canada: Oxford University Press; 2013

[37] Almada AZ. Gender and Caregiving: A Study among Hispanic and Non-Hispanic White Frail Elders. Master's Thesis. Virginia Polytechnic Institute and State University; 2001

[38] Lin FL, Fee HR, Wu HS. Negative and Positive Caregiving Experiences: A Closer Look at the Intersection of Gender and Relationships. The Center for Family and Demographic Research; 2011. pp. 2011-2007. Available from: http://www.bgsu.edu/organizations/cfdr

[39] Papastavrou E, Tsangari H, Kalokerinou A, Papacostas SS, Sourtzi P. Gender issues in caring for demented relatives. Health Science Journal. 2009;**3**:41-53

[40] Parks SH, Pilisuk M. Caregiver burden: Gender and the psychological costs of caregiving. American Journal of Orthopsychiatry. 1991;**61**(4):501-509

[41] VSO. Reducing the burden of HIV and AIDS care on women and girls girls. FOA Policy Brief. Voluntary Service Overseas, VSO. 2006. 23 p. Available from: http://www.vso.org.uk

[42] Kim H, Chang M, Rose K, Kim S. Predictors of caregiver burden in caregivers of individuals with dementia. Journal of Advanced Nursing. 2012;**68**(4):846-855

[43] Flyckt L, Fatouros-Bergman H, Koernig T. Determinants of subjective and objective burden of informal caregiving of patients with psychotic disorders. The International Journal of Social Psychiatry. 2015;**61**(7):684-692. DOI: 10.1177/0020764015573088

[44] Rein G, Lancon C, Simeon M, Duplin S. Caregiver burden in relatives of persons with schizophrenia: An overview of measure instruments. L'Encéphale. 2003;**29**(2):137-147

[45] Platt S. Measuring the burden of psychiatric illness in the family: An evaluation of some rating scales. Psychological Medicine. 1985;**15**:383-393

[46] Phengjard J, Brown MA, Swansen KM, Schepp KG. Family caregiving of persons living with HIV/AIDS in urban Thailand. Thai Journal of Nursing Research. 2002;**6**:87-100

[47] Akpınar B, Küçükgüçlü O, Yener G. Effects of gender on burden among caregivers of Alzheimer's patients. Journal of Nursing Scholarship. 2011, 2011;**43**:248-254. [PubMed] [Google Scholar]

[48] Wallsten S. Effects of caregiving, gender, and race on the health, mutuality, and social supports of older couples. Journal of Aging and Health. 2000;**12**(1):90-111. DOI: 10.1177/089826430001200105

[49] Garlo K, O'Leary JR, Van Ness PH, Fried TR. Burden in caregivers of older adults with advanced illness. Journal of the American Geriatrics

Society. 2010;**58**(12):2315-2322. DOI: 10.1111/j.1532-5415.2010.03177.x

[50] Hughes AM, Jones D. Inpatient Management of the Adult with Advanced HIV Disease: HIV in Site Knowledge Base Chapter. 1998. Available from: http://hivinsite.ucsf.edu/InSite?page=kb-03-03-04#S1X

[51] Cesta T. Family Caregivers: A Key Component of the Discharge Planning Process. Relias Media. 2014. Available from: https://www.reliasmedia.com/articles/118904-family-caregivers-a-key-component-of-the-discharge-planning-process

[52] Tshililo A, Davhana-Maselesele M. Family experiences of home caring for patients with HIV/AIDs in rural Limpopo Province, South Africa. Nursing & Health Sciences. 2009;**11**:135-143

[53] Gholizadeh M, Janati A, Delgoshaei B, Gorji HA, Tourani S. Implementation requirements for patient discharge planning in health system: A qualitative study in Iran. Ethiopian Journal of Health Sciences. 2018; **28**(2):157-168. DOI: 10.4314/ejhs.v28i2.7

[54] Akpan-Idiok PA, Anarado A, N. Caregivers perceptions of benefits from advanced cancer caregiving to patients attending University of Calabar Teaching Hospital, Calabar. International Journal of Cancer Research. 2014;**10**(2):54-64

[55] Turcotte M. Family caregiving: What are the consequences? In: Insights on Canadian Society. 2013

[56] World Health Organization. Mental Health Atlas. 2011. Geneva: World Health Organization. Available from: www.who.int/mental_health/publications/mentalhealth_atlas_2011/

[57] Reinhard S, Given B, Petlick N, Bemis A. In: Hughes RG, editor. Supporting Family Caregivers in Providing Care: Patient Safety and Quality: An Evidence-Based Handbook for Nurses. Rockville (MD): Agency for Healthcare Research and Quality (US); 2008

[58] Thoits P. Social support as coping assistance. Journal of Consulting and Clinical Psychology. 1986;**54**:416-423

[59] Turner S, Street H. Assessing carers' needs: A pilot inquiry. Aging & Mental Health. 1999;**3**:173-178

[60] Federal Ministry of Health Nigeria. National Standard Operating Procedures for Prevention of Mother to Child Transmission (PMTCT) of HIV. Abuja: Federal Ministry of Health; 2011

[61] Becker S. Global perspectives on Children's unpaid caregiving in the family research and policy on 'young Carers' in the UK, Australia, the USA and sub-Saharan Africa. Global Social Policy. 2007;**7**(1):23-50. DOI: 10.1177/1468018107073892

[62] Zarit H. Family care and burden at the end of life. CMAJ. 2004;**170**(12):1811-1812

[63] Canadian Caregiver Coalition. Caregiver's Facts. 2013. Available from: www.parl.gc.ca/Content/HOC/Committee/.../CanadianCaregiverCoalition-e.pdf

[64] Okoye UO. Family care-giving for ageing parents in Nigeria: Gender differences, cultural imperatives and the role of education. International Journal of Education and Ageing. 2012;**2**:139-154

[65] UNAIDS. Caregiving in the Context of HIV/AIDS Joint United Nations Programme on HIV/AIDS. Expert Group Meeting on "Equal Sharing of Responsibilities Between Women and Men, Including Care-Giving in the

Context of HIV/AIDS". United Nations Programme No. EGM/ESOR/2008/BP.4; 2008

[66] Saengtienchai C, Knodel J. UNAIDS Case Study. Parents Providing Care to Adult Sons and Daughters with HIV/AIDS in Thailand. United Nations Programme on HIV/AIDS (UNAIDS) Publishers; 2001

[67] United Nations. We Can End Poverty 2015; MDG 1:Eradicate Extreme Poverty & Hunger. Available from: http://www.un.org/millenniumgoals//poverty.shtml

[68] UNDP. The MDG Report 2013: Assessing Progress in Africa toward the Millennium Development Goals; 2013

[69] Mbirimtengerenji N. Is HIV/AIDS epidemic outcome of poverty in sub-Saharan Africa? Croatian Medical Journal. 2007;**48**:605-617

[70] Allegra CJ. The next generation. Journal of the National Cancer Institute. 2012;**104**(13):961-962

[71] Asuquo EF, Etowa JB, Akpan MI. Assessing women caregiving role to people living with HIV/AIDS in Nigeria. West Africa: SAGE Open; 2017:1-10. DOI: 10.1177/2158244017692013

[72] Takamura T, Williams B. Informal Caregiving: Compassion in Action. An Introductory message from Department of Health and Human Services, USA. 1998. Available from: http://aspe.hhs.gov/daltcp/reports/carebro2.pdf

[73] Abasiubong F, Bassey E, Ogunsemi O, Udobang J. Assessing the psychological well-being of caregivers of people living with HIV/AIDS in Niger Delta region, Nigeria. AIDS Care. 2011;**23**:494-500

[74] Bevans M, Sternberg E. Caregiving burden, stress, and health effects among family caregivers of adult cancer patients. Journal of the American Medical Association. 2012;**307**:398-403

[75] Montgomery R, Rowe J, Kosloski K. Book chapter:Family caregiving. In: Blackburn JA, Dulmus CN, editors. Handbook of Gerontology: Evidence-Based Approaches to Theory, Practice and Policy. New York, NY: JohnWiley; 2006. pp. 426-454

[76] Robison J, Fortinsky R, Kleppinger A, Shugrue N, Porter M. A broader view of family caregiving: Effects of caregiving and caregiver conditions on depressive symptoms, health, work, and social isolation. The Journals of Gerontology. Series B Psychological Sciences and Social Sciences. 2009;**64B**:788-798

[77] Gomo E. Increasing male involvement in home based care to reduce the burden of care on women and girls in Southern Africa, VSO-RAISA in Caregiving in the context of HIV/AIDs, Joint United Nations Programme on HIV/AIDS (UNAIDS). Paper presented at Expert Group meeting of "Equal sharing of responsibilities between men and women including care-giving in the context of HIV/AIFS", United Nations Office in Geneva,6-9 October, 2008; 2008

[78] Family Caregiver Alliance. Women and Caregiving: Facts and Figures. 2003. Avaialble from: http://www.caregiver.org/caregiver/jsp/content_node.jsp?nodeid=892

[79] Cavanaugh JC. Caregiving to adults: A life event challenge. In: Nordhus IH, VandenBos GR, Berg S, Fromholt P, editors. Clinical Geropsychology. Washington, DC: American Psychological Association; 1998. pp. 131-136

[80] Chambers M, Ryan A, Millar SL. Exploring theemotional support needs

and coping strategies of family carers. Journal of Psychiatric and Mental Health Nursing. 2001;**8**:99-106

[81] Rose L. Caring for caregivers: Perceptions of social support. Journal of Psychosocial Nursing and Mental HealthServices. 1997;**35**:17-24

[82] Given B, Wyatt G, Given C, Gift A, Sherwood P, DeVoss D, et al. Burden and depression among caregivers of patient wilt cancer at the end-of-life. Oncology Nursing Forum. 2005;**31**:1105-1117

[83] McKee KJ, Whittick JE, Gilhooly MM, Ballinger BR, Gordon DS, Mutch WJ, et al. The willingness to continue caring in family supporters of older people. Health & Social Care in the Community. 1999;**7**:100-108

[84] Berg-Weger M, McGartland Rubio D, Tebb SS. Depression as a mediator: Viewing caregiver well-being and strain in a different light. Families in Society. 2000;**8**:162-173

[85] Petersen J, Janet SH. The role of gender in educational contexts and outcomes. In: Lynn SL, Bigler RS, editors. Advances in Child Development and Behavior. Vol. 47. 2014. pp. 2-422

[86] Zarit H. Family care and burden at the end of life. Canadian Medical Association Journal. 2002;**170**:1811-1812

[87] Habid T, Rahman S. Psycho-social aspects of AIDS as a chronic illness: Social worker role perspective. AntrocomOnlus. 2010;**6**:79-89

Chapter 9

The Family as Recipient and Provider of Home Care: A Primary Care Perspective

Mira Florea, Aida Puia and Rodica Sorina Pop

Abstract

Advances in modern medicine, effective medication and high-technology interventions contribute to the growth of chronic comorbidities among older people, and many children with chronic diseases that reach adulthood require long-term care at home, provided by formal and informal caregivers and coordinated by primary healthcare professionals. Home caring, performed under different conditions from those of hospital care, requires the involvement of the family that is recipient and provider of home care. This chapter discusses the contribution of family caregivers to personalized home care of dependent children and elderly recipients, coordinated by primary health professionals. Children and youth with special healthcare needs and children abused and neglected require special involvement of family caregivers. The use of digital healthcare for recipients with medical complexity is a modern way to connect home care patients to specialized care, reducing the costs of the hospital care system. However, the burden in home care should be recognized by the general practitioner. Specific interventions are addressed to the unsupportive families and real hidden patients to help maintain their health and functionality. Future family doctors' interprofessional communication skills and resourcefulness should meet the societal changes, and the burden of home care in the modern family is approached from the perspective of academic medicine.

Keywords: family caregiver, home care, recipient, provider, primary healthcare professionals

1. Introduction

The demand for home-based care rises with an ageing population, with elderly people suffering from multiple comorbidities that require long-term management at home [1]. Moreover, due to the advances in modern medicine, efficient medication and high-technology interventions, many children with chronic illnesses reach adulthood, requiring long-term care at home coordinated by family doctors and community nurses. The number of people aged 60 and older is expected to grow from 962 million in 2017 to 21 billion in 2050 in Europe [2].

The proportion of people aged 65 years and older is expected to grow to an average of 28% in the Organisation for Economic Co-operation and Development (OECD) countries in 2050, while in some countries (e.g. Japan, Spain, Portugal, Greece and Korea), a share of 40% is forecasted. China's proportion of older people will triple between 2015 and 2050, and also in the USA, Mexico and Israel, these growing trends will be influenced by higher rates of fertility and migration. Higher age is associated with higher morbidity, which in turn affects care dependency [3, 4]. Prognosis regarding the number of people in need of care shows an increase of 115% in the European Union between 2007 and 2060, and the number of people in need of care in the USA is expected to double from 13 million in 2000 to 27 million in 2050 [5]. Experts anticipate that older adults will comprise 13% of the total population—one in eight people will be 65 or older by 2030 [6].

The healthcare system is changeable and unsteady; the period of hospital admission is limited by the high costs, and the trend is to continue the long-term management by the formal and informal home care providers. The chronically ill patients feel rushed from the hospital and worried because they do not have adequate care in the community, especially in rural areas. Patients are discharged with drainage tubes, urinary wells, nasogastric tubes, open wounds and insufficient pain control, and family members are unprepared for the needed care in these complex contexts. In addition, they face limited money and consequences related to their work and childcare. To meet the current challenges in the home care of the frail elderly and children with disabilities, it is a requirement to strengthen the role of informal caregivers [7].

1.1 Family as a recipient of home care

The family as a recipient of home care has a lot of worries with possible unrealistic expectations. Sometimes, patient's family members are upset, unresponsive or hostile to the home care team. The family is the hidden patient, sometimes acting as a dysfunctional, unsupportive family, with a high perception of the burden of care. Primary care professionals should identify these families that require evaluation and specific interventions to become effective while maintaining their full health status and functionality. Family physicians and community nurses are called upon to build trust, making it clear to the family that they are available to them, explaining the plans of care after discharge, resolving any miscommunication and diminishing concerns about caring for their loved ones at home. These are the persons who they trust, with whom they had the continuity and the relationship. Primary care professionals have an ongoing history with patients, building an agreed relationship over time even in difficult times of an advanced chronic disease or end-of-life care. They need to verify the recipients and his/her family feelings, let them know that they will be listened to and their concerns understood and try to identify an informal home caregiver to work with.

1.2 Family as provider of informal home care

Family caregivers as informal home care providers have an essential role in ensuring the care of the frail recipients at home [7]. Informal caregivers are defined as individuals who are actively and directly involved in the recipient's home care and who repeatedly support and assist with care, without being paid. They provide ongoing assistance with activities of daily living (e.g. toileting, feeding, bathing, walking, clothing) or instrumental activities of daily living (e.g. meal preparation, housecleaning and managing finances), for individuals with a chronic illness or disability [8, 9].

The primary caregivers, most often the family members, are usually people who are not trained in the process of care and are unprepared for facing difficult situations, making the negative impact stronger in the family evolution. The majority of the general population wishes to stay at home in old age and would prefer to receive informal care from their adult children or formal care from home assistance services [10]. However, the decision of family members to take care of a dependent person, and thus fulfilling his/her wish to age in a domestic environment, is influenced by the degree of family relationship and the willingness of family members to be involved in home care [11]. Although, traditionally, in Romania, the primary caregiver was a family member, in recent decades due to migration of active people working abroad, their elderly parents are cared for by friends or neighbours at home. In addition, there is great need to develop home assistance services and community care units for long-term care recipients with multi-morbid chronic diseases. The caregiving experience varies by the diversity of caregiving activities, time commitments and distance. The proximal caregiver provides assistance with personal care, while long-distance caregivers are involved in offering emotional and social support and financial assistance.

The family as provider of informal home care is recognized and valued by the primary healthcare professionals that acknowledge working with family caregivers is the best way to ensure quality outcomes for their recipients. Most physicians (88%) acknowledge seeing better outcomes and higher formal caregiver satisfaction (73%) when they collaborate with families [12]. However, doctors and nurses found that sometimes establishing communication with family caregivers can be challenging. About half of the formal providers (54%) say a recipient having multiple caregivers was a barrier, 44% are not aware who the caregiver is, 44% say there is fluctuation in caregiver involvement, and 39% felt interacting with caregivers was too time-consuming. Among those who felt communication was difficult (20%), most said the inability to reach out to the caregiver was the primary issue [12]. Formal home care providers and informal family caregivers focused on drug administration and meal service, organizing transportation for follow-up visits, discussing the recipient's emotional issues, managing the family caregiver's burden and encouraging more collaboration.

Delegated interventions provided by family caregivers and coordinated by primary care health professionals contribute to a more proactive, personalized and integrated care for recipients with long-term comorbidities [13].

2. International validated tools for the family assessment in primary care

Home care is the health or social service provided by formal and informal caregivers for the recipient who cannot go to the general practitioner (GP) surgery or to the other levels of health services. Eurostat data from 2016 show that 20% of households needed to use professional home care services. The rate of use of home care services is very different: 88% in Luxembourg, 58% in the Czech Republic and only 6% in Romania [14]. Evaluation of the family as recipient and provider of home care comprises four domains: demographic facts, psycho-emotional domain, environment aspects and family burden as caregiver.

2.1 Demographic facts

Information about the family's structure, number of members, education, employment status, living place, family network and members with chronic illness or with disabilities are obtained using a self-administrated questionnaire or an interview. Genogram is a brief tool that should be used in the home care consultation, a system helping to identify the vulnerable recipients in the family. This graphic representation includes all family members, alive and deceased, unrelated persons living in the same place, their relationships, hereditary or recurrent illness, drug addiction and issues related to the elderly or child neglect and abuse [15].

The Resident Assessment for Home Care (RAI-HC) was developed following a high demand for a standardized evaluation of the patient's needs through a comprehensive home care system. This instrument addresses frail elderly and patients with chronic diseases and disabilities. Although a 60-minute duration of the evaluation may be a disadvantage, this tool offers a comprehensive analysis of the recipient, informing the home care provider about demographic characteristics, nutrition, health behaviours, types of diagnosis, functional and cognitive status and health instability (frailty).

The Resident Assessment for Palliative Care (RAI-PC) is an instrument that evaluates the symptoms most commonly seen in palliative care patients: pain, dyspnoea, fatigue, mental capacity, cognition, overall physical tonus and capabilities for self-care.

The needs of the palliative patient, his/her family and the caregivers are constantly changing, which leads to the need to regularly apply RAI-PC, both to the patient and to his/her caregivers.

The shorter duration of the evaluation by RAI-PC is appropriate for the palliative patient and his family. In addition, an important feature of this tool is its quality to evaluate the effectiveness of many types of interventions, establish a comparison between interventions and provide information for cost-effective management of the patient with palliative care needs.

2.2 Psycho-emotional domain

The old age, female gender, long-term provision of home care and type of illness are predictive factors for the emotional stress of the family caregiver [16]. Early identification of high-risk psycho-emotional pressure enables effective interventions of GPs and community nurses. The Family Relationship Index (FRI) is the family relationship assessment tools, developed by Holahan and Moos in 1983. Through its three scales, it explores family cohesion, expressiveness and conflicts, helping the professional home care team and collaboration [17].

2.3 Assessing the need for family support as home care provider

The support needs of family as caregiver refers to the environment/habitat, financial support, help for nursing techniques, the level of preparedness for the caregiver role and educational needs for the caregiving process.

2.3.1 Family social support need

The Oslo Social Assistance Scale (OSS-3) assesses people close to the patient, how much they are concerned about home care and who the recipient would ask for practical help if needed [18]. Another aspect of the social support refers to the financial well-being of the family. In 2006 Prawitz developed the Financial Distress/Financial Well-Being (IFDFW) tool which evaluates the perception and concerns about family financial status. The low score shows the high level of financial distress, leading to an increasing deterioration of health [19].

2.3.2 Preparedness of family for the caregiver role

The Preparedness for Caregiving Scale (PCS) described by Archbold, Stewart, Greenlick and Harvath, in 1990, is an instrument with eight items that ask family caregivers how much they are well prepared for the challenges of caregiving. The lower score signifies the poor preparedness for the caregiver role [20].

2.3.3 Family caregiver burden

The caregiver burden is a negative experience perceived by the person involved in the long-term home care. The Burden Scale for Family Caregivers (BSFC) is a useful tool, assessing the subjective burden perceived by the caregiver in home care. In Romania, GP involved in home care identifies the family caregiver's burden only by a holistic evaluation, without using an instrument for the burden of care assessment. The BSFC instrument started to be used in Romanian primary palliative care research. Measuring the burden of home care allows early interventions for family caregivers and secondary prevention.

3. Interventions provided to the family caregivers by the primary healthcare professionals

3.1 Psycho-educational interventions

The psycho-educational interventions provided to the family caregivers are focused on the preparedness of family for the caregiving role, help for emotional reset, encouragement to identify the positive aspects of this experience, promotion of self-care, respite care and advising for new problem-solving strategies. There are different forms of psycho-educational intervention: individual session face-to-face, focus groups and e-learning programme with an online professional teacher. A useful method is the family meeting, having the following advantages: provides training of caregiver for proper nursing technics, facilitates discussions about the disease' prognosis, updates the home care goals and establishes a concordance between care goals and the recipient's desires. In addition, it is a good moment to share the patient's preferences, to reduce stress, anxiety, depression and emotional changes in end-of-life care [21]. The principles for conducting family meetings are clarifying targets of care, refreshing the knowledge about the disease, anticipating future challenges and offering solutions in accordance with the family needs [22].

3.2 Supportive interventions

Social support is defined as the existence or availability of people on whom individuals or families can rely on difficult times. The support interventions for family caregivers include groups or individual sessions, being conducted by professionals. Group-based support is the most common form wherein the whole family participates, including the patient. In this method experiences are shared, leading to positive changes regarding the personal confidence, acceptance of the family caregiver role and adoption of new coping skills [23]. Applying flexible and individualized forms of support interventions helps reduce the burden of caregivers and increases the knowledge about home care and ability to cope with difficult situations [24].

4. Home care interventions delegated to the family caregivers

4.1 Physical domain

The physical domains of home care such as hygiene of the recipient, proper mobilization of the patient in bed, daily chest massage and oral cavity cleaning are daily medical manoeuvres which are delegated to the family caregiver by the GP. Family caregivers' education about the treatment is mandatory and implies the administration schedule, onset of action, routes of administration and possible side effects. The fulfilment of the treatment plan involves the following interventions: (a) medication administration by different routes (oral, rectal, percutaneous, enteral or using a nasogastric tube) and (b) monitoring of symptom control by the family caregivers. Warnings regarding late-release medications, which require administration at fixed times, and fast-release medications, which are administered when needed, are important. The family caregiver should record in a diary the problems they are experiencing, the side effects of the drugs and the presence of intestinal transit. Some medical interventions can be assigned to a certain family member as long as he/she is well trained and if a safe device is used (e.g. administration of the medication subcutaneously by a microperfuser) and will be supervised by the GP and community nurse.

4.2 Psycho-emotional domain

The psycho-emotional aspect of the home care is burdensome for both the recipient and the family caregiver, affecting the formal home care team as well. Interventions delegated to the family caregiver imply discussions on pleasant topics, keeping in touch with the patient's friends and creating an enjoyable environment. Keeping honesty about the diagnosis, treatment and evolution is a desideratum of communication. Solving family conflicts, establishing good relations between its members and paying attention to people at risk especially for children will complete the care, keeping family members involved in the home care process. Cultural values and spiritual beliefs should be respected.

4.3 Social domain

The social support includes financial assistance, emotional support, information, companionship and self-esteem support. Inadequate social support and social isolation are associated with increased depression [25], cognitive decline, increased pain intensity and increased mortality [26]. The social needs are addressed by the social assistance specialist, and some can be delegated to the patient's family. The family caregiver will create a socially appropriate environment by avoiding isolation and participating in social or religious events and walks, depending on the degree of patient dependence.

5. Home care for children

5.1 Introduction

Defining health like a human right, the United Nations Convention of the Right on the Child (UNCRC) ratifies the importance of the different aspects of child health in all types of care. In 2018 the global under-five mortality rate declines worldwide, but 5.3 million of children died under 5 years due the complications of prematurity, pneumonia or diarrhoea. The care of health especially on ill children is a permanent task for all health system, providers and caregivers. The World Health Organization (WHO) guide "Improving the quality of pediatric care -Operational guide for facility-based audit and review of pediatric mortality" provides data for the improvement, modifies the social, environmental and nutritional risk factors and supports healthcare workers by learning their medical practice [27].

5.2 Home care for healthy children

5.2.1 Planned home birth

The prevalence of home birth is variable by country, from 0.4% in Australia to 3.3% in New Zeeland, with the highest percentage being in the Netherlands (20%) [28].

Even in countries with no tradition in home birth and a low prevalence of planned home birth, mothers show a growing interest for non-medicalization of a natural process. Until recently home birth was widespread, with more than half of the pregnant women giving birth at home in the 1940s. Due to the significant increase in the number of hospital beds and controversies about the safety of home birth and population mobility, the prevalence of planned home birth decreased.

The motivations of the women who desire to give birth at home are related to concern about the high medical interference (induction of labour with oxytocin, peridural anaesthesia and caesarean birth), cultural and religious background, unpleasant previous hospital experiences and the wish to give birth in the family environment [29, 30].

The main concern about out-of-hospital birth comes from the connection between perinatal and neonatal mortalities and the place of childbirth. A meta-analysis based on 14 studies and ~500,000 planned home birth of low-obstetrical risk women demonstrated no statically significant difference regarding perinatal or neonatal mortality between low-risk pregnant women who intend to give birth at home and those who opt for the hospital. All the studies were performed in well-resourced countries, and the midwifes were well-integrated in health system.

The study revealed that multiparous low-obstetrical risk women are more eligible for home birthing than nulliparous [31].

The safety of home birth is possible in countries with well-integrated healthcare programmes, including an educational programme for proper knowledge about low-risk pregnancies and specially trained midwifes. The Dutch midwifery care is one of the best organized systems. The Dutch midwives provide antenatal care and attend home birth. They are trained for the follow-up of low-risk pregnancies and are able to recognize and manage some complications. If women become non-eligible for home birth, they are referred to secondary/tertiary care centres. Their Obstetric Manual (Verloskundig Vademecum) stipulates the agreement to be part in a complex, collaborative team involved in home birth and the clear stratifications of obstetrical risk. The recommendations of the American College of Obstetricians and Gynecologists stipulate that foetal malpresentation, multiple gestation or prior caesarean delivery are absolute contraindications to planned home birth [32]. The optimal candidates for home birth are women who express the option for home birth after being counselled on risks, benefits and alternatives. It is considered that eligible women for home birth are those who have no pre-existing medical and obstetrical conditions, with singleton full-term cephalic foetus having a weight appropriate for gestational age, with spontaneous labour and prior vaginal birth. It is essential not to overlook that home birth may not be a preference of the pregnant woman and can be caused by lack of proper transportation, local maternity facility or insurance/financial resources.

5.2.2 Home care for full-term newborn

One of the characteristics of primary paediatric care in most of the countries is that home care for a healthy newborn starts after discharge with a follow-up medical visit taking place at the family home. The timing of follow-up visits is recommended to be done according to the duration of hospitalization, the discharge medical data and availability of the family and healthcare provider [33]. It is advisable for the healthcare provider to schedule it in such a way as to allow a generous amount of time. The durations of the visit must be appropriate to the complexity of the content of the follow-up visit.

According to the reproductive-maternal-newborn-and-child-health (RMNCH) indicators, alongside a complete physical examination, it is necessary to review some aspect of pregnancy, delivery and period from discharge [34]. It is also important to review the screening tests, to promote breastfeeding, to enhance the interest and to raise awareness regarding immunization. Involving the members of the family (father, grandparents) and observing the communications in the family allow the primary paediatric provider to coordinate a health plan, if needed.

For the newborn and mother, the WHO recommends the use of home-based records in order to improve some aspects of care. These include developing childcare knowledge, nurturing, involvement of the male in the child home care practices and communication between health providers and caregivers. There is not enough evidence in favour of a certain type of home-based record, the efficiency depending on the specific culturalism of a country [35].

The general practitioners' activity, especially the one with interest for child's care, is under a permanent challenge due to misinformation from online media. One of the most popular topics promoted in many countries by social media is the anti-vaccine movement linked to immunization of children and adults.

Social media platforms like Facebook and Instagram have become an important source of medical information for patients, caregivers, healthcare providers and policy-makers, and they must assume responsibility towards their users. The statement released in September 2019 by WHO Director-General Dr Tedros Adhanom Ghebreyesus raises awareness on the importance of social media platforms for spreading such information.

> *The World Health Organization welcomes the commitment by Facebook to ensure that users find facts about vaccines across Instagram, Facebook Search, Groups, Pages and forums where people seek out information and advice.*
>
> *Facebook will direct millions of its users to WHO's accurate and reliable vaccine information in several languages, to ensure that vital health messages reach people who need them the most [36]*

5.2.3 Home care for a healthy preterm baby: neonatal discharge planning

The infants who are born preterm are generally cared for in neonatal intensive care units (NICU), and a discharge planning is necessary for a comprehensive method. Because of the rate of mortality and morbidity, they are considered newborns with high risk after discharge.

Home care for the preterm newborn is coordinated by a complex team of caregivers: physician, paediatric primary care provider/family doctor, nurses, occupational and/or physical therapists, dieticians, pharmacists, parents and social workers. Neonatal discharge planning is developed in four major aspects:

- The complete assessment of the newborn, routine screening and vaccination schedule and, if necessary, planning the follow-up for specific conditions

- Readiness assessment by care providers, including parents and family environment

- Recognition of risk factors and link of the family with community services for support after discharge

- A smooth as possible transition from NICU to primary care and medical home

Respiratory control, maintaining normal temperature (axillar 36.5–37.5°C and rectal temperature 36.6–38°C) in an ambient temperature of 20–22°C, oral feeding skills (breast and/or bottle) and an ascendant parallel growth curve are mandatory for planning the discharge of the preterm infant.

A complete routine screening must be performed before discharge, and ophthalmological, hearing and prematurity anaemia screening must be included in the follow-up programme. The schedule of vaccine is planned according to the chronological age of preterm infant and follows the same schedule of a full-term newborn. Before discharge it is mandatory to observe the preterm infants for a minimum period of 90–120 minutes while sitting in a car safety seat because of frequent oxygen desaturation and episodes of apnoea, hypotonia or bradycardia. Families/caregivers should be trained by hospital staff regarding the proper position in the car safety seat [37, 38].

The parents/primary care providers of preterm infants planned to be discharged from NICU must prove competency in daily care regarding breastfeeding/bottle feeding, care for the infant's skin and genitalia and the way the baby is bathed and clothed. It is necessary for the parents/caregivers to demonstrate some basic medical knowledge on the possible signs of illness, like changes in pattern of feeding or sleep, significance of dry diapers or modifications of the stool aspect. The caregivers must be able to monitor the temperature of preterm baby, evaluate the respiratory pattern and skin colour and assess the muscular tonus. It is important to educate the parents/caregivers about the safe sleep position for preterm infants as they must sleep alone on a plan surface and in a supine position [39]. The readiness of parents to care for newborns discharged from NICU should be assessed in order to improve the discharge preparation process. A parental and nurse survey demonstrated that iterative improvements of the discharge preparation process lead to an increase in family self-assessment of discharge readiness and in nurse assessment of the family's emotional discharge readiness [40].

5.3 Home care for children with special healthcare needs

5.3.1 Children and youth with special healthcare needs (CYSHCN)

The definition of this category of children has become more comprehensive during time, and now it is accepted that CYSHCN are those "who have or are at increased risk of developing a chronic physical, developmental, behavioral, or emotional condition and require health and related services of a type or amount beyond that usually required by children" [41]. More than a quarter of families have at least one child with special healthcare needs. Data from the 2016–2017 National Survey of Children's Health (NSCH) indicate that 18.8% of children <18 years of age in the USA have special healthcare needs, with 13.2% of children being medically complex.

In Western Europe non-communicable diseases (NCDs) for children under 15 represent almost 75% of the total diseases related with disability-adjusted life years (DALYs). In the first month of life, complications due to prematurity are the leading cause of death and DALYs, the second cause being congenital anomalies, which then holds the leading place until the age of 4 years. Some of these causes of death or DALYs for children are largely preventable as they are especially due to road injury, drug and alcohol use, smoking and poverty [42].

The framework of care for CYSCHN comprises the Standards for Systems of Care for Children and Youth with Special Health Care Needs, version 2.0 [43]. It is necessary to coordinate all the parts of care, comprising family professional partnership, medical home, insurance and financing and early and continuous assessment of needs. All these elements have to be culturally and linguistically appropriate for an optimal understanding and acceptance. The primary care provider and/or paediatric subspecialist evolving in an integrated team of care has to encourage the children and their families in self-management of issue of health and seeking advice for a good quality of life, healthy behaviors throughout all stages of life. Cooperation with the other caregivers involved in the care process must ensure an efficient and prompt sharing of information inside the team.

Care mapping for family and professional caregivers is available in some medical units, and designing a care map provides a valuable work tool.

Primary and preventive care is similar for CYSCHN and children without special needs. The routine healthcare maintenance comprises the vaccinations, routine screening and surveillance, assessment of visual and hearing impairment, behaviour and mental health problems, maltreatment, neglect and dental care.

An anticipated guidance for CYSCHN and their family should include information about the possible complication of disease, the short and long prognostic of illness and the manner in which the disease may affect the child's development, behaviour and potential to accomplish daily activities and family life.

The professional caregivers can enlighten children and the family about the possibility of illness exacerbation or relapse, changes in treatment or future procedures. The family of a child with special health needs, especially his siblings, is in risk to develop psychosocial functional stress and hence requires surveillance [44].

The partnership between caregivers, patient and his family centred by medical, social, developmental, behavioural, educational and financial needs of CYSHCN defines the concept of care coordination [45]. The plan of care must consider the patient and family health goals, a list of barriers, an inventory of medical supplies, home nursing, therapy plans, contact information for all caregivers, feeding plans and educational support. Home care services are more frequently provided to CYSHCN by the members of family and/or different types of caregivers.

5.3.1.1 Chronic lung and pulmonary vascular diseases

Home care for children with chronic lung disease, pulmonary hypertension with or without congenital cardiovascular malformation, metabolic disease, children's interstitial lung disease (ChILD) or haematological disorders has multiple benefits for the child and his family. Among them are the improvement of psychological aspects of the child's development, avoiding the family caregivers' burnout syndrome and a lower cost than hospitalization. The need of children with chronic hypoxaemia for home oxygen therapy (HOT) may be assessed by pulse oximetry. This is an important conclusion of the Clinical Practice Guidelines of the American Thoracic Society who strongly recommends HOT for children with cystic fibrosis and severe hypoxaemia, bronchopulmonary dysplasia with chronic hypoxaemia and pulmonary hypertension without congenital heart disease. HOT is conditionally recommended for children who cannot support positive airway pressure therapy for sleep breathing disorders with severe nocturnal hypoxaemia. For ChILD complicated with severe hypoxaemia, HOT is strongly recommended, while for ChILD with mild chronic hypoxaemia, dyspnoea or sleep desaturation, HOT is conditionally recommended. The chronic untreated hypoxaemia influences the growth parameters, the neurodevelopment milestones achievement and the architecture of sleep. Some studies even relate hypoxaemia with brief resolved unexplained events (BRUEs) [46].

5.3.1.2 Home care for children with cerebral palsy

Cerebral palsy is defined as a "group of permanent disorders of the development of movement and posture that cause activity limitations that are attributed to nonprogressive disturbances that occurred in the developing fetal or infant brain. The motor disorders of CP are often accompanied by disturbances of sensation, perception, cognition, communication, and behavior and by epilepsy and secondary musculoskeletal problems" [47].

In the neonatal period, successive evaluations have to be performed; some abnormality in muscle tonus, coordination, reflex and posture must be assessed and referred to the neurologist if needed. Primary care providers (physicians, physician assistants and nurse practitioners) are expected to develop an interventional plan according with the family structure, resources and possible target.

5.3.1.3 Home care for children with congenital heart disease (CHD)

Congenital heart disease is the most common congenital anomaly. Due to surgery and advanced palliative therapies, the survival of children with special needs has increased. The American Academy of Pediatrics (AAP) and the American College of Cardiology (ACCA) reviewed the current literature and provided a policy statement whose purpose was to highlight the role of primary care providers in the management of patients with CHD and their families during all phases of life.

The role of primary care providers was emphasized by the chronological approach of life stages of children with CHD. Parental counselling, support and coordination of care cover all stages of life, while prenatal diagnosis, predictive of neonatal need, early diagnosis of CHD, nutrition, growth and development, immunizations and academic and future career support are specific for specific periods of life.

Some particular requirements are important for the care of child with CHD: special immunizations (seasonal respiratory syncytial virus, influenza, vaccination for close contacts), nutrition and feeding issues (optimal growth velocity), obesity, practicing a sport and transition to adult care (especially for girls: appropriate contraception, teenage pregnancy) [48].

5.3.2 Child abuse and neglect

Child abuse and neglect is a complex and hypersensitive issue. Child maltreatment is a public health problem with lifetime health impact for children and their families [49]. Child maltreatment is defined by the World Health Organization as "all forms of physical and/or emotional ill-treatment, sexual abuse, neglect or negligent treatment or commercial or other exploitation, resulting in actual or potential harm to the child's health, survival, development or dignity in the context of a relationship of responsibility, trust or power" [50]. Children who have experienced maltreatment are at greater risk to evidence antisocial conduct, aggressive behaviour and substance abuse as a coping mechanism [51]. Chronic stress in early childhood alters the function and structure of the developing brain [52], influences the immune system function [53] and increases inflammatory markers [54], associated with physical and mental health disorders [55, 56]. Abuse and neglect of a child may take many forms. Physical abuse is an intentional injury caused by a parent or a caregiver upon a child. Physical child abuse can lead to serious physical injury, the most common form of abuse being bruising, but it can lead to severe fractures or even death [57, 58].

Sexual abuse is an exploitation of a child in any sexual manner. It is not restrained to physical contact such vaginal, oral or anal sex between an adult and a child and may include noncontact abuse, such as exhibitionism, fondling a child's genitals, masturbation in front of the child or forcing him to masturbate, sexual harassment by obscene phone calls or text messages and child pornography and prostitution [59].

Child marriage is considered a disguised form of sexual abuse, and it also represents a violation of children's rights. The boys are also concerned, but girls remain disproportionately affected. Poverty, lack of education, regional customs, tradition and religions can be a pressure that leads to child marriage. Child marriage is most common in developing countries, but it happens even in developed countries as many countries' laws allow children under 18 to marry upon parental consent or public authority. This practice denies children of their right for childhood, education or having their own opinion about sexuality and reproduction. Child marriage is linked to early pregnancy, health risks like sexually transmitted infections, obstetric fistula and maternal mortality.

Emotional abuse is a behaviour model that affects a child's emotional development and his health outcome. It is more challenging than physical or sexual abuse, being often difficult to diagnose. Emotional abuse can lead to anxiety, depression, low self-esteem, post-traumatic stress disorder and suicidal tendency.

Medical child abuse or factitious disorder imposed on another (previously called Munchausen syndrome by proxy) is an unnecessary and a potentially harmful treatment received by a child due to a caregiver seeking medical help for exaggerated or made-up symptoms of the child in his or her care [60]. It should be suspected if the child has frequent, unexplained health issues and multiple hospital admissions. The most common form when a mother induces an illness to her child consists in symptoms that usually occur only in her presence and may not be objectivized during the medical evaluation [61]. Neglect is very difficult to conceptualize, being an omission behaviour, and consists in failure of a parent or a caregiver to address the basic needs of a child. It can include physical necessities like food, hygiene, clothing, shelter or protection, educational (schooling and education) and medical neglect defined as a failure to provide necessary medical, dental or mental healthcare for the child [62].

Refusing vaccination can also be considered "medical neglect".

Child maltreatment provides a significant challenge for medical providers. Practitioners have an important role in prevention and recognition of neglect and abuse and assessment and treatment of children at risk. Once the condition is suspected, they are obligated to report it. Programmes of prevention and intervention aim for early recognition and intervention to protect children's wellbeing.

The primary approach is addressed to the general population by an anticipatory guidance for parents and care providers and by implementing media content and school programmes to educate the population about signs and behaviour of child abuse and neglect.

The secondary approach is addressed to families if risk factors such as poverty, low education, substance abuse, mental health issues, family conflict or violence, social isolation, neighbourhood disadvantage and violence are present. The purpose of intervention is to encourage positive interaction between parent and children and to break down the coercive cycle [63].

Families with abused or neglected children may benefit from a tertiary approach. To assess these cases, the multidisciplinary team should consist of therapist, social workers, police, general practitioner, paediatrician and teachers. An individual plan best suited to the family needs (e.g. individual therapeutic interventions, home visiting, family behaviour therapy, social integration) has to be established. If the intervention fails, foster care system may be considered. In this case certain challenges need to be acknowledged: managing challenging behaviour, interacting with biological families and even guiding children into adoption.

5.4 Worldwide tendencies: community health worker (CHW), misinformation, and telemedicine in home-based care for children

The community health worker, named as such in the USA and defined as a front-line public health worker who is a trusted member of the community, is present under different names in several European countries [64]. This trusting relationship enables the worker to serve as an intermediary between health/social services and the community to facilitate access to services and improve the quality and cultural competence of service delivery [65]. Preventive maternal and child health (MCH) interventions delivered by CHWs through home visiting have improved important maternal and child outcomes. Efforts are targeted towards early prenatal care, breastfeeding, reduction of maternal morbidity and perinatal mortality and appropriate childhood immunizations. Home visiting interventions lead to a decreased incidence of preterm birth and low birthweight [66]. By having a common language, a similar socioeconomic status and understanding life experiences of their clients, CHWs are accepted by vulnerable and disenfranchised groups. Being integral contributors in collaborative health-based and community-based teams, CHWs improve comprehensive care and contribute to health improvements and cost savings [66].

Misinformation has reached an unprecedented level in the digital age. Forums, blogs and other alternative news sources facilitate fake news or inaccurate information penetration. Health information at every level, from ordinary people to researchers and policy-makers, is troubled by misinformation. It can contain false narratives and lead to poor decision-making and dangerous behaviours [67].

The Internet is a rapidly evolving territory. Intentionally or unintentionally misleading or provocative information may have serious consequences [68].

A research performed on 210 subjects showed, as expected, that people use search engines to learn about serious or highly stigmatic conditions, but surprisingly, an important amount of sensitive health information is sought and shared via social media [69]. The term telemedicine meaning “healing at a distance” was introduced in 1970 [70].

An international Group Consultation on WHO’s Telemedicine Policy adopted the following definition for health telematics: “Health telematics is a composite term for health-related activities, services and systems, carried out over a distance by means of information and communication technologies, for the purpose of global health promotion, disease control and healthcare, as well as education, management and research for health” [71].

Telemedicine can be synchronous or asynchronous. Synchronous or “real-time” care consists in a bidirectional audio-visual videoconferencing between a patient and a more or less remote healthcare provider. Asynchronous or “store-and-forward” care comprises the transmission of medical information to a distant provider.

Telemedicine in children may be useful in improving paediatric concussion care in remote areas and communities [70]. Although international guidelines recommend urgent medical assessment after a concussion [72], a study on 126,654 children and youth showed that, at best, only one third of youth sought medical follow-up and obtained clearance to return to sport activities [73].

In many countries, including Romania, patients living in remote rural areas face numerous geographic, socioeconomic and cultural barriers in accessing primary and specialized healthcare services. Considering the fact that especially in these areas medical assessment and clearance for youth with concussion falls upon primary care providers, telemedicine would improve results and ease the pressure of malpractice.

Telemedicine and telehealth devices can improve and facilitate care in children with medical complexity. A single-centre nonblinded randomized clinical trial based on tracheostomy status demonstrated that the group utilizing a telehealth device obtained better results. Thus, at a device connectivity of 96% of the time and image and sound quality acceptable in 98% of visits, hospitalization rate was lower in the telehealth group [74].

Improvement of care in children with complex medical conditions has increased survival, contributing to a continuously rising percentage of paediatric population with chronic healthcare needs. The highest prevalence of children with special healthcare needs (19.8%) is estimated to be in the USA [75].

Introduced mainly to reduce the need for urgent care leading to recurrent emergency department visits and hospital admissions, synchronous digital health technologies are expected to improve parental caregiver outcomes such as quality of life, psychological health, satisfaction with care and social support. As expected, the majority of the papers on this topic originate from the USA and Australia. The explanations lie in the higher economic level but also in the necessity to cover by telemedicine remote areas with few inhabitants [76]. Feasibility-related outcomes were conducted on haematology/oncology/palliative care populations, autism spectrum disorder, asthma or mental health issues and included assessing acute clinical issues, providing psychosocial support, facilitating case conferences, providing routine care and follow-up, delivering therapy and monitoring progress and adherence acceptability [76].

The technical problems encountered were, as expected, both human related and technology related.

The programmes were aiming to provide patient care or replace in-person assessments. Telemedicine was delivered by a multidisciplinary team or nurses with various levels of expertise.

The positive results consisted of decreases in hospitalizations, quicker recovery and reductions in unplanned hospitalizations. No significant changes were recorded in emergency department visits or hospital admissions and in health-related quality of life. Family members reported overall high satisfaction scores with digital health interventions, and parents perceived availability of digital health to be "very important" in assisting them in managing their child's condition at home [77]. Some of the programmes actively involved families in the development, testing and refinement of the intervention. The results were encouraging, with the development of educational materials that were acceptable and useful to parents [76]. An important issue in telemedicine is the evaluation of the technologies available to families. A response bias may be linked to the gap existing between Caucasian and minority populations. Some interventions supplied equipment or internet services to families [78]. Technical issues, affecting digital health interventions, consisting mainly in disruption in connectivity did not alter overall satisfaction for clinicians, management and patients [79]. Even if most of the studies reported a favourable feedback, digital health was not always appropriate. Therapists had difficulty engaging with younger children with hearing loss during videoconferencing appointments, social workers preferred in-person appointments to facilitate a personal connection with patients, and some parents considered that face-to-face demonstrations of clinical skills were mandatory for optimal treatment fidelity [70]. Funding is an issue affecting digital health because of the restrictions related to reimbursement. Up to 36% of booked telehealth appointments are not billed by a faulty system [80].

The use of digital health to care for children with medical complexity is a modern way to connect patients, some in remote areas, to expert care from health professionals while lowering the expenses and avoiding potential harms of the hospital-based care system.

6. Family caregivers for home care recipients with advanced non-cancer diseases

Conditions as congestive heart failure, end-stage renal disease, chronic obstructive pulmonary disease, liver failure and dementia represent the non-malignant life-threatening illnesses which require a complex home care. The different trajectories of functional decline are useful for the home care providers, helping them to tailor strategies and make a better plan of care. Lunney identified four theoretical trajectories of chronic illnesses: sudden death, cancer death or terminal phase, death from organ failure and frailty and dementia [81]. In cancer, the clinical status of the patients is acceptable until the disease does not respond to the treatment and the rapid decline makes easier to predict the terminal stage. In non-oncological chronic diseases, the trajectory is different with several deteriorations and improvements of the clinical state and a slow decline line. In dementia or general frailty, the illness trajectory has a gradual and prolonged decline. The trajectory of renal failure disease may be that of a steady decline, with the rate of this decline varying according to the underlying renal pathology and other comorbidities [82]. Sometime the issues of caring for patients with non-oncological illnesses is more difficult than for patients with cancer because the prevalence of symptoms is higher and there is a prolonged trajectory of decline.

Patients with non-oncological illnesses as opposed to patients with cancer are older and have many comorbidities and cognitive impairment. The barriers in home care assistance for the recipients with non-cancer illnesses include less predictable trajectory, the lack of knowledge regarding the care needs of end-stage period, the low use of and late referral to palliative care [83], the possible overwhelm of the palliative care services, the necessity of knowledge in different specialties and the necessity of training in the areas of symptom control [84], and prognostication in non-malignant disease tends to be less accurate than in cancer [85]. These recipients require a multidisciplinary home care team, because they have a multidimensional area of caring. The involvement of the family caregivers is valuable and implies management of digestive problems, balance of fluid and food intake, nutritional status and care of bedsores. Needs such as: fall risks, self-care capacity, instrumental activities of daily living, dementia, fecal and urinary incontinence are difficult to solve [86]. Compared with cancer patients, the non-malignant patient's needs are more complex: moderate and severe neurological issues, psychiatric problems, needs for assistance with defecation and bladder function and moderate and severe deterioration of vigilance (somnolent and comatose) [87]. A higher proportion of non-cancer patients was discharged and died at home, and the proportion of readmitted patients to the hospital was less than for oncological patients [87].

7. Integration of basic palliative care in the Romanian general practice

The majority of the incurable ill patients can be treated within primary care health professionals, and 10–15% will be in need of specialist palliative care (PC) [88]. Family physicians' role in primary palliative care and cooperation between specialist palliative care services should become stronger. Palliative care has expanded since its relevance for non-oncological diseases has been widely acknowledged and integration of PC at an earlier stage in the disease process has been shown to be beneficial [89].

The real palliative care extent in primary care is underestimated since the estimates of an average care by family doctor for three to four patients with PC needs per quarter do not appropriately reflect care for patients with non-oncological conditions [90]. There is a predominance of non-oncological chronic multi-morbid patients such as cardiovascular or pulmonary diseases in need of PC in general practice, and these recipients require a valuable involvement of the informal caregivers from their families [91]. Despite the widely acknowledged importance of family doctors' engagement in primary PC [92], difficulties and even barriers were identified in the delivery of home-based PC in practice in our country as well as in the high-developed countries [88].

In a project developed in Romania in 2013–2016 by the Hospice of Hope, Brasov, with the financial support from the Swiss contribution to the enlarged European Union, barriers and ways to integrate a pilot model of basic palliative care in the healthcare system were identified [93]. Hospice of Hope, Brasov, is a Romanian non-profit organization, Centre of Excellence in PC for Eastern Europe and Central Asia, and one of the seven globally recognized models of palliative care. It develops palliative care at national and international levels through information, by improving the legislation in the field and through educational programmes dedicated to professionals, recipients of PC and family as provider of home-based PC.

The impediments in the delivery of primary palliative care refer to:

- Structural barriers (e.g. family physicians and community nurses' shortage due to high emigration rates of junior doctors and nurses and unequal distribution of primary care offices in rural versus urban areas)

- Knowledge barriers (e.g. lack of skills and clinical routine in providing PC, practical obstacles in palliative training due to distance from the training centre and lack of substitute in the medical office)

- Service barriers (e.g. lack of palliative care services for home care in some regions of the country, insufficient reimbursement of these services in the public healthcare system).

Nationally, approximately 150,000 people with oncological diagnosis and other incurable diseases need home-based palliative care every year, but less than 7% of them benefit in a timely manner. During the project, the model of basic palliative care was tested in 4 pilot counties, on 26 family doctors trained for 6 months to provide palliative services to a number of 138 oncological patients treated at home. A guide of basic palliative care was developed and offered to the family doctors, contributing to the replication of the model in other counties and to the training of the community nurses and informal caregivers.

Adopting the model of providing basic palliative care through family doctors can increase in the coming years, contributing to the palliative care needs assessment after diagnosing the incurable disease, not only in the end of life, and through specific interventions to increase the quality of life of these recipients in the community.

Basic or primary palliative care includes the following:

- Communicating the diagnosis and reasonable possibilities of treatment at home, identifying the treatment goals in agreement with the recipient and his/her family, controlling the symptoms of low to medium complexity and maintaining the functions and capacity for self-care

- Involving the family caregivers in the home care, in making decisions regarding the treatment, and preferred place of death

- Treatment of symptoms due to chemo- and radiotherapy and their complications

- The burden of care assessment and interventions to protect the health of the family caregiver

- Clarification of aspects related to obtaining socioeconomic rights for people diagnosed with incurable disease

The family caregivers' role in the management of spiritual pain caused by feelings of helplessness of life with disease is essential. It needs to be recognized and addressed by the primary healthcare professionals, offering psychological and spiritual support and elevating the self-esteem of recipient from the stable stage onwards.

Providing home-based palliative care that maximizes the self-determination of patients depending on patient-centred needs and preferences through communication is important. Prioritizing the home care needs may differ depending on individual perspectives which make mediation of different opinions through open communication between home care multidisciplinary team, recipient and family caregiver to be pivotal. With increasing aging population, keeping living and functioning the chronically ill on long term with current means of treatment, it is anticipated that the proportion of people who should receive PC will increase considerably [89, 94, 95]. An intervention package for the primary PC, such as that proposed in Germany in a study protocol of a research study of the organizational health services with three mixed methods [88], tailored to each country in its context of healthcare, should enable primary healthcare professionals to provide primary PC to their recipients in accordance with their professional standards that address barriers and involve family caregivers in the home care of loved ones.

8. Future family doctors' resourcefulness to meet the societal changes and the burden of home care in the modern family: academic medicine perspective

Due to demographic changes, with increasing number of people in need of care and societal changes (decreased family size, more geographically dispersed families, erosion of barriers that previously could have kept couples together during difficult times, erosion of bonds between family generations, increasing number of people living alone), informal care structures are affected by considerable challenges [96]. In addition, the increase of urbanization, the rural-urban movement and the international migration profoundly affect the family structure and its involvement in providing long-term home care and providing a supportive environment.

Family caregivers involved in home care often face the challenge of balancing caregiving and job responsibilities. Involving older adults in caring for the elderly and children with disabilities and integrating informal caregivers, such as friends and neighbours, is valuable and requires strong intergenerational solidarity in the community. However, in low- and middle-income countries, chronic patients who seek support for maintaining independence and quality of life are often faced with a lack of health and social services, especially in rural areas, or in-home care with poor quality.

The availability of both in-home services (such as personal care and home healthcare) and community services (such as day programmes, congregate meals and social centres) enables a growing percentage of older recipients to delay or even avoid institutional care [97]. The shortage of formal and qualified caregivers presents a challenge for the future regarding the structure and organization of long-term care for most countries. The increasing number of care-dependent people leads to a high economic burden for most healthcare systems [98]. In order to support and facilitate family caregivers in their role of nursing, it is important to be carefully coordinated and their burden of care assessed by the comprehensive trained primary care health professionals.

Family physicians need a set of specific competences to perform well in interprofessional teams, and these competences should be achieved by graduating from a medical school [99]. Most medical schools have components of communication skills in the curriculum, but there are no clear standards for competence in communication skills, and the approach of interprofessional communication in the care team is limited. Beyond standardization of communication skills curricula, it is also necessary to verify primary care physicians' proficiency in interpersonal and interprofessional skills.

In some residency programmes, residents receive 360-degree evaluations which go beyond the typical assessment performed by the supervising attending physicians [100]. Such evaluations help residents better understand how they are viewed by those with whom they work and by those for whom they care. Family medicine residents' assessments are requested from the attending physicians and nurses and from the patients themselves who complete questionnaires from their perspective on the interaction of the resident doctor with the recipient and his family, obtaining 360-degree feedback from all those who have interacted with the resident functions as a valuable teaching tool in family medicine residency programme. Observations gained from multiple perspectives are believed to be more valid than individual opinion, and sharing them will likely have a positive effect on the development of physician trainees in family medicine and his future involvement in home care provision.

Academic medicine seeks to enhance training introducing new curricular areas dedicated to the development of interprofessional communication skills and resourcefulness in managing difficult circumstances in medical profession [101]. Future primary healthcare professionals, especially family doctors, should provide more comprehensive home care to their recipients, maintaining their independence and offering expected years of life free of disability.

Author details

Mira Florea, Aida Puia* and Rodica Sorina Pop
Family Medicine Department, University of Medicine and Pharmacy "Iuliu Hatieganu", Cluj-Napoca, Romania

*Address all correspondence to: draidapuia@gmail.com

References

[1] Malpas PJ, Mitchell K. "Doctors shouldn't underestimate the power that they have": NZ doctors on the care of the dying patient. The American Journal of Hospice & Palliative Care. 2017;**34**(4):301-307. DOI: 10.1177/1049909115619906

[2] United Nations. World Population Aging Highlights. 2020. Available from: http://www.un.org/en/development/desa/population/publications/pdf/ageing/WPA2017_Highlights.pdf [Accessed: 20 January 2020]

[3] Koller D, Schön G, Schäfer I, Glaeske G, van den Bussche H, Hansen H. Multimorbidity and long-term care dependency—A five-year follow-up. BMC Geriatrics. 2014;**14**(1):70. DOI: 10.1186/1471-2318-14-70

[4] Divo MJ, Martinez CH, Mannino DM. Aging and the epidemiology of multimorbidity. The European Respiratory Journal. 2014;**44**(4):1055-1068. DOI: 10.1183/09031936.00059814

[5] U.S. Department of Health and Human Services, and U.S. Department of Labor. The Future Supply of Long-term Care Workers in Relation to the Aging Baby Boom Generation: Report to Congress. Washington, DC: Office of the Assistant Secretary for Planning and Evaluation; 2003. Available from: https://aspe.hhs.gov/basic-report/future-supply-long-term-care-workers-relation-aging-baby-boom-generation [Accessed: 15 January 2020]

[6] Lopez AD, Mathers CD, Ezzati M, Jamison DT, Murray CJL, editors. Global Burden of Disease and Risk Factors. Washington, DC: World Bank; 2006. Available from: www.dcp2.org/pubs/GBD [Accessed: 24 January 2008]

[7] Plöthner M, Schmidt K, de Jong L, et al. Needs and preferences of informal caregivers regarding outpatient care for the elderly: A systematic literature review. BMC Geriatrics. 2019;**19**:82. DOI: 10.1186/s12877-019-1068-4

[8] Roth DL, Fredman L, Haley WE. Informal caregiving and its impact on health: A reappraisal from population-based studies. Gerontology. 2015;**55**(2):309-319. DOI: 10.1093/geront/gnu177

[9] Better Health While Aging. What are Activities of Daily Living (ADLs) & Instrumental Activities of Daily Living (IADLs)? 2018. Available from: https://betterhealthwhileaging.net/what-are-adls-and-iadls/ [Accessed: 20 December 2019]

[10] Karsch-Völk M, Landendörfer P, Linde K, Egermann A, Troeger-Weiß G, Schneider A. Medizinische und kommunale Herausforderungen einer alternden Gesellschaft im ländlichen Bereich. Gesundheitswesen. 2012;**74**(07):410-415. DOI: 10.1055/s-0031-1286272

[11] Pinquart M, Sörensen S. Spouses, adult children, and children-in-law as caregivers of older adults: A meta-analytic comparison. Psychology and Aging. 2011;**26**(1):1-14. DOI: 10.1037/a0021863

[12] Skufca L. Primary Care Providers' Experiences With Family Caregivers. Washington, DC: AARP Research; 2019. DOI: 10.26419/res.00273.001

[13] NHS England. Transforming Primary Care: Safe, Proactive, Personalised Care for Those Who Need it Most. London: Department of Health; 2014. Available from: http://bit.ly/1fl76ua [Accessed: 19 January 2020]

[14] European Comission. 1 in 5 Households in Need in the EU Use Professional Homecare Services [Internet]. 2018. Available from:

https://ec.europa.eu/eurostat/web/products-eurostat-news/-/DDN-20180228-1?inheritRedirect=true& [Accessed: 31 January 2020]

[15] O'Connor KJ, Ammen S. Play Therapy Treatment Planning and Interventions. The Ecosystem Model and Workbook. 2nd ed. Academic Press; 2013. 336 p. eBook ISBN: 9780080920214

[16] Kim Y, Schulz R. Family caregivers' strain: Comparative analysis of cancer caregiving with dementia, diabetes and frail elderly caregiving. Journal of Aging and Health. 2008;**20**:483. DOI: 10.1177/0898264308317533

[17] Hoge RD, Andrews DA, Faulkner P, Robinson D. The family relationship index: Validity data. Journal of Clinical Psychology. 1989;**45**(6):897-903. DOI: 10.1002/1097-4679(198911)45:6<897:aid-jclp2270450611>3.0.co;2-t

[18] Kocalevent R, Berg L, Beutel ME, et al. Social support in the general population: Standardization of the Oslo social support scale (OSSS-3). BMC Psychology. 2018;**6**:31. DOI: 10.1186/s40359-018-0249-9

[19] Prawitz A, Garman ET, Sorhaindo B, O'Neill B, Kim J, Drentea P. Incharge financial distress/financial well-being scale: Development, administration, and score interpretation. Journal of Financial Counseling and Planning. 2006;**17**(1). Available from: https://ssrn.com/abstract=2239338). DOI: 10.1037/t60365-000

[20] Archbold PG, Stewart BJ, Greenlick MR, Harvath T. Mutuality and preparedness as predictors of caregiver role strain. Research in Nursing and Health. 1990;**13**:375-384. DOI: 10.1002/nur.4770130605

[21] Lautrette A, Darmon M, Megarbane B, et al. A communication strategy and brochure for relatives of patients dying in the ICU. The New England Journal of Medicine. 2007;**356**:469-478. DOI: 10.1056/NEJMoa063446]

[22] Hudson P, Quinn K, O'Hanlon B, Aranda S. Family meetings in palliative care: Multidisciplinary clinical practice guidelines. BMC Palliative Care. 2008;7:12. DOI: 10.1186/1472-684X-7-12

[23] Chiu M, Wei G, Lee S, Choovanichvong S, Wong F. Empowering caregivers: Impact analysis of Family Link Education Programme (FLEP) in Hong Kong, Taipei and Bangkok. The International Journal of Social Psychiatry. 2013;**59**(1):28-39. DOI: 10.1177/0020764011423171

[24] Ewertzon M, Hanson E. Support interventions for family members of adults with mental illness: A narrative literature review. Issues in Mental Health Nursing. 2019;**40**(9):768-780. DOI: 10.1080/01612840.2019.1591547

[25] Golden J, Conroy RM, Bruce I, Denihan A, Greene E, Kirby M, et al. Loneliness, social support networks, mood and wellbeing in community-dwelling elderly. International Journal of Geriatric Psychiatry. 2009;**24**(7):694-700. DOI: 10.1002/gps.2181

[26] Holt-Lunstad J, Smith TB, Layton JB. Social relationships and mortality risk: A meta-analytic review. PLoS Medicine. 2010;**7**:e1000316. DOI: 10.1371/journal.pmed.1000316

[27] World Health Organization. Improving the Quality of Paediatric Care: An Operational Guide for Facility-based Audit and Review of Paediatric Mortality [Internet]. 2018. Available from: https://www.who.int/maternal_child_adolescent/documents/improving-quality-paediatric-care/en [Accessed: 20 January 2020]

[28] Zielinski R, Ackerson K, Kane LL. Planned home birth: Benefits, risks, and opportunities. International Journal of Women's Health. 2015;7:361-377. DOI: 10.2147/IJWH.S55561

[29] Lindgren HE, Rådestad IJ, Christensson K, Wally-Bystrom K, Hildingsson IM. Perceptions of risk and risk management among 735 women who opted for a home birth. Midwifery. 2010;**26**(2):163

[30] Boucher D, Bennett C, McFarlin B, Freeze RJ. Staying home to give birth: Why women in the United States choose home birth. Midwifery Womens Health. 2009;**54**(2):119

[31] Hutton EK, Reitsma A, Simioni J, Brunton G, Kaufman K. Perinatal or neonatal mortality among women who intend at the onset of labour to give birth at home compared to women of low obstetrical risk who intend to give birth in hospital: A systematic review and meta-analyses. EClinicalMedicine. 2019;**25**: 59-70. DOI: 10.1016/j.eclinm.2019.07.005

[32] Committee Opinion No 697 Summary: Planned home birth. Obstetrics & Gynecology. 2017;**129**(4): 779-780. DOI: 10.1097/AOG.0000000000002015

[33] Shakib J, Buchi K, Smith E, Korgenski K, Young PC. Timing of initial well-child visit and readmissions of newborns. Pediatrics. 2015;**135**(3): 469-474 [Epub: 2 February 2015]

[34] World Health Organization. State of Inequality Reproductive, Maternal, Newborn and Child Health [Internet]. 2015. Available from: https://www.who.int/docs/default-source/gho-documents/health-equity/state-of-inequality/state-of-inequality-reproductive-maternal-new-born-and-child-health [Accessed: 2 February 2020]

[35] World Health Organization. WHO Recommendations on Home-based Records for Maternal, Newborn and Child Health [Internet]. 2018. Available from: https://www.who.int/maternal_child_adolescent/documents/home-based-records-guidelines/ [Accessed: 29 January 2020]

[36] World Health Organization. Vaccine Misinformation: Statement by WHO Director-General on Facebook and Instagram [Internet]. 2019. Available from: https://www.who.int/news-room/detail/04-09-2019-vaccine-misinformation-statement-by-who-director-general-on-facebook-and-instagram [Accessed: 3 February 2020]

[37] Bull Marilyn J, Engle WA. The committee on injury, violence, and poison prevention and the committee on fetus and newborn. Safe transportation of preterm and low birth weight infants at hospital discharge. Pediatrics. 2009;**123**(5):1424-1429. DOI: 10.1542/peds.2009-0559

[38] Policy Statement. Safe transportation of preterm and low birth weight infants at hospital discharge. Pediatrics. 2009;**123**(5):1424-1429 [Internet] Available from: http://pediatrics.aappublications.org/content/123/5/1424.full [Accessed: 6 February 2020]

[39] Task Force on Sudden Infant Death Syndrome. SIDS and other sleep-related infant deaths: Updated 2016 recommendations for a safe infant sleeping environment. Pediatrics. 2016;**138**(5):e20162938. DOI: 10.1542/peds.2016-2938

[40] Gupta M, Pursley DM, Smith VC. Preparing for discharge from the neonatal intensive care unit. Pediatrics. 2019;**143**(6):e20182915. DOI: 10.1542/peds.2018-2915

[41] Kuo DZ, Turchi RM. UpToDate [Internet]. 2020. Available from: https://www.uptodate.com/contents/children-and-youth-with-special-health-care-needs [Accessed: 7 February 2020]

[42] Ingrid W, McKee M, editors. European Child Health Services and Systems: Lessons Without Borders [Internet]. 2013. Available from: http://www.euro.who.int/__data/assets/pdf_file/0003/254928/

European-Child-Health-Services-and-Systems-Lessons-without-borders.pdf [Accessed: 7 February 2020]

[43] Lucile Packard Foundation for Children's Health. Standards for Systems of Care for Children and Youth with Special Health Care Needs, Version 2.0 [Internet]. 2017. Available from: https://www.lpfch.org/publication/standards-systems-care-children-and-youth-special-health-care-needs [Accessed: 7 February 2020]

[44] Roberts RM, Ejova A, Giallo R, Strohm K, Lillie M, Fuss B. A controlled trial of the SibworkS group program for siblings of children with special needs. Research In Developmental Disabilities. 2015;**43-44**:21. [Epub: 4 July 2015]

[45] Council on Children with Disabilities and Medical Home Implementation Project Advisory Committee. Patient- and family-centered care coordination: A framework for integrating care for children and youth across multiple systems. Pediatrics. 2014;**133**(5):e1451–e1460. DOI: 10.1542/peds.2014-0318

[46] Hayes D Jr, Wilson KC, Krivchenia K, Hawkins SMM, Balfour-Lynn IM, Gozal D, et al. Home oxygen therapy for children an official american thoracic society clinical practice guideline. American Journal of Respiratory and Critical Care Medicine. 2019;**199**(3):e5-e23. DOI: 10.1164/rccm.201812-2276ST

[47] Rosenbaum P, Paneth N, Leviton A, Goldstein M, Bax M, Damiano D, et al. A report: The definition and classification of cerebral palsy. Developmental Medicine and Child Neurology. Supplement. 2007;**109**:8-14

[48] Lantin-Hermoso MR, Berger S, Bhatt AB, Julia R, Morrow R, Freed MD, et al. The care of children with congenital heart disease in their primary medical home. Pediatrics. 2017;**140**(5):e20172607. DOI: 10.1542/peds.2017-2607

[49] Middlebrooks JS, Audage NC. The Effects of Childhood Stress on Health Across the Lifespan. Atlanta, GA: Centers for Disease Control and Prevention, National Center for Injury Prevention and Control; 2008. [Internet] Available from: http://stacks.cdc.gov/view/cdc/6978 [Accessed: 7 February 2020]

[50] Krug EG, Dahlberg Linda L, Mercy JA, Zwi AB, Lozano R. editors. World Report on Violence and Health. Geneva. [Internet]. 2002. 331p. Available from: https://www.who.int/violence_injury_ prevention/violence/world_report/en/ [Accessed: 7 February 2020]

[51] Leeb RT, Paulozzi L, Melanson C, Simon T, Arias I. Child Maltreatment Surveillance: Uniform Definitions for Public Health and Recommended Data Elements, Version 1.0. Atlanta, GA: Centers for Disease Control and Prevention, National Center for Injury Prevention and Control; 2008. [Internet] Available from: www.cdc.gov/violenceprevention/pdf/CM_Surveillance-a.pdf [Accessed: 6 February 2020]

[52] Shonkoff JP, Garner AS. The lifelong effects of early childhood adversity and toxic stress. Pediatrics. 2012;**129**:e232-e246

[53] Bierhaus A, Wolf J, Andrassy M, Rohleder N, Humpert PM, Petrov D, et al. A mechanism converting psychosocial stress into mononuclear cell activation. Proceedings of the National Academy of Sciences of the United States of America. 2003;**100**(4):1920-1925. pmid: 12578963

[54] Poulton R, Caspi A, Milne BJ, Thomson WM, Taylor A, Seras MR, et al. Association between children's experience of socioeconomic disadvantage and adult health: A life-course study. Lancet. 2002;**360**(9346):1640-1645. pmid: 12457787

[55] Michopoulos V, Powers A, Gillespie CF, Ressler KJ, Jovanovic T. Inflammation in fear- and anxiety-based disorders: PTSD, GAD, and beyond. Neuropsychopharmacology. 2017;**42**:254-270

[56] Muneer A. Bipolar disorder: Role of inflammation and the development of disease biomarkers. Psychiatry Investigation. 2016;**13**:18-33

[57] Hoehn EF, Wilson PM, Riney LC, Ngo V, Bennett B, Duma E. Identification and evaluation of physical abuse in children. Pediatric Annals. 2018;**47**(3):e97-e101. DOI: 10.3928/19382359-20180227-01

[58] Leventhal JM, Thomas SA, Rosenfield NS, Markowitz RI. Fractures in young children: Distinguishing child abuse from unintentional injuries. American Journal of Diseases of Children. 1993;**147**:87-92

[59] Beitchman JH, Zucker KJ, Hood JE, daCosta GA, Akman D. A review of the short-term effects of child sexual abuse. Child Abuse and Neglect. 1991;**15**(4):537-556. DOI: 10.1016/0145-2134(91)90038-F

[60] Meadow R. Munchausen syndrome by proxy the hinter-land of child abuse. Lancet. 1977;**310**(2):343-345. DOI: 10.1016/S0140-6736(77)91497-0

[61] Flaherty EG, MacMillan HL, American Academy of Pediatrics Committee on Child Abuse and Neglect. Caregiver-fabricated illness in a child: A manifestation of child maltreatment. Pediatrics. 2013;**132**:590-597

[62] Schilling S, Christian CW. Child physical abuse and neglect. Child and Adolescent Psychiatric Clinics of North America. 2014;**23**(2):309-319. DOI: 10.1016/j.chc.2014.01.001

[63] Lunkenheimer E, Lichtwarck-Aschoff A, Hollenstein T, Kemp CJ, Granic I. Breaking down the coercive cycle: How parent and child risk factors influence real-time variability in parental responses to child misbehavior. Parenting. 2016;**16**(4):237-256. DOI: 10.1080/15295192.2016.1184925

[64] Roman G, Rodica G, Angela-Mariana E, Andrada-Viorica P. Determinanti ai calitatii vietii pacientilor de etnie roma din prespectiva mediatorilor sanitari (Determinants of the quality of life of roma patients from the perspective of health mediators). Quality of Life/Calitatea Vietii. 2012;**23**(3):209-238

[65] APHA. Community Health Workers. 2019. Available from: https://www.apha.org/apha-communities/member-sections/community-healthworkers [Accessed: 29 January 2020]

[66] Sabo S, Butler M, McCue K, Wightman P, Pilling V, Celaya M. Rumann Sara Evaluation protocol to assess maternal and child health outcomes using administrative data: A community health worker home visiting programme. BMJ Open. 2019;**9**:e031780. DOI: 10.1136/bmjopen-2019-031780

[67] Introne J, Gokce Yildirim I, Iandoli L, DeCook J, Elzeini S. How people weave online information into pseudoknowledge. Social Media + Society. 2018;**4**(3):205630511878563. DOI: 10.1177/2056305118785639

[68] http://reports.weforum.org/global-risks-2013/risk-case-1/digital-wildfires-in-a-hyperconnected-world/ [Accessed: 2 February 2020]

[69] De Choudhury M, Morris M, White R. Seeking and sharing health information online: Comparing search engines and social media. In: CHI '14: Proceedings of the Conference on Human Factors in Computing Systems. 2014. pp. 1365-1376. DOI: 10.1145/2556288.2557214

[70] Ellis MJ, Russell K. The potential of telemedicine to improve pediatric concussion care in rural and remote communities in Canada. Frontiers in Neurology. 2019;**29100**:840. DOI: 10.3389/fneur.2019.00840

[71] WHO. A Health Telematics Policy in support of WHO's Health-For-All strategy for Global Health Development: Report of the WHO Group Consultation on Health Telematics, 11-16 December, Geneva, 1997. Geneva: World Health Organization; 1998. Available from: https://apps.who.int/iris/handle/10665/63857 [Accessed: 4 February 2020]

[72] McCrory P, Meeuwisse W, Dvorak J, Aubry M, Bailes J, Broglio S, et al. Consensus statement on concussion in sport-the 5(th) international conference on concussion in sport held in Berlin, October 2016. British Journal of Sports Medicine. 2017;**51**:838-847. DOI: 10.1136/bjsports-2017-097699

[73] Fridman L, Scolnik M, Macpherson A, Rothman L, Guttmann A, Grool AM, et al. Annual trends in follow-up visits for pediatric concussion in emergency departments and physicians' offices. Journal of Pediatrics. 2018;**192**:184-188. DOI: 10.1016/j.jpeds.2017.09.018

[74] Notario PM, Gentile E, Amidon M, Angst D, Lefaiver C, Webster K. Home-based telemedicine for children with medical complexity. Telemedicine Journal and E-Health. 2019;**25**(11):1123-1132. DOI: 10.1089/tmj.2018.0186. [Epub: 30 January 2019]

[75] U.S. Department of Health and Human Services, Health Resources and Services Administration (HRSA), Maternal and Child Health Bureau (MCHB). Who Are Children with Special Health Care Needs? Available from: https://www.childhealthdata.org/docs/drc/whoarecshcn_09-10-21-13-final.pdf [Accessed: 1 February 2020]

[76] Bird M, Li L, Ouellette C, Hopkins K, McGillion MH. Carter N, Use of synchronous digital health technologies for the care of children with special health care needs and their families: Scoping review. JMIR Pediatrics and Parenting. 2019;**2**(2):e15106. DOI: 10.2196/15106

[77] Cady RG, Kelly AM, Finkelstein SM, Looman WS, Garwick AW. Attributes of advanced practice registered nurse care coordination for children with medical complexity. Journal of Pediatric Health Care. 2014;**28**(4):305-312. DOI: 10.1016/j.pedhc.2013.06.005

[78] Looman WS, Hullsiek RL, Pryor L, Mathiason MA, Finkelstein SM. Health-related quality of life outcomes of a telehealth care coordination intervention for children with medical complexity: A randomized controlled trial. Journal of Pediatric Health Care. 2018;**32**(1):63-75. DOI: 10.1016/j.pedhc.2017.07.007

[79] Katalinic O, Young A, Doolan D. Case study: The interact home telehealth project. Journal of Telemedicine and Telecare. 2013;**19**(7):418-424. DOI: 10.1177/1357633x13506513

[80] Jury SC, Walker AM, Kornberg AJ. The introduction of web-based video-consultation in a paediatric acute care setting. Journal of Telemedicine and Telecare. 2013;**19**(7):383-387. DOI: 10.1177/1357633x13506530

[81] Lunney JR, Lynn J, Foley DJ, Lipson S, Guralnik JM. Patterns of functional decline at the end of life. Journal of the American Medical Association. 2003;**289**(18):2387-2392. DOI: 10.1001/jama.289.18.2387

[82] Murtagh FEM, Preston M, Higginson I. Patterns of dying: Palliative care for non-malignant disease. Clinical Medicine. 2004;**4**(1):39-44. DOI: 10.7861/clinmedicine.4-1-39

[83] Chen M-L. Inequity of palliative care for non-cancer patients. The Journal of

Nursing Research. 2019;**27**(2):1-2. DOI: 10.1097/JNR.0000000000000324

[84] Traue DC, Ross JR. Palliative care in non-malignant diseases. Journal of the Royal Society of Medicine. 2005;**98**:503-506

[85] Fox JM. Doubts about a particularly high nephrotoxicity of combination analgesics. Nephrology, Dialysis, Transplantation. 1999;**14**:2966-2968

[86] Lee J, Park Y, Lim K, Lee A, Lee H, Lee JE. Care needs of patients at the end of life with a non-cancer diagnosis who live at home. The Journal of Nursing Research. 2019;**27**(2):e10. DOI: 10.1097/jnr.0000000000000277

[87] Stiel S, Heckel M, Seifert A, Frauendorf T, Hanke RM, Ostgathe C. Comparison of terminally ill cancer- vs. non-cancer patients in specialized palliative homecare in Germany—A single service analysis. BMC Palliative Care. 2015;**14**:34. DOI: 10.1186/s12904-015-0033

[88] Ewertowski H, Tetzlaff F, Stiel S, Schneider N, Jünger S. Primary palliative care in general practice—Study protocol of a three-stage mixed-methods organizational health services research study. BMC Palliative Care. 2018;**17**:21. DOI: 10.1186/s12904-018-0276-6

[89] Gott M, Seymour J, Ingleton C, Gardiner C, Bellamy G. 'That's part of everybody's job': The perspectives of health care staff in England and New Zealand on the meaning and remit of palliative care. Palliative Medicine. 2012;**26**(3):232-241. DOI: 10.1177/0269216311408993

[90] Kratel U. Fortschritte in der ambulanten Palliative Care-Versorgung in Deutschland—Eine Bestandsaufnahme. Deutsche Zeitschrift für Onkologie. 2014;**46**(01):8-15. DOI: 10.1055/s-0033-1357616

[91] Gagyor I, Luthke A, Jansky M, Chenot JF. End of life care in general practice: Results of an observational survey with general practitioners. Schmerz. 2013;**27**(3):289-295. DOI: 10.1007/s00482-013-1324-z

[92] Thomas K, Free A. The gold standards framework is pivotal to palliative care. Guidelines in Practice. 2006;**9**:29-39

[93] http://www.studiipaliative.ro/proiecte/abordare-paliativa-prin-medicii-de-familie-srcp/ [Accessed: 20 Januaery 2020]

[94] Sepulveda C, Marlin A, Yoshida T, Ullrich A. Palliative care: The World Health Organization's global perspective. Journal of Pain and Symptom Management. 2002;**24**(2):91-96. DOI: 10.1016/S0885-3924(02)00440-2

[95] Strukturen und regionale Unterschiede in der Hospiz-und Palliativversorgung [Internet]. Bertelsmann-Stiftung. 2015. Available from: https://www.bertelsmannstiftung.de/fileadmin/files/BSt/Publikationen/GrauePublikationen/Studie_VV__FCG_Versorgungsstrukturen-palliativ.pdf

[96] Plöthner M, Schmidt K, de Jong L, et al. Needs and preferences of informal caregivers regarding outpatient care for the elderly: A systematic literature review. BMC Geriatrics. 2019;**19**: Article number: 82. DOI: 10.1186/s12877-019-1068-4

[97] Hokenstad MC. Older persons in a changing society: Report to the United Nations Department of Economic and Social Affairs Division for Social Policy and Development. 2006. www.un.org [Accessed: 15 February 2020]

[98] Kok L, Berden C, Sadiraj K. Costs and benefits of home care for the elderly versus residential care: A comparison using propensity scores. The European

Journal of Health Economics. 2015;**16**(2):119-131. DOI: 10.1007/s10198-013-0557-1

[99] Prediger S, Fürstenberg S, Berberat PO, et al. Interprofessional assessment of medical students' competences with an instrument suitable for physicians and nurses. BMC Medical Education. 2019;**19**:46. DOI: 10.1186/s12909-019-1473-6

[100] Oktay C, Senol Y, Rinnert S, Cete Y. Utility of 360-degree assessment of residents in a Turkish academic emergency medicine residency program. Turkish Journal of Emergency Medicine. 2019;**17**(1):12-15. DOI: 10.1016/j.tjem.2016.09.007

[101] Florea M. Work-family balance within the medical profession: An exploratory study. Letter to the editor. Acta Médica Portuguesa. 2020;**33**(2): 150-153. DOI: 10.20344/amp.13213

Section 4

Symptoms and Medications in Palliative Care

Chapter 10

Chemotherapy-Induced Nausea and Vomiting

Elisabetta Di Liso

Abstract

Chemotherapy-induced nausea and vomiting is a common adverse effect in cancer patients that not only impacts quality of life, but also treatment outcomes. The prevalence of nausea and vomiting is related to several factors, including the emetogenicity of the chemotherapy regimen, the dose and rate of administration of the chemotherapy agents, various environmental triggers and patient-related factors. The pathogenesis involves multiple organ systems, central nervous system, gastrointestinal tract and neurotransmitters. Clinical management should include a complete assessment of nausea and vomiting to investigate the possible etiology and the pharmacologic approach should involve agents that target each of these pathways and neurotransmitters. Various national guidelines provide recommendations for the prevention and management of CINV and combining these evidence-based strategies into clinical practice is crucial l to improve morbidity and quality-of-life outcomes among cancer patients.

Keywords: nausea, vomiting, chemotherapy, radiotherapy, risk of emesis, management

1. Introduction

Nausea and vomiting (N/V) represents a primary issue in oncology requiring effective management for both prevention and treatment. Although in cancer patients several causes, such as opioid medications, can induce N/V, it is mainly related to antitumoral therapy. Chemotherapy-induced nausea and vomiting (CINV) is the most common and intolerable adverse event with negative impact on quality of life and treatment's adherence and efficacy. It is important to notice that large literature is available about N/V related to standard chemotherapy and little literature about new antitumoral therapies such as tyrosine kinase inhibitors, monoclonal antibodies and immunotherapeutic agents, instead. Management of N/V in cancer patients should begin with a complete assessment including evaluation of intensity and timing of appearance. To determine whether N/V is related to treatment (chemotherapy, radiation) or is independent of cancer treatment should be the second step. Various national and international antiemetic guidelines have been developed for the prevention of chemotherapy- and radiotherapy-induced nausea and emesis. The prevention of CINV is crucial to improve patients' confidence and compliance to treatments and the clinical management include both pharmacologic and nonpharmacologic therapies. This chapter addresses the epidemiology, clinical features, risk factors, mechanisms, and management of CINV.

2. Epidemiology

CINV involves about 60–80% of patients with cancer increasing the risk of patients' discomfort and chemotherapy's discontinuation [1]. The prevention of CINV is mainly important in reducing morbidity and total healthcare costs, as well as increasing the quality of care in patients receiving emetogenic chemotherapy. Patients experiencing CINV may refuse treatment, request or require dose reductions or seek alternative therapy options. Acute CINV may be prevented in 50% to 90% of patients using effective preventive strategies [2]. In a large European observational study, 1000 patients who had received guideline antiemetic treatment had significantly better CINV control than those who did not receive guideline treatment. The complete control rates were 60% versus 51%, respectively; however, the overall adherence to guidelines was just 29% [3].

Radiotherapy-induced nausea and vomiting (RINV) is one of the most common side effects during radiation, from which about 50% to 80% of the patients undergoing radiotherapy will suffer [4].

3. Clinical presentation

Cancer patients often experience N/V together but not necessarily. It is possible to experience nausea without emesis or emesis without nausea. The events of nausea and vomiting are generally protecting reflexes to rid intestine and stomach of toxic substances.

Nausea is described as a subjective and diffuse feeling of unease and discomfort often perceived as an urge to vomit. It can be considered a prodromal phase to the act of vomiting. It is characterized by sickness in the stomach, epigastrium and/or throat. Vomiting or emesis means the expulsion of stomach contents beyond the mouth and is accompanied by shivering and salivation.

The use of single agent cisplatin led to classify CINV into five types: acute, delayed, anticipatory, breakthrough and refractory according to the timing of appearance and in the absence of effective antiemetic prevention [5]. Acute CINV occurs within 24 hours of the chemotherapy administration, while delayed CINV occurs after 24 hours and could persist for 2–3 weeks after the administration of chemotherapy. Chemotherapeutic agents such as cisplatin, carboplatin, cyclophosphamide, anthracyclines are generally related to delayed CINV [6]. Anticipatory CINV involves patients who had already experienced N/V and occurs prior to the impending administration of chemotherapy triggered by the just thinking of it through a sensorial way (sight, smell). The incidence of anticipatory CINV has decreased in recent years because of the improved strategies for controlling acute and delayed emesis. Breakthrough CINV is vomiting and/or nausea that occurs within five days of chemotherapy administration after the use of guideline directed prophylactic antiemetic agents. This type of CINV usually requires immediate treatment or requires "rescue" with additional antiemetics. Refractory CINV is defined as vomiting and/or nausea occurring after chemotherapy in subsequent chemotherapy cycles after guideline directed prophylactic antiemetic agents have failed in earlier cycles (**Table 1**).

Patients with CINV should be assessed with a visual analog scale (0 to 10, with 0 no nausea and 10 maximum nausea). The frequency, severity, time of appearance and any associated activities (meals, drugs) should be requested. Recent treatment with chemotherapy and/or radiation therapy should then be noted with evaluation of single agent or combination of chemotherapy. The physical examination should include a complete assessment of the abdomen in order to identify a possible

	Clinical presentation and physiopathology
Acute CINV	Within 24 hours of initial administration of chemotherapy. Mainly by 5-HT3 release from the enterochromaffin cells
Delayed CINV	After 24 hours of initial administration of chemotherapy to 2–3 weeks. Mainly by substance P release, disruption of the blood–brain barrier and disruption of the gastrointestinal motility.
Anticipatory CINV	After a previous cycle of chemotherapy. Triggered by taste, smell, sight, thoughts of a previous CINV.
Breakthrough CINV	Within 5 days of initial administration of chemotherapy.
Refractory CINV	After chemotherapy despite prophylactic antiemetic agents

Table 1.
Clinical presentation and physiopathology of CINV.

organic cause of the emesis such as gastritis, bowel obstruction, an inflammatory process. A complete neurologic examination should also be performed to determine the search focal neurologic signs suggesting intracranial hypertension or meningeal carcinosis. Weight loss, appetite, anorexia, and/or cachexia should be evaluated to investigate the possible etiology of N/V and to help the differential diagnosis.

4. Risk factors

The occurrence of CINV can depend on several factors. The risk factors for CINV are both patient- and treatment-related. The most common patient-related risk factors are age, gender, previous motion sickness and/or pregnancy-related N/V and previous CINV. Patients younger than 50 years, females, patients with a history of previous motion sickness and/or pregnancy-related N/V have a greater

High-risk of emesis (>90%)	Moderate-risk of emesis (30–90%)	Low-risk of emesis (10–30%)	Minimal-risk of emesis (<10%)
Carmustine	Procarbazine	Bortezomib	Bevacizumab
Cisplatin	Carboplatin	Cetuximab	Bleomycin
Cyclophosphamide	Cyclophosphamide	Docetaxel	Busulfan
Dacarbazine	Cytosine arabinoside	Etoposide	Capecitabine
Mechlorethamine	Doxorubicin	5-fluorouracil	Chlorambucil
Streptozotocin	Epirubicin	Gemcitabine	Fludarabine
	Ifosfamide	Lapatinib	Vinblastine
	Irinotecan	Methotrexate	Vincristine
	Oxaliplatin	Mytomicin	Vinorelbine
	Melphalan	Mitoxantrone	
		Paclitaxel	
		Pemetrexed	
		Topotecan	
		Trastuzumab	

Table 2.
Classification of antitumoral therapy according to the risk of emesis.

risk of experiencing CINV. Instead, a previous history of high alcohol consumption is associated with a lower risk of CINV [7–9].

Treatment-related factors and emetogenicity of chemotherapeutic regimens are also relevant. Chemotherapeutic agents are related to various risk of emesis depending on mechanism of action, dose, route and administration in single or combined way. The intrinsic emetogenicity of chemotherapy is the crucial factor to guide the choose of antiemetic treatment. In 2004 an expert consensus conference proposed a classification of chemotherapeutic agents in four categories according to emetogenic potential: high, moderate, low and minimal risk [10]. In the high-risk category, more than 90% could experience CINV without an antiemetic prophylaxis. In the moderate-risk category the potential experience of CINV involves 30–90% of patients. In the low- and minimal risk less than 30% and 10% respectively of cancer patients experience CINV (**Table 2**) [11].

5. Physiopathology

The mechanisms of emesis are not well defined. The physiopathology of CINV includes both central nervous and peripheral system pathways and it is different in acute, delayed and anticipatory setting. The mechanisms inducing CINV have gradually been investigated over the past 60 years. In the 1950s the first hypothesis by Wang and Borison was the existence of a central site called 'vomiting center' located in the medulla processing all the afferent impulses to generate emesis [12]. The presence of some neuronal areas located within medulla coordinating the emetic reflex is now a more realistic hypothesis. All the neuronal cells involved in the series of events occurring during CINV have been called 'central pattern generator' [13]. Three primary components have been found out in the physiopathology of CINV: chemoreceptor trigger zone (CTZ), abdominal vagal afferents and neurotransmitters. After exposure to chemotherapy, the emetic reflex involves two primary sources of afferent input to neuronal areas: abdominal vagal afferents and area postrema, a structure located in the caudal end of the fourth ventricle [14, 15]. 5-hydroxytryptamine 3 (5-HT3), neurokinin-1 (NK1) and cholecystokinin-1 receptors located in the terminal ends of the vagal afferents are close to enteroendocrine cell into the gastrointestinal mucosa of the proximal small intestine. Chemotherapeutic agents stimulate enteroendocrine cells to release some mediators such as 5-hydroxytryptamine, substance P and cholecystokinin which bind to the specific receptors on the close vagal fibers. The afferent impulse reaches the dorsal brain stem through the nucleus of the solitary tract. Among the various receptors, 5-HT3 are considered the most active in acute emesis. In summary, in acute CINV chemotherapeutic agents release free radicals stimulating enterochromaffin cells in the peripheral gastrointestinal tract with subsequent release of serotonin. Serotonin binds 5-HT3 receptors through intestinal vagal afferent nerves and nucleus of the solitary tract and reaches the central nervous system. In delayed CINV the physiologic way is similar but involves less frequently 5-HT3 and more frequently NK1 receptors respectively. In delayed CINV chemotherapeutic agents induce the release of substance P from the neuronal cells in the central and peripheral nervous system. Substance P binds NK1 receptors in the nucleus of solitary tract and led the afferent impulse to central nervous system.

The second pathway potentially involved in the emetic reflex include area postrema. In this region of the brain the blood–brain barrier is more permeable so it is accessible to afferent impulses in either blood or cerebrospinal fluid. This area has commonly been called 'chemoreceptor trigger zone'. This region has afferent and efferent connections with underlying structures, the subnucleous gelatinosus and nucleus of solitary tract, receiving vagal afferent fibers from the gastrointestinal mucosa. Metabolites and peptides released under the effect of chemotherapeutic agents can also induce emesis binding at this site.

The clinical role of neurotransmitters has been longer investigated in the past 30 years. The first interest was focused on dopamine, more recently on 5-HT and substance P. Dopaminergic antagonists are the first investigated antiemetic agents [16]. The 5-HT3 receptor antagonists are currently the single most effective class of antiemetics for prevention and treatment of acute CINV. These receptors are located both in central sites such as area postrema and nucleus of solitary tract and in peripheral sites such as vagal afferents. The blockage of 5-HT3 receptor is the most effective mechanism of antiemetic treatment. NK1 receptors are also located both in area postrema and nucleus of solitary tract and in the gastrointestinal mucosa. This evidence suggests that NK1 receptor antagonists plays a central role in prevention and treatment of CINV similar to 5-HT3 receptor antagonists. Endocannabinoids have been more recently investigated as relevant neurotransmitters inducing N/V. The endogenous cannabinoids are agonistic antiemetic agents. Synthetic cannabinoids have been recently evaluated to treat refractory CINV.

Anticipatory CINV occurs as a response to a previous experience of CINV. A sensory feeling related to the first administration of chemotherapy led the patient to associate that feeling with N/V. Subsequent exposure to that feeling triggers the response of N/V. Anticipatory CINV can be effectively avoided with an adequate prevention of acute and delayed CINV [7, 17–19].

6. Management

Antiemetic guidelines are published by all the cancer organizations including American Society of Clinical Oncology (ASCO), the National Comprehensive Cancer Network (NCCN), the European Society of Medical Oncology (ESMO) and the Multinational Association of Supportive Care in Cancer (MASCC). There are some differences among the guidelines particularly in the choice of the preferred 5-HT3 receptor antagonist and the use of cannabinoids. The general scheme for antiemetic protocols is similar for the various guidelines.

Prevention of CINV is the primary treatment to avoid subsequent episodes of CINV and anticipatory CINV. Due to physiopathology of CINV, 5-HT3 and NK1 receptor antagonists are the main classes of drugs Management include also both pharmacologic and nonpharmacologic agents such as steroids, dopamine antagonists, benzodiazepines, cannabinoids, antipsychotics. The primary issue is the prevention and treatment of moderately and highly emetogenic chemotherapy.

6.1 5-HT3 antagonists

Selective 5-HT3 receptor antagonists have revolutionized the management of CINV. They are indicated in preventing and treating N/V induced by chemotherapy with moderate and high emetic potential. The 5-HT3 receptor antagonists include both first-generation drugs such as ondansetron (Zofran), dolasetron (Anzemet) and granisetron (Kytril) with half-life between 3–9 hours and second-generation drugs such as palonosetron (Aloxi) with half-life of approximately 40 hours. According to their half-life they are used in different indication with more use in acute CINV for first-generation drugs and delayed CINV for second-generation drugs. The first-generation antiemetic drugs are equivalent in efficacy [20–22] and they have few adverse events. The most common adverse events of 5-HT3 receptor antagonist include headache, constipation, transient high levels of hepatic enzymes and QT prolongation [23]. The oral and intravenous formulation are therapeutically equivalent [24]. The first-generation drugs are more active in acute CINV and appear little active and modest active in delayed N/V induced by cisplatin and moderately emetogenic chemotherapeutic agents, respectively. The second-generation 5-HT3 receptor antagonist has a longer half-life and a greater binding affinity for the specific receptor. Three randomized prospective trials compared palonosetron with a first-generation antiemetic drug in patients receiving moderately and highly emetogenic chemotherapy. The noninferiority of palonosetron in term of complete response was demonstrated [25–27]. Some international guidelines consider palonosetron the preferred 5-HT3 antagonist for moderate emetogenic chemotherapy regimens but there are no prospective trials demonstrating the superiority of palonosetron compared to first-generation agents.

6.2 NK1 antagonists

In the past 10 years, antiemetic treatment has greatly advanced with the availability of NK1 receptor antagonists. The NK1 receptor antagonists are the most recent class of antiemetic agents and include aprepitant (emend) fosaprepitant (ivemend), rolapitant (varuby) and netupitant (akynzeo). Aprepitant was the first approved agent in the class and is formulized as oral drug. In acute CINV the NK1 receptor antagonists are usually administered in combination with a 5-HT3 receptor antagonists and dexamethasone. 3-days aprepitant can also be administered in delayed CINV [28]. Three randomized prospective trials compared the combination of ondansetron plus dexamethasone plus aprepitant versus ondansetron and dexamethasone in patients receiving highly emetogenic chemotherapy. Aprepitant was administered before chemotherapy and continued along with dexamethasone. The addition of aprepitant led to an approximate 50% reduction in the risk of emesis or need for rescue medications [29–31]. These evidences underline the crucial role of aprepitant in the management of CINV induced by highly emetogenic chemotherapy. A randomized prospective trial investigated the use of aprepitant in moderately emetogenic chemotherapy in almost a thousand of patients with breast cancer. A significantly higher rate of complete response in the aprepitant group was reported [32]. Fosaprepitant is an intravenous NK1 receptor antagonist. In is a water-soluble phosphoryl prodrug of aprepitant converted to aprepitant within 30 minutes after administration. A randomized double-blind study reported that a single dose of fosaprepitant after ondansetron and dexamethasone was noninferior to a standard aprepitant 3-days regimen in preventing CINV in more than 2 thousand patients receiving cisplatin [33]. This evidence suggests that a single dose of fosaprepitant enhances the antiemetic effects provided by conventional 5-HT3 receptor agonists and corticosteroid therapy over conventional therapy alone and may provide a level of efficacy similar to that of the recommended 3-days aprepitant regimen. Rolapitant is a highly selective competitive long-acting NK-1 receptor antagonist demonstrating efficacy in randomized phase III trials. A single oral dose of rolapitant was effective in preventing delayed CINV compared with placebo, when each was used in combination with a 5-HT3 receptor antagonist plus dexamethasone in patients receiving highly or moderately emetogenic chemotherapy [34]. Netupitant is formulated with palonosetron in a fixed-dose combination. Complete response rates during the acute and delayed CINV were significantly higher with single-dose netupitant plus palonosetron than with single-dose palonosetron in highly and moderately emetogenic chemotherapy in phase II and III trials [35].

The most common adverse events of NK1 receptor antagonists are fatigue, hiccups, dyspepsia and diarrhea. The use of aprepitant requires the evaluation of potential drug interaction due to its mechanism of action moderately inhibiting cytochrome CYP3A4. In particularly, aprepitant is related to an increase of plasma dexamethasone levels. Dexamethasone dose should be reduced when used in combination with aprepitant. Some antitumoral agents are also metabolized by CYP3A4 with the risk of increased toxicity when administered in combination with aprepitant. Aprepitant is also a weak inducer of the cytochrome CYP450. In patient receiving warfarin in combination with aprepitant the international normalized ratio (INR) decreases by 15% [36]. Rolapitant is well tolerated and its most common adverse events include neutropenia and dizziness. It inhibits CYP2D6 and it is metabolized by CYP3A4 so CYP3A4 inducers can reduce rolapitant blood levels and efficacy. The most common adverse events of netupitant include asthenia, dyspepsia, erythema and neutropenia. It is contraindicated in patients with severe renal and hepatic failure and it is an inhibitor of CYP3A4 as aprepitant [37–40].

6.3 Steroids

The antiemetic use of corticosteroids dates to the 1980s although the mechanism of efficacy is not yet clear. Dexamethasone is the most effective corticosteroid and it is widely used in combination with other antiemetic drugs both in acute and delayed CINV. In N/V induced by low emetogenic chemotherapy it could also be effectively used as single antiemetic agent (**Table 3**).

6.4 Other antiemetic treatments

A lot of agents including dopamine receptor antagonists, phenothiazines, cannabinoids, olanzapine are currently used to treat CINV induced by low emetogenic potential. Dopamine receptor antagonists such as metoclopramide and butyrophenones were most commonly used in past years and they could still be administered in combination with other antiemetic agents or in low-risk CINV. The efficacy of metoclopramide improves with increasing doses. Dopamine antagonists exhibit many adverse events and the most serious is represented by extrapyramidal symptoms. Dopamine antagonists may be considered when breakthrough CINV occurs. Currently breakthrough CINV is managed with an agent from a drug class that was not used in the prophylactic regimen. The phenothiazines are rarely administered in CINV and mainly in CINV induced by low emetogenic effect or as salvage therapy in breakthrough emesis. Antipsychotics such as olanzapine are sometimes prescribed in CINV not responding to conventional antiemetics. Olanzapine antagonizes several neurotransmitter receptors involved in the antiemetic reflex and it has been reported effective in preventing both and delayed CINV. No robust data comparing olanzapine with other antiemetic agents is available [41, 42]. In clinical practice olanzapine is often added to the standard three-drugs combination but it does not replace any of them. Olanzapine may be considered for the treatment of breakthrough and refractory CINV in addition to a change in the prophylactic antiemetic regimen. The most common adverse events of olanzapine include fatigue, sedation, headache, dry mouth, hyperglycemia, diarrhea.

In CINV with low and moderate emetic potential, synthetic cannabinoids have been recently evaluated. The two known cannabinoid receptors are CB1 and CB2. Blocking of CB1 and CB2 results in emesis. Cannabinoids act as an agonist on the CB1 receptors, resulting in their pharmacologic effect [43]. The use of these agents with a lower therapeutic index is not recommended as first-line treatment for prevention of CINV and should be reserved for patients refractory to or intolerant of standard antiemetics. Evidence remains insufficient for a recommendation regarding medical marijuana for the prevention of nausea and vomiting in patients with cancer who receive chemotherapy or radiation therapy.

Antiemetic agent	Dose	
	Acute CINV	*Delayed CINV*
Ondansetron	8 mg or 0.15 mg/kg day 1 (intravenous) 24 mg day 1 for high-risk (oral) 8 mg twice daily day 1 for moderate-risk (oral)	8 mg twice daily days 2–3 (oral)
Dolasetron	100 mg or 1.8 mg/kg day 1 (intravenous) 100 mg day 1 (oral)	100 mg days 2–3 (oral)
Granisetron	1 mg or 0.01 mg/kg day 1 (intravenous) 2 mg day 1 (oral)	1 mg twice daily days 2–3 (oral)
Palonosetron	0.25 mg day 1 (intravenous)	
Aprepitant	125 mg day 1 (oral)	80 mg days 2–3 (oral)
Fosaprepitant	115 mg day 1 (intravenous)	80 mg days 2–3 (oral)
Rolapitant		
Netupitant		
Dexamethasone	12 mg day 1 (intravenous) with aprepitant 12 mg day 1 (oral) with aprepitant	8 mg days 2–4 for high risk (oral) with aprepitant 8 mg days 2–3 for moderate-risk (oral) with aprepitant
	20 mg day 1 for high-risk (intravenous) without aprepitant 8 mg day 1 for moderate-risk (intravenous) without aprepitant 20 mg day 1 for high-risk (oral) without aprepitant 8 mg day 1 for moderate-risk (oral) without aprepitant	8 mg twice daily days 2–4 for high risk (oral) without aprepitant 8 mg days 2–3 for moderate-risk (oral) without aprepitant
Metoclopramide	1–2 mg/kg day 1 (intravenous)	1–2 mg/kg 2 hours after chemotherapy (intravenous) 0.5 mg/kg every 6 hours days 2–4 (oral)
Prochlorperazine	5–10 mg day 1 (intravenous) 5–10 mg day 1 (oral)	5–10 mg every 6 hours (oral)
Dronabinol	5 mg/mq (oral)	5 mg/mq every 2–4 hours (oral)
Nabilone	1–2 mg (oral)	1–2 mg twice daily (oral)
Olanzapine	5 mg for 2 days before chemotherapy (oral) 10 mg day 1 (oral)	10 mg days 2–4 (oral)

Table 3.
Management of CINV.

Two commercial forms of synthetic cannabinoids have been approved by Food and Drug Administration (FDA) with CINV indication: nabilone and dronabinol in 2005 and 2016, respectively. Studies with dronabinol and nabilone were performed in the 1970s and 1980s, before the approval of 5-HT3 receptor antagonists, and often included a placebo arm. Tramer et al. published a meta-analysis on the use of cannabinoids for CINV control. The investigators analyzed data from 30 randomized controlled studies from 1975 to 1997; 16 studies were with nabilone, 13 with dronabinol, and 1 with intramuscular levonantradol. Of the 30 studies,

10 used a placebo as the comparator, and prochlorperazine was prescribed in 12 trials. Other antiemetic controls included metoclopramide, chlorpromazine, thiethylperazine, haloperidol, domperidone, and alizapride. The authors found that cannabinoids were more effective with moderately emetogenic chemotherapy regimens than all of the active controls, but were not more effective with very high or low emetogenic regimens. More side effects were associated with the cannabinoid treatment, and patients were more likely to withdraw from therapy [44]. A 2015 meta-analysis evaluated the role of cannabinoids in chemotherapy induced nausea and vomiting. 51 trials included in the analysis were conducted between 1975 and 1991 and none involved comparisons with current antiemetic regimens. The authors concluded that cannabis-based medications may be useful for treating refractory CINV. However, methodological limitations of the trials limit any conclusions [45]. Nabilone and dronabinol are orally active synthetic cannabinoid approved for the treatment of CINV in patients who have not experienced adequate response to conventional antiemetic treatments. The restriction is related to the side effects spectrum of this agents. Some of these adverse events are seen as beneficial to the patient. Events such as a feeling of being high or euphoria and drowsiness are seen as potentially beneficial side effects of this agent. Other side effects that are not considered beneficial and are more problematic include ataxia, anxiety, disorientation, hallucinations, depression, and psychosis. Adverse events may persist for a variable and unpredictable period, with adverse psychiatric reactions persisting 48 to 72 hours after the last dose. Orthostatic hypotension has been reported. Use of synthetic oral cannabinoids should be limited to the management of breakthrough and refractory CONV and they have no place as a first-line treatment for CINV.

In the anticipatory CINV benzodiazepines are the treatment of choice due to their antianxiety property [17]. Lorazepam or alprazolam are the most used agents in the prevention and management of anticipatory emesis in combination with standard antiemetic strategies.

Alternative treatments should also be considered particularly for the anticipatory CINV. Behavioral approaches include hypnosis, muscle relaxion, music therapy, acupuncture or acupressure [46]. Evidence remains insufficient for a recommendation for or against the use of ginger, acupuncture/acupressure and other complementary or alternative therapies for the prevention of nausea and vomiting in patients with cancer. The role of ginger in the prevention of CINV has been evaluated evaluated in two trials and a meta-analysis. The first trial compared powdered ginger plus standard of care versus standard of care alone in 60 patients treated with anthracycline-based chemotherapy experienced severe CINV during previous cycles. Patients in the ginger arm reported less severe nausea and fewer vomiting episodes on days 2, 3, and 5. No adverse events were attributable to ginger [47]. The second trial compared three doses of ginger versus placebo in more than 500 patients receiving a 5-HT3 inhibitor and dexamethasone. The two lower doses of ginger produced the largest reductions in nausea intensity [48]. A 2013 systematic review evaluated four trials and reported that ginger did not have a significant effect on the incidence of acute nausea, acute vomiting, or delayed vomiting [49].

The use of acupuncture has been evaluated in 70 patients who were randomly assigned to receive acupuncture in cycle 1 and ondansetron in cycle 2, or the reverse. All patients also received dexamethasone for 3 days. Complete response from 0 to 24 hours was similar with the two treatments, but acupuncture produced higher complete response rates from 24 to 120 hours. Constipation and insomnia were less common with acupuncture than with ondansetron [50]. Two trials evaluated acupressure wristbands and found no significant benefit against nausea and vomiting when wristbands were added to standard antiemetic treatment among patients treated with chemotherapy [51, 52].

6.5 Radiotherapy-induced N/V

Few randomized controlled clinical trials have evaluated the prevention or treatment of N/V associated with radiotherapy. As for CINV, RINV is classified according to the emetogenic risk of radiation (**Table 4**).

Patients experiencing high-emetic-risk radiation therapy should be received a two-drug combination of a 5-HT3 receptor antagonist and dexamethasone before each fraction and on the day after each fraction if radiation therapy is not planned for that day. Optimal frequency and duration of prophylactic 5-HT3 receptor antagonist therapy and prophylactic dexamethasone therapy for high-emetic-risk single-fraction or multiple-fraction radiation are unclear. Previous studies administered prophylactic 5-HT3 receptor antagonist therapy for durations longer than, equal to, and shorter than the duration of radiation therapy. Randomized studies comparing these approaches are lacking [53, 54].

Patients receiving moderate-emetic-risk should be treated with a 5-HT3 receptor antagonist before each fraction, with or without dexamethasone before the first five fractions. Optimal frequency and duration of prophylactic 5-HT3 receptor antagonist therapy for moderate-emetic-risk, single-fraction or multiple-fraction radiation therapy are unclear. Guidelines recommend prophylaxis before each fraction with careful monitoring of patients during radiation therapy schedules that span multiple weeks to detect symptoms experienced during interspersed days when radiation therapy and prophylaxis are not administered and to balance the benefits and toxicities of prolonged 5-HT3 receptor antagonist therapy. A study that involved moderate-emetic-risk radiation therapy demonstrated a benefit for a number of secondary end points by adding prophylactic dexamethasone therapy to prophylactic 5-HT3 receptor antagonist therapy before the first five fractions [55].

Patients treated with low- and minimal-emetic-risk radiation therapy should receive rescue therapy with a 5-HT3 receptor antagonist, dexamethasone, or a dopamine receptor antagonist.

Patients who are treated with concurrent radio-chemotherapy should receive antiemetic therapy that is appropriate for the emetic risk level of antineoplastic agents, unless the risk level of the radiation therapy is higher [56].

One trial evaluated the addition of fosaprepitant to palonosetron and dexamethasone among women who received low-emetic-risk pelvic radiation and concurrent weekly cisplatin.36 The other trial compared fosaprepitant with olanzapine—each given with palonosetron and dexamethasone—among patients with head and neck or esophageal cancers who received radiation therapy and concurrent cisplatin and fluorouracil.

A systematic review of RINV reported that the clinical trial designs varied considerably in the methodologies, endpoints, and outcome measures employed with

High-risk of emesis (>90%)	Moderate-risk of emesis (30–90%)	Low-risk of emesis (10–30%)	Minimal-risk of emesis (<10%)
Total body irradiation	Upper abdomen, craniospinal irradiation	Brain, head and neck, thorax, pelvis irradiation	Extremities, breast irradiation

Table 4.
Classification of radiotherapy according to the risk ok emesis.

great difficult to conclude definitive recommendations [57]. Most of the patients will be suggested to take the antiemetic by the international antiemetic guidelines. A MASCC/ESMO consensus systematic review recently evaluated 18 publications. The only fully published randomized studies in prevention of RINV were two negative studies in acupuncture and green tea, respectively. No data to support new recommendations for antiemetic prophylaxis in RINV was available. The serotonin receptor antagonists are still the corner stone in antiemetic prophylaxis of nausea and vomiting induced by high and moderate emetic risk radiotherapy. The emetogenicity of craniospinal radiotherapy was reclassified from low to moderate emetic level along with some other minor changes [58]. Further investigations are warranted to explore RINV prophylaxis in single fraction, multiple fractions and concomitant chemo-radiotherapy.

Although the mechanisms of acupuncture are not completely clear yet, a plenty of high-quality clinical trials have been conducted to evaluate the efficacy and safety of this therapy and reported that acupuncture could reduce nausea and vomiting induce by chemotherapy and radiotherapy with less side effects [50, 59, 60]. Neural mechanism like stimulating the secretion of endogenous opioid endorphin has been proved one of mechanisms of acupuncture therapeutical effect, but for RINV relative neural mechanisms have not been found yet [61].

7. Conclusions

CINV represents a common adverse event of chemotherapy with potentially significant negative impact on quality of life for patients and their families. Prevention and management of CINV is crucial to increase patients' compliance and adherence to antitumoral treatments.

7.1 High-risk of emesis

The combination of a 5-HT3 receptor antagonist, dexamethasone and aprepitant before chemotherapy is currently the recommended strategy for chemotherapy with high- and moderate-risk of emesis. More robust data is available for cisplatin-based chemotherapy and anthracycline plus cyclophosphamide regimen, less robust data is available for other agents. Approximately 90% of patients receiving cisplatin-based chemotherapy and anthracycline plus cyclophosphamide regimen develop delayed emesis. These patients should receive a regimen with one of 5-HT3 receptor antagonists plus 3-days oral aprepitant plus dexamethasone on days 2 to 4 to avoid delayed emesis.

7.2 Moderate-risk of emesis

For moderate-risk agents different from and anthracycline plus cyclophosphamide regimen, a combination of a 5-HT3 receptor antagonist and dexamethasone should be administered before chemotherapy. Patients with moderate risk of emesis have moderate potential for delayed emesis. These patients should be treated with a 5-HT3 receptor antagonist or dexamethasone alone on days 2 and 3.

7.3 Low-risk of emesis

For patients receiving chemotherapy with low-risk of emesis, a single dose of dexamethasone or a dopaminergic before chemotherapy is currently recommended. No routine prevention for delayed emesis is recommended.

Risk of emesis		Antiemetic strategy	
		Acute CINV	**Delayed CINV**
Minimal		None	None
Low		Dexamethasone or dopamine antagonist	None
Moderate	Anthracycline plus cyclophosphamide	5-HT3 receptor antagonist plus dexamethasone plus aprepitant	Dexamethasone days 2–4 plus aprepitant days 2–3
	Other regimens	5-HT3 receptor antagonist plus dexamethasone	5-HT3 receptor antagonist or dexamethasone days 2–3
High		5-HT3 receptor antagonist plus dexamethasone plus aprepitant	Dexamethasone days 2–4 plus aprepitant days 2–3

Table 5.
Management of RINV.

7.4 Minimal-risk of emesis

No routine prevention for acute and delayed CINV is generally indicated for chemotherapy with minimal-risk of emesis (**Table 5**).

Strategies to prevent and manage CINV represents a major challenge. In the last 20 years, more effective and well-tolerated antiemetic agents have been introduced in the clinical practice. Selective 5-HT3 receptor antagonist, NK1 antagonist receptors and steroids are currently the most effective combination. This antiemetic strategy achieved an excellent control of CINV in over 80% of patients with an excellent side-effect profile. The further goal should be the management of patients with refractory CINV impacting on therapeutic adherence.

Author details

Elisabetta Di Liso
Department of Oncology, Unit of Oncology 2, Veneto Institute of Oncology IOV – IRCCS, Padua, Italy

*Address all correspondence to: elisabetta.diliso@iov.veneto.it

References

[1] Sommariva S, Pongiglione B, Tarricone R. Impact of chemotherapy-induced nausea and vomiting on health-related quality of life and resource utilization: A systematic review. Crit Rev Oncol Hematol 2016 Mar;99:13-36.

[2] Van Laar ES, Desai JM, Jatoi A. Professional educational needs for chemotherapy-induced nausea and vomiting (CINV): multinational survey results from 2388 health care providers. Support Care Cancer 2015 Jan;23(1):151-157.

[3] Aapro M, Molassiotis A, Dicato M, Pelaez I, Rodriguez-Lescure A, Pastorelli D, et al. The effect of guideline-consistent antiemetic therapy on chemotherapy-induced nausea and vomiting (CINV): the Pan European Emesis Registry (PEER). Ann Oncol 2012 Aug;23(8):1986-1992.

[4] Feyer PC, Maranzano E, Molassiotis A, Roila F, Clark-Snow RA, Jordan K, et al. Radiotherapy-induced nausea and vomiting (RINV): MASCC/ESMO guideline for antiemetics in radiotherapy: update 2009. Support Care Cancer 2011 Mar;19 Suppl 1:S5-14.

[5] Tavorath R, Hesketh PJ. Drug treatment of chemotherapy-induced delayed emesis. Drugs 1996 Nov;52(5):639-648.

[6] Roila F, Donati D, Tamberi S, Margutti G. Delayed emesis: incidence, pattern, prognostic factors and optimal treatment. Support Care Cancer 2002 Mar;10(2):88-95.

[7] Jordan K, Jahn F, Aapro M. Recent developments in the prevention of chemotherapy-induced nausea and vomiting (CINV): a comprehensive review. Ann Oncol 2015 Jun;26(6):1081-1090.

[8] Hesketh PJ, Aapro M, Street JC, Carides AD. Evaluation of risk factors predictive of nausea and vomiting with current standard-of-care antiemetic treatment: analysis of two phase III trials of aprepitant in patients receiving cisplatin-based chemotherapy. Support Care Cancer 2010 Sep;18(9):1171-1177.

[9] Molassiotis A, Aapro M, Dicato M, Gascon P, Novoa SA, Isambert N, et al. Evaluation of risk factors predicting chemotherapy-related nausea and vomiting: results from a European prospective observational study. J Pain Symptom Manage 2014 May;47(5):839-848.e4.

[10] Roila F, Hesketh PJ, Herrstedt J, Antiemetic Subcommitte of the Multinational Association of Supportive Care in Cancer. Prevention of chemotherapy- and radiotherapy-induced emesis: results of the 2004 Perugia International Antiemetic Consensus Conference. Ann Oncol 2006 Jan;17(1):20-28.

[11] Grunberg SM, Warr D, Gralla RJ, Rapoport BL, Hesketh PJ, Jordan K, et al. Evaluation of new antiemetic agents and definition of antineoplastic agent emetogenicity--state of the art. Support Care Cancer 2011 Mar;19 Suppl 1:S43–S47.

[12] WANG SC, BORISON HL. The vomiting center; a critical experimental analysis. Arch Neurol Psychiatry 1950 Jun;63(6):928-941.

[13] Koga T, Fukuda H. Neurons in the nucleus of the solitary tract mediating inputs from emetic vagal afferents and the area postrema to the pattern generator for the emetic act in dogs. Neurosci Res 1992 Aug;14(3):166-179.

[14] Andrews PL, Davis CJ, Bingham S, Davidson HI, Hawthorn J, Maskell L. The abdominal visceral innervation and the emetic reflex: pathways, pharmacology, and plasticity.

Can J Physiol Pharmacol 1990 Feb;68(2):325-345.

[15] Miller AD, Leslie RA. The area postrema and vomiting. Front Neuroendocrinol 1994 Dec;15(4):301-320.

[16] Saller R, Hellenbrecht D. High doses of metoclopramide or droperidol in the prevention of cisplatin-induced emesis. Eur J Cancer Clin Oncol 1986 Oct;22(10):1199-1203.

[17] Roila F, Molassiotis A, Herrstedt J, Aapro M, Gralla RJ, Bruera E, et al. 2016 MASCC and ESMO guideline update for the prevention of chemotherapy- and radiotherapy-induced nausea and vomiting and of nausea and vomiting in advanced cancer patients. Ann Oncol 2016 Sep;27(suppl 5):v119-v133.

[18] Rapoport BL. Delayed Chemotherapy-Induced Nausea and Vomiting: Pathogenesis, Incidence, and Current Management. Front Pharmacol 2017 Jan 30;8:19.

[19] Roscoe JA, Morrow GR, Aapro MS, Molassiotis A, Olver I. Anticipatory nausea and vomiting. Support Care Cancer 2011 Oct;19(10):1533-1538.

[20] del Giglio A, Soares HP, Caparroz C, Castro PC. Granisetron is equivalent to ondansetron for prophylaxis of chemotherapy-induced nausea and vomiting: results of a meta-analysis of randomized controlled trials. Cancer 2000 Dec 1;89(11):2301-2308.

[21] Jordan K, Hinke A, Grothey A, Voigt W, Arnold D, Wolf HH, et al. A meta-analysis comparing the efficacy of four 5-HT3-receptor antagonists for acute chemotherapy-induced emesis. Support Care Cancer 2007 Sep;15(9):1023-1033.

[22] Jordan K, Hinke A, Grothey A, Schmoll HJ. Granisetron versus tropisetron for prophylaxis of acute chemotherapy-induced emesis: a pooled analysis. Support Care Cancer 2005 Jan;13(1):26-31.

[23] Rao KV, Faso A. Chemotherapy-induced nausea and vomiting: optimizing prevention and management. Am Health Drug Benefits 2012 Jul;5(4):232-240.

[24] American Society of Clinical Oncology, Kris MG, Hesketh PJ, Somerfield MR, Feyer P, Clark-Snow R, et al. American Society of Clinical Oncology guideline for antiemetics in oncology: update 2006. J Clin Oncol 2006 Jun 20;24(18):2932-2947.

[25] Gralla R, Lichinitser M, Van Der Vegt S, Sleeboom H, Mezger J, Peschel C, et al. Palonosetron improves prevention of chemotherapy-induced nausea and vomiting following moderately emetogenic chemotherapy: results of a double-blind randomized phase III trial comparing single doses of palonosetron with ondansetron. Ann Oncol 2003 Oct;14(10):1570-1577.

[26] Eisenberg P, Figueroa-Vadillo J, Zamora R, Charu V, Hajdenberg J, Cartmell A, et al. Improved prevention of moderately emetogenic chemotherapy-induced nausea and vomiting with palonosetron, a pharmacologically novel 5-HT3 receptor antagonist: results of a phase III, single-dose trial versus dolasetron. Cancer 2003 Dec 1;98(11):2473-2482.

[27] Aapro MS, Grunberg SM, Manikhas GM, Olivares G, Suarez T, Tjulandin SA, et al. A phase III, double-blind, randomized trial of palonosetron compared with ondansetron in preventing chemotherapy-induced nausea and vomiting following highly emetogenic chemotherapy. Ann Oncol 2006 Sep;17(9):1441-1449.

[28] Basch E, Hesketh PJ, Kris MG, Prestrud AA, Temin S, Lyman GH. Antiemetics: american society of

clinical oncology clinical practice guideline update. J Oncol Pract 2011 Nov;7(6):395-398.

[29] Poli-Bigelli S, Rodrigues-Pereira J, Carides AD, Julie Ma G, Eldridge K, Hipple A, et al. Addition of the neurokinin 1 receptor antagonist aprepitant to standard antiemetic therapy improves control of chemotherapy-induced nausea and vomiting. Results from a randomized, double-blind, placebo-controlled trial in Latin America. Cancer 2003 Jun 15;97(12):3090-3098.

[30] Hesketh PJ, Grunberg SM, Gralla RJ, Warr DG, Roila F, de Wit R, et al. The oral neurokinin-1 antagonist aprepitant for the prevention of chemotherapy-induced nausea and vomiting: a multinational, randomized, double-blind, placebo-controlled trial in patients receiving high-dose cisplatin--the Aprepitant Protocol 052 Study Group. J Clin Oncol 2003 Nov 15;21(22):4112-4119.

[31] Schmoll HJ, Aapro MS, Poli-Bigelli S, Kim HK, Park K, Jordan K, et al. Comparison of an aprepitant regimen with a multiple-day ondansetron regimen, both with dexamethasone, for antiemetic efficacy in high-dose cisplatin treatment. Ann Oncol 2006 Jun;17(6):1000-1006.

[32] Warr DG, Hesketh PJ, Gralla RJ, Muss HB, Herrstedt J, Eisenberg PD, et al. Efficacy and tolerability of aprepitant for the prevention of chemotherapy-induced nausea and vomiting in patients with breast cancer after moderately emetogenic chemotherapy. J Clin Oncol 2005 Apr 20;23(12):2822-2830.

[33] Grunberg S, Chua D, Maru A, Dinis J, DeVandry S, Boice JA, et al. Single-dose fosaprepitant for the prevention of chemotherapy-induced nausea and vomiting associated with cisplatin therapy: randomized, double-blind study protocol--EASE. J Clin Oncol 2011 Apr 10;29(11):1495-1501.

[34] Heo YA, Deeks ED. Rolapitant: A Review in Chemotherapy-Induced Nausea and Vomiting. Drugs 2017 Oct;77(15):1687-1691.

[35] Keating GM. Netupitant/Palonosetron: A Review in the Prevention of Chemotherapy-Induced Nausea and Vomiting. Drugs 2015 Dec;75(18):2131-2141.

[36] Depre M, Van Hecken A, Oeyen M, De Lepeleire I, Laethem T, Rothenberg P, et al. Effect of aprepitant on the pharmacokinetics and pharmacodynamics of warfarin. Eur J Clin Pharmacol 2005 Jul;61(5-6):341-346.

[37] Rapoport B, Chua D, Poma A, Arora S, Wang Y, Fein LE. Study of rolapitant, a novel, long-acting, NK-1 receptor antagonist, for the prevention of chemotherapy-induced nausea and vomiting (CINV) due to highly emetogenic chemotherapy (HEC). Support Care Cancer 2015 Nov;23(11):3281-3288.

[38] Schwartzberg LS, Modiano MR, Rapoport BL, Chasen MR, Gridelli C, Urban L, et al. Safety and efficacy of rolapitant for prevention of chemotherapy-induced nausea and vomiting after administration of moderately emetogenic chemotherapy or anthracycline and cyclophosphamide regimens in patients with cancer: a randomised, active-controlled, double-blind, phase 3 trial. Lancet Oncol 2015 Sep;16(9):1071-1078.

[39] Takahashi T, Nakamura Y, Tsuya A, Murakami H, Endo M, Yamamoto N. Pharmacokinetics of aprepitant and dexamethasone after administration of chemotherapeutic agents and effects of plasma substance P concentration on chemotherapy-induced nausea and

vomiting in Japanese cancer patients. Cancer Chemother Pharmacol 2011 Sep;68(3):653-659.

[40] AaproM,KarthausM,SchwartzbergL, Bondarenko I, Sarosiek T, Oprean C, et al. NEPA, a fixed oral combination of netupitant and palonosetron, improves control of chemotherapy-induced nausea and vomiting (CINV) over multiple cycles of chemotherapy: results of a randomized, double-blind, phase 3 trial versus oral palonosetron. Support Care Cancer 2017 Apr;25(4):1127-1135.

[41] Navari RM, Einhorn LH, Loehrer PJ S, Passik SD, Vinson J, McClean J, et al. A phase II trial of olanzapine, dexamethasone, and palonosetron for the prevention of chemotherapy-induced nausea and vomiting: a Hoosier oncology group study. Support Care Cancer 2007 Nov;15(11):1285-007-0248-5. Epub 2007 Mar 21.

[42] Navari RM, Einhorn LH, Passik SD, Loehrer PJ S, Johnson C, Mayer ML, et al. A phase II trial of olanzapine for the prevention of chemotherapy-induced nausea and vomiting: a Hoosier Oncology Group study. Support Care Cancer 2005 Jul;13(7):529-534.

[43] Parker LA, Rock EM, Limebeer CL. Regulation of nausea and vomiting by cannabinoids. Br J Pharmacol 2011 Aug;163(7):1411-1422.

[44] Tramer MR, Carroll D, Campbell FA, Reynolds DJ, Moore RA, McQuay HJ. Cannabinoids for control of chemotherapy induced nausea and vomiting: quantitative systematic review. BMJ 2001 Jul 7;323(7303):16-21.

[45] Smith LA, Azariah F, Lavender VT, Stoner NS, Bettiol S. Cannabinoids for nausea and vomiting in adults with cancer receiving chemotherapy. Cochrane Database Syst Rev 2015 Nov 12;(11):CD009464. doi(11):CD009464.

[46] Kamen C, Tejani MA, Chandwani K, Janelsins M, Peoples AR, Roscoe JA, et al. Anticipatory nausea and vomiting due to chemotherapy. Eur J Pharmacol 2014 Jan 5;722:172-179.

[47] Arslan M, Ozdemir L. Oral intake of ginger for chemotherapy-induced nausea and vomiting among women with breast cancer. Clin J Oncol Nurs 2015 Oct;19(5):E92–E97.

[48] Ryan JL, Heckler CE, Roscoe JA, Dakhil SR, Kirshner J, Flynn PJ, et al. Ginger (Zingiber officinale) reduces acute chemotherapy-induced nausea: a URCC CCOP study of 576 patients. Support Care Cancer 2012 Jul;20(7):1479-1489.

[49] Lee J, Oh H. Ginger as an antiemetic modality for chemotherapy-induced nausea and vomiting: a systematic review and meta-analysis. Oncol Nurs Forum 2013 Mar;40(2):163-170.

[50] Enblom A, Johnsson A, Hammar M, Onelov E, Steineck G, Borjeson S. Acupuncture compared with placebo acupuncture in radiotherapy-induced nausea--a randomized controlled study. Ann Oncol 2012 May;23(5):1353-1361.

[51] Genc A, Can G, Aydiner A. The efficiency of the acupressure in prevention of the chemotherapy-induced nausea and vomiting. Support Care Cancer 2013 Jan;21(1):253-261.

[52] Molassiotis A, Russell W, Hughes J, Breckons M, Lloyd-Williams M, Richardson J, et al. The effectiveness and cost-effectiveness of acupressure for the control and management of chemotherapy-related acute and delayed nausea: Assessment of Nausea in Chemotherapy Research (ANCHoR), a randomised controlled trial. Health Technol Assess 2013 Jun;17(26):1-114.

[53] Dennis K, Jamani R, McGrath C, Makhani L, Lam H, Bauer P, et al. A

systematic review of methodologies, endpoints, and outcome measures in randomized trials of radiation therapy-induced nausea and vomiting. Support Care Cancer 2017 Jun;25(6):2019-2033.

[54] Abbott B, Ippoliti C, Bruton J, Neumann J, Whaley R, Champlin R. Antiemetic efficacy of granisetron plus dexamethasone in bone marrow transplant patients receiving chemotherapy and total body irradiation. Bone Marrow Transplant 1999 Feb;23(3):265-269.

[55] National Cancer Institute of Canada Clinical Trials Group (SC19), Wong RK, Paul N, Ding K, Whitehead M, Brundage M, et al. 5-hydroxytryptamine-3 receptor antagonist with or without short-course dexamethasone in the prophylaxis of radiation induced emesis: a placebo-controlled randomized trial of the National Cancer Institute of Canada Clinical Trials Group (SC19). J Clin Oncol 2006 Jul 20;24(21):3458-3464.

[56] Hesketh PJ, Kris MG, Basch E, Bohlke K, Barbour SY, Clark-Snow RA, et al. Antiemetics: American Society of Clinical Oncology Clinical Practice Guideline Update. J Clin Oncol 2017 Oct 1;35(28):3240-3261.

[57] Dennis K, Jamani R, McGrath C, Makhani L, Lam H, Bauer P, et al. A systematic review of methodologies, endpoints, and outcome measures in randomized trials of radiation therapy-induced nausea and vomiting. Support Care Cancer 2017 Jun;25(6):2019-2033.

[58] Ruhlmann CH, Jahn F, Jordan K, Dennis K, Maranzano E, Molassiotis A, et al. 2016 updated MASCC/ESMO consensus recommendations: prevention of radiotherapy-induced nausea and vomiting. Support Care Cancer 2017 Jan;25(1):309-316.

[59] Zhang Y, Lin L, Li H, Hu Y, Tian L. Effects of acupuncture on cancer-related fatigue: a meta-analysis. Support Care Cancer 2018 Feb;26(2):415-425.

[60] Ezzo JM, Richardson MA, Vickers A, Allen C, Dibble SL, Issell BF, et al. Acupuncture-point stimulation for chemotherapy-induced nausea or vomiting. Cochrane Database Syst Rev 2006 Apr 19;(2):CD002285. doi(2):CD002285.

[61] Shi Y, Xu T, Chen Q, Wu J, Zhong Y, Song S, et al. Acupuncture for radiotherapy-induced nausea and vomiting: A systematic review protocol. Medicine (Baltimore) 2019 Jun;98(24):e16027.

Chapter 11

Assessment and Management of Pain in Palliative Care

Sonika Charak, Robin George Thattil, Chandra Mohan Srivastava, Prabhu Prasad Das and Manish Shandilya

Abstract

Palliative care is an essential component in any disease management. Pain assessment acts as the connecting link between the nerves, brain and spinal cord. Classification and assessment of the pain have great significance in controlling the pain-related symptoms. Pain is broadly divided into three types nociceptive, neuropathic and mixed depending upon the damage caused. Nociceptive pain is caused due to the stimulation of the pain receptors in the tissues and is further divided into visceral and somatic depending on the pain site. Neuropathic pain arises when the nervous system gets damaged or start dysfunctioning. Cancer pain assessment includes several factors like the site, intensity, syndrome, timing and temporal variation of pain. Edmonton staging system for cancer pain prognostic is widely used for pain management includes emotional/psychological distress cognitive impairment caused by pain. A comprehensive understanding of pain assessment will help in enhancing the quality of life of the patients.

Keywords: Pain assessment, Pain management, Nociceptive, Neuropathic, Opioids

1. Introduction

Pain is broadly defined as the unpleasant sensations in the body resulting due to the complex experience of various factors like physical, psychological and emotional [1]. Pain is subjective as pain tolerance differs from person to person. Pain cannot be quantified as it is associated with the effective as well as sensory components. Most cancer patients claim pain as the most common symptom and are quite dreaded, a major cause of anxiety [1]. Palliative care is an essential component in disease management. Good pain management is an important step towards palliative care. First of all, it is very important to understand the cause of pain, then assessment and manage pain, finally reassessment and monitoring the factors resulting in the pain. Managing and correct assessment of these symptoms are important for the wellbeing of the person to whom palliative care is being given.

It is very important to note that palliative care is intended to provide quality life by symptom control. To accomplish this, it is must to classify and assess the effects of pain. Pain is classified into various categories depending upon the duration, location, intensity and etiology of the pain (**Figure 1**). Pain can be acute or chronic depending on the duration of the pain. Acute pain is not long-lasting

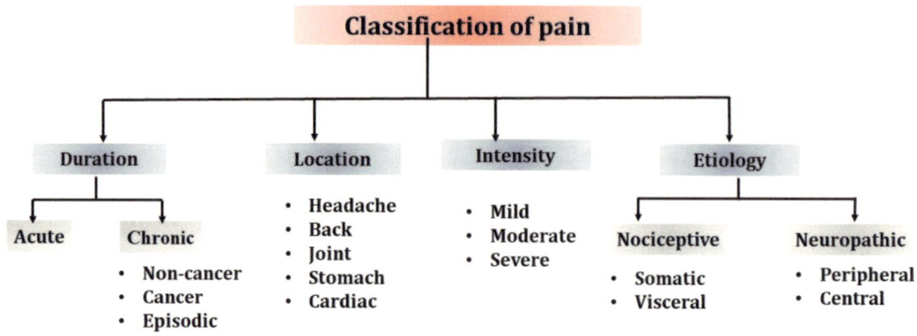

Figure 1.
Classification of pain.

as it gets resolved within a short duration whereas pain that cannot be resolved within six months is considered chronic pain. Chronic pain is further of three types: non-cancer, cancer and episodic. The intensity of pain ranges from mild to severe. Pathophysiology is mostly done by the utilization and knowledge of the damage caused to the tissue (nociceptive) and nerve (neuropathic) or could be unlocalized (visceral) or break-through that was given by the International Association for the Study of Pain (IASP) [2, 3]. It is noteworthy that pain can be physical as well as emotional. European Association for Palliative Care (EAPC) conducted an extensive review on the management of the use of pain assessment tools in palliative care research [3–5]. The newly revised version of cancer pain prognostics has included emotional/psychological distress, cognitive impairment caused by pain in the Edmonton staging system for cancer pain [4]. This improvement in pain prognostics has been able to be predictive than the previous methods used by IASP [3]. There are methods for the staging and progression of cancer like TNM Classification of Malignant Tumors (TNM). Unfortunately, there is no consensus on a single standardized tool for pain assessment [6]. The reason behind this is the varied nature of cancer and its malignancy and different perceptive and tolerance of pain in patients [6, 7]. Also, to blame is less predictability of the nature of tools available, as sometimes the mechanisms are not well known. To work on this problem, an extensive literature study on the physical, medical, psychological background and education on self-awareness/acceptance of pain should be deemed feasible.

2. Cause of pain

2.1 Nociceptive pain

It is also known as momentary pain. It is a form of acute pain caused by the triggering of nociceptive nerve receptors. This triggering occurs as a result of damaging chemicals or inflammation in the region [8]. A great example will be hitting your head on the table or stubbing your toe. Generally, nociceptive pain location is local. This type of pain gets notified by the nociceptors present throughout the skin and the internal organs. They can detect any chemical or physical damage send through the nervous system for immediate action [9]. There are two types of nociceptors as suggested by F. Cervero in 1985; one of them works for the fast transmission of pain called A-delta fibers whereas another one that slowly transmits pain is C–fibers [8]. The unmyelinated structure of C-fibres detects sudden pain while A-delta fibers detect pain arising due to noxious elements or mechanical stress [8]. Increased abnormal sensitivity to the pain or chemical stimulus is named hyperalgesia caused by inflammation in the area [8–10].

Nociceptive pain is divided into two components:

- Somatic
- Visceral

2.1.1 Somatic pain

This type of pain arises from the stimulation of the nerve cells in the tissue such as skin, bones muscles, etc. due to damage [11]. Based on the site of cause the person can have superficial or surface-level deep somatic pain in bone or tendons and this type of pain comes in a flash as the injury is sustained [9, 11]. Due to the two varied nature of this pain person suffering from superficial pain will have an easier go at finding and pinpointing the pain rather than the deep somatic pain which is much harder to pinpoint as it diffuses easily and tends to radiate.

2.1.2 Visceral pain

Visceral pain occurs in cases when the person suffers from damage to the internal organs such as the intestine etc. The sensation of pain can be caused by damage to the tissue by external force or extensive pressure caused due to oncological reasons or infection in the abdominal organs [4, 8, 12]. This pain is not easy to pinpoint as the patient feels dull and as if squeezing most of the time due to the scarcity of the nociceptors [4]. Feeling in the area of damage detected by the nociceptors present in the abdominal cavity and on the organs it doesn't have a sharp onset visceral pain [8]. This effect is also termed as viscero-somatic convergence where the pain signal transported by afferent nerves converge with the nerves that are transferring pain from the say skin area can cause side effects such as nausea vomiting etc. [12].

2.2 Non-nociceptive pain

2.2.1 Neuropathic pain

This type of pain is characterized by the damage or improper function/misfiring of the neurons. The IASP defines neuropathic pain "pain initiated or caused by a primary lesion or dysfunction in the peripheral or central nervous system. A study by Martin, L. A., & Hagen, N. A. (1997) broadly classified them into peripheral and central neuropathic pain. Peripheral neuropathic pain has many sub iterations depending on the nerves involved. In a case study done by them, it was stated that out of 72 patients, six of whom had benign tumors, suffered central neuropathic pain [13]. This study concludes that the nerves that get damaged will start firing erratically with or without any nociceptive signal. Patients suffering from such chronic pain have reported that they experience pain constantly and are shooting in nature [13]. The pain can be triggered by a small number of stimuli or even without any stimuli. Multiple reports and studies suggest that hyperactivity of damaged neurons and further release of neurotransmitters, inducers, modulators, increase the effect [2, 10, 14]. Also, it is noted that the person's immune response to the pain releases cytokines which also elevate the neuropathic pain. Diseases such as diabetes, chronic back pain, alcohol consumption, cancer stroke are some reasons for this type of pain. The sympathetic nervous system can lead to the increased sensitivity of the nerves. The release of hormones during flight/fight response increases awareness and due to this the nerves also get more sensitized leading to such pain suggested by Gierthmühlen, J. and R. Baron in 2016 [10].

2.2.2 Psychological effect on pain

Psychological factors are the major players in how the patient perceive the pain. Factors such as initial awareness, emotional status, interpretation and processing of pain and coping strategy play an important role in the perception of the pain [15]. Research on the effect of psychology and mental state by S.J. Linton and W.S. Shaw defines that initial detection of pain plays a crucial role in building up the psychological effects of it [16]. It is noted that pain needs attention and it is mostly under our conscious control. If the pain is deemed a threat, the autonomous nervous system kicks in, and also for later stages the object is likely to be avoided. Emotional state and interpretation can play a major role in sensitization and interpretation of pain [16]. Pain behaviour can be linked to how the person interprets the pain while suffering from it like verbal or non-verbal action and also after suffering from pain like the patient may start avoiding the source of stimuli as it generates the fear response. Negative thoughts about life such as anxiety, depression and fear can negatively affect the perception of pain and this may consequence in not only increasing the intensity but also prolonging the pain. Studies such as in S.J. Linton and W.S. Shaw in 2011 have shown 52% of people suffer from such a negative emotional state during pain [16]. Patients with imminent fear of the future also fall in this category and this all consequences in poor rehabilitation of the patient [15]. The next stage comes to coping with the pain, it has been seen that painful stimuli trigger the flight response with epinephrine released that can greatly affect the sensation of pain [15, 16]. It can be inferred by this that in both cases, the sensation seems to be more tolerable as the person either avoids pain or confronts the source. The other method that seems to work is having a relaxed state of mind. Effects such as phantom limb pain are still considered to be a psychological phenomenon [17, 18]. Even though the limb does not exist, the pain is still perceived. In all, pain is greatly affected by the mental state of the person, but it has to be well understood and more studied.

3. Tools for analysing pain intensity

Pain intensity is subjective from person to person hence a common ground is picked which either in pictorial form or in the form of a questionnaire is communicated between the patient and the caregiver where the caregiver gets an idea of the situation and can plan before the treatment. These pain intensity tools play a major role in the assessment of pain and the tools used to analyze. There are many tools, but few are used quite often such as the McGill pain questionnaire, Wong-baker face pain scale, (**Figure 2**) visual analogue and numerical scales (**Figure 3**). Much of them work in a similar method by presenting the patient with a pictorial or a numerical based scale that the person can relate to and the person can pinpoint on which part of the scale he/she thinks the pain suffered stands [7].

3.1 Unidimensional pain assessment tools

The unidimensional assessment tool consists of mainly 2 categories which include the visual analogue scale or numerical rating scale and the pictorial rating

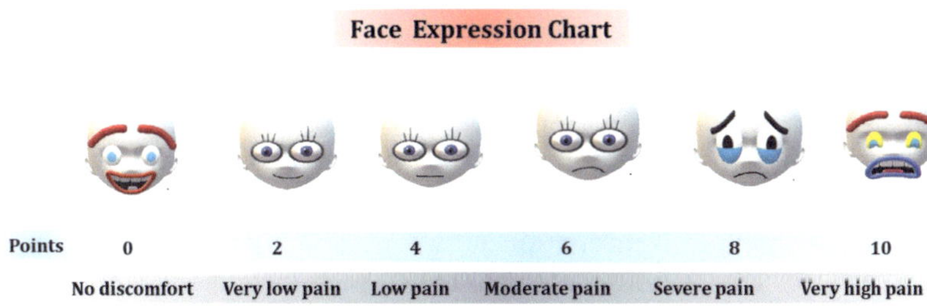

Figure 2.
Visual analogue pain intensity scale. Patient has to pin-point on where their pain stands on the scale [7].

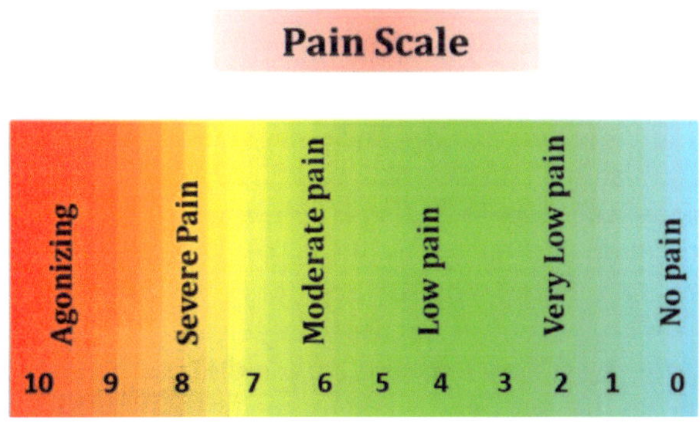

Figure 3.
Wong-baker face pain scale. The physician and the patient can look and state which expression they feel matches the scale. Ages 3 and above [7].

scale. These may or may not include verbal descriptions of the pain such as - moderate, severe, or less pain. In the visual analogue and the numerical method of scaling, a patient is asked to choose and mark the word or the number they compare/relate their pain to [17, 19]. The other method is utilizing the pictorial representation (**Figure 2**) such as faces which utilizes the comical representation of the reactions suffered during pain this method is best suited for children as it is difficult for them to translate a sensory experience to a spot on the scale example of such pictorial scale is Wong-baker face pain scale which utilizes 6 facial expressions describing the severity of pain [7].

The drawback of these methods is that these methods rely on the opinion of the patient and the opinion may vary due to different pain tolerance limits in different patients to the same pain sources [7]. Tolerance of a patient can be judged for a specific area using a dolorimeter which uses heat, electricity, or pressure to analyze the sample area's sensitivity and this can be later noted for further scaling [7].

3.2 Multi-dimensional pain assessment tools

As the name implies this type of tool assesses a patient on different levels/dimensions compared to the unidimensional pain assessment method. The Multi-dimensional method includes an assessment of more features such as the impact of pain, quality of pain and phenotype of pain for example to determine whether the person is suffering from neuropathic pain or not [19]. These tools utilize different types of the questionnaire to achieve its goal such as determining the impact and screening of the pain.

These include:

Brief Pain Inventory (BPI).
McGill Pain Questionnaire (MPQ).
Neuropathic Pain Scale (NPS).
Pain Quality Assessment Scale (PQAS).
Leeds Assessment of Neuropathic Symptoms and Signs (LANSS).
Neuropathic Pain Questionnaire (NPQ).
Douleur Neuropathique en 4 Questions (DN4) [20, 21].

3.2.1 Brief Pain Inventory (BPI)

BPI was developed by Collaborating Centre for Symptom Evaluation in Cancer Care, a team of WHO [22]. This is a method incorporated to assess self-reported pain severity and any interference in daily functioning, used in both clinical and research settings and is widely utilized and recognized in cancer pain assessment it is being self-administered and easy to access [7, 20, 23, 24]. It was approved and translated into many languages including Hindi, Spanish, Brazilian, etc. [22]. The subject is asked to fill up nine questions like if they have been feeling pain recently, location of the pain (a pictorial representation of both dorsal and ventral side of the human body which the subject can use to highlight the area of distress), pain intensity/severity during different intervals and other questions may include the effect of the drugs like an opioid taken for medication for pain management and lastly how pain affects your mood and your daily routine [25]. The scoring is divided into two categories that are pain severity and pain interference with a score of 0–10 where zero being no pain and ten being severe [25]. Similar scaling is done for interference also the final scoring is 0–40 and 0–70 respectively [25]. Multiple studies suggest that this two-dimensional tool (BPI) is quite adequate and is a capable method in analyzing pain intensity and pain interference caused due to neuropathic and nociceptive pain. In cancer pain assessment such as in a study conducted with 199 patients who underwent radiotherapy and results showed that there is a good correlation with an increase in pain intensity and its interference in the daily routine after radiotherapy [22].

3.2.2 Neuropathic Pain Scale (NPS)

As the name suggests it is a scale that is utilized for the differentiation in the neuropathic and non-neuropathic pain developed by Galer and Jensen [26, 27]. This scale contains 11 items for judging the qualitative and quantitative aspects of pain [20]. These items include pain intensity and its effect some items help in determining the features of the neuropathic pain such as sharpness, sensitivity, etc., and also how deep the pain is [28]. These items help in drawing a more accurate picture of the location and the quality of the pain widely utilized in the diagnosis of multiple sclerosis [20, 27, 28].

3.2.3 Pain Quality Assessment Scale (PQAS)

It is also a multidimensional scaling tool with questions that are explained descriptively such as sensitivity etc. In case of severity of pain, a numerical rating from 1 to 10 with ten being severe pain. The patient is advised to fill up/mark answers to the questions based on 20 items. These queries were recently revised by Mark P. Jensen in a cognitive revision test of the items to make them more understandable by the patients [21].

3.2.4 Leeds Assessment of Neuropathic Symptoms and Signs (LANSS)

LANSS was developed to address the less reliability of the NPS in neuropathic pain. This tool has a self-reportable version similar to BPI called S-LANASS with seven elements each weighted differently and is readily used in cancer pain assessment [20, 26, 27, 29]. Five questions mostly deal with yes or no questions for the severity, location, sensitivity, duration, etc. The last two questions are activity-based and require certain diagnostic actions such as gentle touching/rubbing the painful area [26, 29, 30]. These help in deducing if there is any nerve dysfunction, the final scoring is given by 24 [26, 29]. If the person receives a general score of less than 12 the pain is designated in the nociceptive section if the scoring is greater than 12 then the person falls in the category of neuropathic or Pain of Predominantly Neuropathic Origin (POPNO) [29, 30]. Originally designed by Michael Bennett has now been translated to many languages such as German Turkish, Chinese and even in Malayalam. It confirms the validation of this tool 101 chronic pain suffering patients were brought of which fifty patient were nociceptive and fifty-one were neuropathic the test concluded with a Cohen's Kappa 0.743(is a statistical analysis to test the reliability of a test with a range of −1 to +; generally >0.70 values are considered substantial) with 89.5% sensitivity [29, 31].

3.2.5 Neuropathic Pain Questionnaire (NPQ)

This is another method for judging and differentiating neuropathic pain from non-neuropathic pain [20]. A test regarding the validation on 528 chronic pain suffering patients of which 149 of them with neuropathic symptoms they were asked to fill up the NPQ with 12 items with the last 2 related effect of pain [32]. It was noted that it had a very low-reliability rate (66% sensitivity only) because of which it is not much popular as compared to the others [20, 30, 32]. Hence, it has been mainly used in the initial screening of neuropathic pain [20].

3.2.6 Douleur Neuropathique 4 Questions (DN4)

A ten-item scaling method utilized in the characterization of neuropathic pain has 4 questions that are simple to attempt with validated cognitive tests to prove its understandability to the patients it is administered to [21]. It has been translated into many languages and has a sensitivity of 83% [20].

3.2.7 McGill Pain Questionnaire (MPQ)

McGill pain questionnaire established by Dr. Melzack and Torgerson in 1971 at McGill University in Montreal, Canada is widely used in assessment tools for monitoring the intensity of pain [7]. Many studies have been conducted on the questionnaire such as by B Nicholson suggesting that it is a documentation method that utilizes the patient's experience like how he feels the pain, duration site, etc. [3, 7, 14]. A survey done by P. Kumar et al. showed that a total of 297 patients who underwent MPQ reported that it was qualitatively and quantitatively satisfying [7]. It gives multiple choices that help in identifying and in relating the pain suffered by the patient and these can be later compared with changes in a longer period of monitoring the patient [7, 14]. Not only that it also gives a human diagram to point out wherein the body the pain exists. With questions such as where your pain is? Is it internal or external? And the multiple-choice for how the pain changes with time, with this it seems to be quite regarded and efficient in diagnosing pain and related ailments [14].

4. Methods of pain assessment (pain assessment tools)

Assessment is the rigorous process of documentation, self-knowledge and interpretation. The need for cancer pain assessment during and after the treatment at the end-of-life stage is very important. Many contributing factors may affect the diagnosis of the source of the pain. Due to the varied nature complexity in the classification of pain, there is no consensus on a common pain assessment tool. This is to be noted and a common effective method should be there to evaluate the pain and its history in the patient. Since the pain assessed is in the boundary of cancer, the method to stage malignancy and its type is measured by TNM classification of cancer. Since its discovery, it has been proficiently helping in the further planning of treatment to be provided. With the staging ranging from 1 to 4 with the fourth being severe [3, 6]. TNM staging plays an important role in the assessment of the pain as it can convey information about size, if it is malignant or if it has spread into the lymph [6]. Similarly, widely used pain assessment tools are

- International Association for the Study of Pain -IASP assessment tool for chronic pain taxonomy
- Edmonton classification system for cancer pain -ECS-CP
- Cancer pain prognostic scale-CPPS [3].
- Alberta breakthrough pain assessment tool [33–36].

4.1 International Association for the Study of Pain (IASP)- Assessment Tool for Chronic Pain Taxonomy

It is a symptom sign-based type of deducing the effects of chronic pain in the patient. It is the list of diseases that provide information and classification of pain. Studies on the basis of the location of occurrence the pain, where it is present in the body. Next comes how the patient feels the pain like it is pinching, radiating or may be flickering in nature or does it change as time passes. This helps the clinical person to deduce the type of pain whether neuropathic or nociceptive and also possible organ system that is affected by the pain by deducing if it is visceral or somatic. The last consideration taken is the intensity of the pain [3, 14]. To extract this information, the patient is asked to fill up a questionnaire such as the McGill pain questionnaire which deals with [7, 14]. The problem with such classification of pain is that it is not predictive in similar aspects to TNM which is predictive and can give an idea on how to plan the treatment [3, 6]. Due to much-received criticism, changes were done in 2011 namely, the International Classification of Disease 11th revision (ICD -11) was for chronic pain groups such as chronic cancer pain involving the use of visceral and neuropathic pain and also adding continuous pain and episodic pain (pain that comes and goes) [2].

The IASP classification of chronic pain is done by using these following groups/ domains

Domain 1-The site where the pain occurs
Domain 2-Organ systems that get affected due to pain
Domain 3-Temporal characteristics deal with the frequency of pain
Domain 4-Intensity of the pain and time passed since its onset
Domain 5-Pain etiology [3].

4.2 Cancer pain prognostics scale

It is a numerical-based scale for characterizing and for running prognostic assessment of the condition and it is more predictive as compared to the previous ones. It is based on the scores ranging from 0 to 17, where the higher the scoring on this scale the good/better the prognosis and better chances of pain relief. Hence, this is a very useful tool in determining poor prognostics amongst patients [2]. This scaling has added features compared to IASP assessment for pain such as

Domain 1-Worst of pain
Domain 2- Emotional well-being of the patient
Domain 3- Pain characteristics
Domain 4- Daily opioid consumption [3].

Where scaling for worst pain is given from 1 to10, for emotional well-being is judged by using Functional Assessment of Cancer Therapy (FACT-G) and the daily opioid dose is monitored for greater than 60 mg consumption as its higher levels of it will make it difficult to control pain and person seems to be more tolerant [3].

4.3 Edmonton classification system for cancer pain (ECS-CP)

To improve on the IASP system of classification for chronic pain, there is a better versed and more widely accepted method of classification called ECS-CP (Edmonton Classification System for Cancer Pain) also is incorporated in the multisite of European Palliative Care Research Collaborative (EPCRC) [3, 4]. It is a more rigorous and user-friendly system of pain classification compared to the previous iterations for classifying pain. Additional descriptive features for pain classification are also incorporated such as the patient's emotional wellbeing. Other than this it incorporates seven components to evaluate the patient as suggested by Bruera E.[4]:

Domain 1-Mechanism of pain
Domain 2- Characteristics
Domain 3- Cognitive function
Domain 4- Previous opioid use
Domain 5-Psychological distress
Domain 6- Tolerance
Domain 7-History of such related pain [2, 4, 37].

Hence it is implied that this is better for further prognosis and pain treatment as this not only keeps check on the emotional/psychological distress but also considers the patient history of having difficulties in the same area or maybe similar types of pain [2, 4, 37]. Also, to be noted that it also checks whether if there is any case of taking opioids and if due to pain there is any cognitive impairment in the concerned patient though their involvement is still debated in the process of pain assessment in the newer version of this model. This method of assessment and prognosis of pain has widely been reviewed and validated in many studies and there is still improvement going on.

ECS-CP questionnaire categories are further dived into subcategories such as the understanding mechanism of pain it can be divided into the following subcategories (**Table 1**) [4]. These can be denoted by a letter such as N for the

S.No	Mechanism Of Pain (M)	Your Response	Characteristics Of Pain (C)	Your Response	Cognitive Function (F)	Your Response	Psychological Distress (P)	Your Response	Past History Of Addictive Abuse (A)	Your Response
1	Nociceptive Pain		Incident Pains		Normal Functioning		No Distress		Yes, Present	
2	Neuropathic Pain		Non- Incident Pains		Abnormal Functioning		Distress Present		Not Present	
3	No Pain Felt		No Incident Pains							
	Specify if, Psychological distress is present: ____ Specify if, Past history of addictive abuse: ____ *Result: M__C__F__P__A__*									

Table 1.
ECS-CP questionnaire.

category and subcategory can be in small caps alphabetic or numerical, the lower sub-feature as seen provides more information higher the chances of good prognosis. Similarly, for the rest of the groups depending on the new version such as opioid intake, tolerance, they are also divided into subcategories according to their function [2, 4].

4.4 Alberta breakthrough pain assessment tool (ABPAT)

ABPAT was developed by Alberta Cancer Board and the Alberta Cancer Foundation. It is an emerging tool for pain prognostics and works under the boundaries of assessing breakthrough pain. This method was developed by a knowledgeable panel of the reviewer by utilizing the Delphi process and conducting many patient's think-aloud interviews [34, 36]. Breakthrough pain is generally categorized as a sudden increase or flaring of existing chronic pain such as in cases of cancer or joint-related problems [33]. It is reported that breakthrough pain in cancer patients, its occurrence is about 40–93%, hence quite common as it has come up quite a lot of times that no standardized assessment tool exists so the goal of Alberta breakthrough pain assessment tool was to provide a standardized format for research purposes [34]. Using the opinion of experts in this field reaching a consensus a questionnaire of 17 questions was put out. Next came the validation of this process, whether the patients were understanding what they have been asked to fill up so that the researcher added the think-aloud to judge the comprehensive and cognitive understanding of the people participating in the survey (**Figure 4**). This helped in the revaluation of their question by rigorous feedback from the participants and adding any changes in between.

The format of questions participants was asked:

- Relationship to the baseline pain
- Location and intensity of pain
- Quality, duration and frequency of pain
- Predictability of pain
- Response to medication [34].

This was well evaluated in a study conducted that was mentioned by Sperlinga R. where approximately 90% of the participants said that the questions were understandable and 80% said that it is a good tool for the breakthrough problem [35]. The validation and reviewing of the results were done both nationally and internationally such as in UK, Australia, Middle-East, Israel and North America and many respondents that participated in the survey were from medical nursing fields [34].

4.4.1 Why pain arises?

Pain is the 3rd most common symptom of cancer and reportedly has many reasons for the cause of pain from cancer [38]. It winds up being the patient-related factors such as, the location of the tumor, the neural system and the tissue being affected, stage of cancer its malignancy etc. People also suffer from pain related discomfort while going through the treatment of cancer which includes surgery for the removal of the tumor from the affected area, chemotherapy and radiotherapy

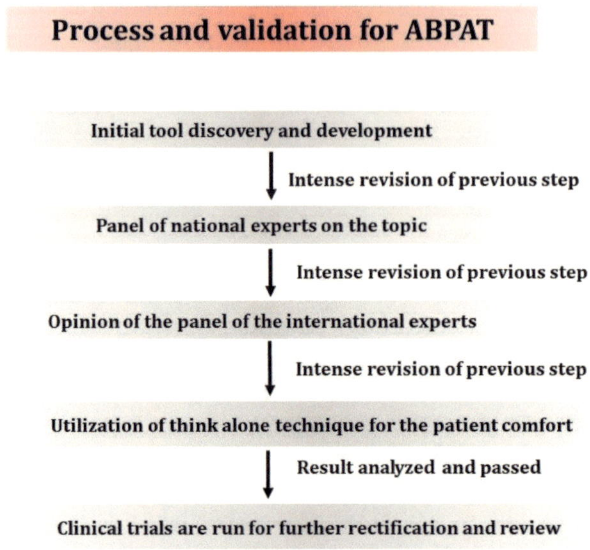

Figure 4.
Flowchart representing research design for ABPAT [34].

that the patient may be undergoing for managing cancer [39]. Hence cancer pain can be broadly divided into two categories

1. Pain caused due to tumor

2. Pain caused while undergoing treatment

Tumor related cancer pain mainly occurs due to excessive pressure on the nearby tissue or bone (Cancer-induced bone pain) and nerve causing the sensation of pain. Also, this can lead to blockages to a certain area and bodily mechanism of transport of nutrients, causing tissue damage which can cause both nociceptive pain and neuropathic pain if the nerves are damaged [38, 40]. Inflammatory responses can also be a major player in destroying affected areas such as in a study related to pancreatic cancer. It was noted that due to inflammation transient receptor potential cation channel gets activated which in turn activates Substance P (SP) and Calcitonin Gene-Related Peptide (CGRP) two neurotransmitters that transfer pain signals to dorsal root ganglia [38]. In the case of cancer-induced bone pain, cancer cells release RANKL (Receptor activator of nuclear factor kappa-B ligand) which increases the reabsorption of the bone by osteoclasts degrading the bone and sensitizing pain nerves [41, 42]. Drugs that are used in the treatment of neoplastic disease(chemotherapy) such as Bortezomib, Cisplatin, Vincristine, etc. although are widely used and effective but have a big downside of causing peripheral neuropathy by damaging sensory neurons, dorsal root ganglia and neurons present in the spinal cord [40]. Surgical procedures cause side effects in many cases and may have minor damage to the operated area. This can lead to neuralgia due to damaged nerve or in one study on myofascial pain syndrome caused after post breast cancer surgery. The neuromuscular damage after breast cancer surgery in the thoracic area stays contracted in pressure and is sensitive to myofascial trigger points [39, 43]. Even patients who are undergoing radiotherapy for head neck cancer have reported that radiotherapy results in other problems like mucositis in their buccal cavity and their throat and esophageal tract with severe lesioning [44]. These studies suggest that cancer pain can not only be caused by the tumor but also by the treatment that the person is undergoing.

4.4.2 Treatment and management

The best and widely accepted treatment in cancer pain is the utilization of opioids which are predominantly used for symptomatic treatment of pain [45]. Opioids function by binding to opioid binding receptors such as (mu, kappa, delta, and sigma) and these ligands and receptors are present throughout the body. Opioids function as inhibitory agents during excitation and in turn decreases the release of excitatory neurons [46]. Morphine is the most well-known among opioids [41]. These opioids such as buprenorphine, codeine, fentanyl, methadone, oxycodone, and tramadol are given in various methods such as oral, intravenous injection or drip, etc. The amount of dosage to be given is determined by the body-weight of the subject [46]. Various drugs have their benefits like fentanyl which can be used for rapid action in cases of oral administration it is also good for delivering transdermally including opioid buprenorphine [45]. Other methods include the administration of corticosteroids for anti-inflammatory effects. In the USA, this method is used against inflammation caused by cancer and related treatments in palliative care [47]. Similarly, the utilization of aspirin as a non-steroidal drug is also widely administered [47]. Recently due to much increase in cancer pain research, the analgesic abilities of marijuana (cannabinoids) are also being looked upon as a potential drug for pain mitigation. Another drug "oliceridine" which was recently approved in 2020 for cancer pain management in adults was found to have fewer side effects as it also activates G- coupled protein receptor based μ-opioid receptor and has therefore an analgesic effect with tolerance comparable to morphine [42, 48]. In cases where analgesic medicines are deemed ineffective, gabapentin or pregabalin are recommended for low dosage use.

Although opioids are well suited and effective against nullifying the effects of pain. Although, it has been well documented that if abused, they do have detrimental effects on the patient with higher doses having the possibility of addiction and then withdrawal from the drugs. Short-term effects still include nausea, vomiting, breathing difficulties and many more [46, 49]. This was validated by a study done by Kata V. on opioid abuse stating that in 2016 one of the top causes of accidental death in the U.S was opioid drug overdosing [49]. In the same study, it was also noted that due to breakthrough cancer pain requiring short-acting opioids and are required in frequent doses compared to long-acting opioids this can cause overdosing of the patient leading to complications [49]. A long-proposed idea is the use of non-opioids and non-steroidal anti-inflammatory drugs. In a study conducted by Janette Vardy and Meera Agar, they mentioned that multiple studies and research on more than 2000 patients were conducted and these patients were administered with acetaminophen [50]. It was noted that at various doses of acetaminophen ranging from 500–1000 mg, there was significant reduction in pain and there was no ill effect about the same. Furthermore, nonsteroidal anti-inflammatory drugs can become toxic in patients with cardiovascular and GI tract issues, indicating that even they have to be administered only after checking for these ailments on the patients [50]. For further research, proper mitigated administration of these pain repressing drugs should be followed.

5. Conclusion

Still, pain assessment remains quite challenging to the caregivers. The reasons being first there is no consensus available or a format that speaks a common language to the masses. Pain acts differently in individuals and even though two people suffer from the same ailments their pain tolerance will be affected by many environmental and genetic factors. Differences in the site, the comprehension and pinpointing of the pain, the varied nature in intensity and the change in the same intensity due to previous/ongoing emotional turmoil, rendering the use of the same type of method for each obsolete. Many of the assessment tools are either disregarded or are still under heavy reviewing by peers. Some such as the IASP tool for assessment are unable to predict the future movement of pain symptoms and their debilitating effect. Though the ECS-CP, CPPS and ABPAT can predict to some extent they are not on par with the basic TNM staging of cancer. The intensity of the pain is very subjective and will vary from patient to patient.

The major problem of pain assessment is the subjective nature. The addition of emotional and psychological effects has been shown to produce more correlation between the subjective and the documented results and this will help in predicting the future pathway, the pain may take. Though this has been accomplished by the commonly accepted ECS-CP & CPPS but extensive review and research should be conducted such as in ABPAT with international validation (though it is still on-going). Also, assessment tools rather than being rigid can be multi-dimensional and include more domains specifically catering to the patient. This will not only provide a proper prognostic to the patient, but the caregiver will also be more prepared to administrate the required amount of analgesic /opioids to not only treat pain symptoms but also preventing any such overdosing of the drugs. And maybe increase the administration of drug alternatives that are not addictive such as non-opioids and nonsteroidal anti-inflammatory drugs. Hence, hopefully, this multi-dimensional pain assessment method might able to provide a smoother life during the patient's palliative care stage.

Acknowledgements

Sonika Charak is thankful to National Brain Research Centre for providing financial assistance. Chandra Mohan Srivastava and Manish Shandilya would like to acknowledge the support provided by Amity University Haryana for financial assistance.

Conflict of interest

The authors declare no conflict of interest.

DOI: http://dx.doi.org/10.5772/intechopen.96676

Author details

Sonika Charak[1], Robin George Thattil[2], Chandra Mohan Srivastava[2], Prabhu Prasad Das[3] and Manish Shandilya[2]*

1 National Brain Research Centre, Manesar, Gurugram, Haryana, India

2 Amity School of Applied Sciences, Amity University Haryana, Gurugram, Haryana, India

3 ACOAST, Amity University Haryana, Gurugram, Haryana, India

*Address all correspondence to: shandilya.manish7@gmail.com

References

[1] Brescia, F.J., et al., *Pain, opioid use, and survival in hospitalized patients with advanced cancer.* 1992. **10**(1): p. 149-155.

[2] Caraceni, A. and M.J.C. Shkodra, *Cancer pain assessment and classification.* 2019. **11**(4): p. 510.

[3] Hjermstad, M.J., et al., *Assessment and classification of cancer pain.* 2009. **3**(1): p. 24-30.

[4] Bruera, E., et al., *The Edmonton staging system for cancer pain: preliminary report.* 1989. **37**(2): p. 203-209.

[5] Hølen, J.C., et al., *Pain assessment tools: is the content appropriate for use in palliative care?* 2006. **32**(6): p. 567-580.

[6] Woodard, G.A., K.D. Jones, and D.M. Jablons, *Lung cancer staging and prognosis*, in *Lung Cancer*. 2016, Springer. p. 47-75.

[7] Kumar, P. and L.J.I.J.o.P. Tripathi, *Challenges in pain assessment: Pain intensity scales.* 2014. **28**(2): p. 61.

[8] Cervero, F.J.P.T.o.t.R.S.o.L.B., Biological Sciences, *Visceral nociception: peripheral and central aspects of visceral nociceptive systems.* 1985. **308**(1136): p. 325-337.

[9] Woolf, C.J.B.J.o.A., *Somatic pain--pathogenesis and prevention.* 1995. **75**(2): p. 169-176.

[10] Gierthmühlen, J. and R. Baron. *Neuropathic pain*. in *Seminars in Neurology*. 2016. Thieme Medical Publishers.

[11] Lewis, T.J.B.M.J., *Study of somatic pain.* 1938. **1**(4023): p. 321.

[12] Cervero, F.J.V.p.L., *Laird JM.* 1999. **353**: p. 2145-2148.

[13] Martin, L.A., N.A.J.J.o.p. Hagen, and s. management, *Neuropathic pain in cancer patients: mechanisms, syndromes, and clinical controversies.* 1997. **14**(2): p. 99-117.

[14] Nicholson, B.J.T.C.j.o.p., *Taxonomy of pain.* 2000. **16**(3 Suppl): p. S114-7.

[15] Adams, N., J. Ravey, and D.J.P. Taylor, *Psychological models of chronic pain and implications for practice.* 1996. **82**(2): p. 124-129.

[16] Linton, S.J. and W.S.J.P.t. Shaw, *Impact of psychological factors in the experience of pain.* 2011. **91**(5): p. 700-711.

[17] Khanna, R., A. Kumar, and R.J.I.J.o.P. Khanna, *Brief pain inventory scale: An emerging assessment modality for orofacial pain.* 2015. **29**(2): p. 61.

[18] Kaur, A. and Y.J.C.J.o.T. Guan, *Phantom limb pain: A literature review.* 2018. **21**(6): p. 366-368.

[19] Jaaniste, T., et al., *Why unidimensional pain measurement prevails in the pediatric acute pain context and what multidimensional self-report methods can offer.* 2019. **6**(12): p. 132.

[20] May, S. and M.J.F.m.r. Serpell, *Diagnosis and assessment of neuropathic pain.* 2009. **1**.

[21] Jensen, M.P., et al., *Cognitive testing and revision of the Pain Quality Assessment Scale.* 2013. **29**(5): p. 400-410.

[22] Kumar, S.P.J.I.j.o.p.c., *Utilization of brief pain inventory as an assessment tool for pain in patients with cancer: a focused review.* 2011. **17**(2): p. 108.

[23] Keller, S., et al., *Validity of the brief pain inventory for use in documenting the outcomes of patients with noncancer pain.* 2004. **20**(5): p. 309-318.

[24] Erdemoglu, A. and R.J.A.N.S. Koc, *Brief Pain Inventory score identifying and*

discriminating neuropathic and nociceptive pain. 2013. **128**(5): p. 351-358.

[25] Cleeland, C., *The brief pain inventory user guide. Houston, TX: Author*. 2009.

[26] Bennett, M.J.P., *The LANSS Pain Scale: the Leeds assessment of neuropathic symptoms and signs.* 2001. **92**(1-2): p. 147-157.

[27] Fishbain, D.A., et al., *Can the neuropathic pain scale discriminate between non-neuropathic and neuropathic pain?* 2008. **9**(2): p. 149-160.

[28] Rog, D.J., et al., *Validation and reliability of the Neuropathic Pain Scale (NPS) in multiple sclerosis.* 2007. **23**(6): p. 473-481.

[29] Anzar, S., C. Koshy, and K.M.J.I.j.o.p.c. Abraham, *Validation of the Malayalam version of Leeds assessment of neuropathic symptoms and signs pain scale in cancer patients in the Regional Cancer Centre, Thiruvananthapuram, Kerala, India.* 2017. **23**(3): p. 293.

[30] Bennett, M.I., et al., *Using screening tools to identify neuropathic pain.* 2007. **127**(3): p. 199-203.

[31] McHugh, M.L.J.B.m., *Interrater reliability: the kappa statistic.* 2012. **22**(3): p. 276-282.

[32] Krause, S.J. and M.-M.J.T.C.j.o.p. Backonja, *Development of a neuropathic pain questionnaire.* 2003. **19**(5): p. 306-314.

[33] Caraceni, A., et al., *Breakthrough pain characteristics and syndromes in patients with cancer pain. An international survey.* 2004. **18**(3): p. 177-183.

[34] Hagen, N.A., et al., *The Alberta Breakthrough Pain Assessment Tool for cancer patients: a validation study using a delphi process and patient think-aloud interviews.* 2008. **35**(2): p. 136-152.

[35] Sperlinga, R., et al., *A lberta B reakthrough P ain A ssessment T ool: A validation multicentre study in cancer patients with breakthrough pain.* 2015. **19**(7): p. 881-888.

[36] Williams, P.L. and C.J.J.o.a.n. Webb, *The Delphi technique: a methodological discussion.* 1994. **19**(1): p. 180-186.

[37] Arthur, J., et al., *Assessing the prognostic features of a pain classification system in advanced cancer patients.* 2017. **25**(9): p. 2863-2869.

[38] Koulouris, A.I., et al., *Pain in patients with pancreatic cancer: prevalence, mechanisms, management and future developments.* 2017. **62**(4): p. 861-870.

[39] Jung, B.F., et al., *Neuropathic pain following breast cancer surgery: proposed classification and research update.* 2003. **104**(1): p. 1-13.

[40] Cope, T., et al., *Channelopathy contributes to proprioceptive deficits following chemotherapy.* 2014. **596**: p. 90-107.

[41] Falk, S., K. Bannister, and A.H.J.B.j.o.p. Dickenson, *Cancer pain physiology.* 2014. **8**(4): p. 154-162.

[42] Marcin, C.J.F., *Recent advances in understanding and managing cancer pain.* 2017. **6**.

[43] Lacomba, M.T., et al., *Incidence of myofascial pain syndrome in breast cancer surgery: a prospective study.* 2010. **26**(4): p. 320-325.

[44] Mirabile, A., et al., *Pain management in head and neck cancer patients undergoing chemo-radiotherapy: Clinical practical recommendations.* 2016. **99**: p. 100-106.

[45] Bausewein, C., et al., *Palliative care of adult patients with cancer.* 2015. **112**(50): p. 863.

[46] Wiffen, P.J., et al., *Opioids for cancer-related pain in children and adolescents.* 2017(7).

[47] Roxburgh, C. and D.C.J.B.j.o.c. McMillan, *Cancer and systemic inflammation: treat the tumour and treat the host.* 2014. **110**(6): p. 1409-1412.

[48] Calo, G. and L. David, *Approval of oliceridine (TRV130) for intravenous use in moderate to severe pain in adults.* 2020.

[49] Kata, V., et al., *Opioid addiction, diversion, and abuse in chronic and cancer pain.* 2018. **12**(2): p. 124-130.

[50] Vardy, J. and M.J.J.o.c.O. Agar, *Nonopioid drugs in the treatment of cancer pain.* 2014.

Chapter 12

Effects of Antipsychotic Medication on Mortality in Long-Term Care Home Residents

Michael John Stones, Jason Randle and Peter Brink

Abstract

This chapter examines mortality in long-term care home (LTCH) residents as associated with the use antipsychotic medication when combined with other psychotropic medications. The data at census-level pertain to all new admissions to long-term care homes (LTCH) in Ontario, Canada, during a given financial year (i.e., over 20,000 LTCH residents). The observations include comprehensive assessment upon admission and at quarterly intervals thereafter for a maximal period of 1-year after the initial assessment. The mortality data derive from three linked databases, with mortality classified as death within 90 days of the final assessment. The findings indicate that combinations of concurrent daily usage of antipsychotic medication with daily usage of other psychotropic medications (particularly antidepressants and analgesics) are associated with relatively low mortality, whereas intermittent usage (e.g. *pro re nata*; as needed) is associated with relatively high mortality.

Keywords: mortality, medication, psychotropic, antipsychotic, analgesic, antidepressant, anxiolytic, hypnotic, aging, elderly, gerontology, long-term care, dementia

1. Introduction

This chapter builds upon findings from retrospective studies described in a previous chapter by Stones, Worobetz, Randle, Marchese, Fossum, Ostrum and Brink [1]. Those studies examine associations between mortality in long-term care home (LTHC) residents in the Canadian province of Ontario and the reported use of psychotropic medications. Regulations in Section 155 of the Canadian province of Ontario's *Long-Term Care Homes Act* of 2007 specifies that the residents of LTCH should be (1) 18+ years of age; (2) insured under the *Health Insurance Act*; (3) in need of 24-hours on-site nursing care, or (4) frequent daily assistance with activities of daily living (ADL), or (5) on-site monitoring or supervision in order to ensure safety and well-being. Alternative terms for LTCH in other dominions and countries include nursing homes and homes for the aged. Such homes contrast with supportive housing and continuing care hospitals that respectively provide lesser or greater levels of health care provision.

The impetus for what became our research program concerns the allegedly harmful effects of antipsychotic medication on mortality and medical conditions that potentially precipitate mortality. Although the research we describe in this chapter relates specifically to the effects of antipsychotics, our overall research program evolved to focus more generally on associations between mortality and the reported usage of any type of psychotropic medication. The latter includes not only antipsychotics but also anxiolytics, analgesics, antidepressants and hypnotics. The primary instrumentation deployed in these studies is the Resident Assessment Instrument 2.0 (RAI 2.0). This tool provides standardized clinical assessment and good data quality [2], with widespread adoption throughout the world. The measure of psychotropic usage on the RAI 2.0 is the number of days of delivery during the week preceding an assessment.

The findings described in the earlier chapter indicate strongest associations with mortality for intermittent usage of 1–6 days per week when compared with no use or daily use. These findings are significant for each type of psychotropic medication in both univariate and multivariate analyses, where the latter attempts to control for potentially confounding effects and interactions. We refer to intermittent prescribing as *pro re nata* (PRN, or 'as needed') prescription in order to be consistent with recent regulatory initiatives to curb hazardous effects associated with 'as needed' prescribing practices [3].

In contrast to augmented mortality with PRN prescribing, our earlier findings indicate lower mortality associated with daily usage of antidepressant and antipsychotic medications when compared to an absence of usage. The findings on daily usage of antipsychotic medication depart from expectations in the existing literature of its hazardous effects on mortality. This finding is also surprising because the database is among the most all-encompassing of any used in previous studies. It includes consensus level, yearly incidence data on all new admissions to all LTCHs in Ontario (i.e., over 20,000 new admissions to over 600 LTCHs during a given year, with each resident followed up for 1-year). The purpose of the research in this chapter is to explore reasons for this discrepancy.

1.1 Caregiving for behavioral and psychological symptoms of dementia

The context of our research concerns caregiving for residents of long-term care homes with behaviors that generally fall under the rubric of behavioral and psychological symptoms of dementia (BPSD). A consensus conference of the International Psychogeriatric Association in 1976 defined BPSD as "symptoms of disturbed perception, thought content, mood or behavior that frequently occur in patients with dementia" [4]. These symptoms include physical aggression, loud vocalization, restlessness, agitation, wandering, anxiety, depressive mood, hallucinations, and delusions [5]. Not all residents with dementia exhibit such symptoms, which usually emerge during the middle and later stages of the illness. Previous estimates indicate that BPSD characterizes nearly 40% of residents in Ontario's LTCHs [1].

By far the most frequent treatment for residents of LTCHs is chemical management. Of the five types of psychotropic medication, the main purposes are to alleviate pain and discomfort (i.e., analgesics), depression (i.e., antidepressants), anxiety (i.e., anxiolytics), sleeplessness (i.e., hypnotics) and BPSD (i.e., antipsychotics). The two categories of antipsychotic medication are termed *typical* and *atypical*. The latter were introduced in attempt to intent reduce adverse side-effects associated with the former [6].

The first columns in **Figure 1**, which is adapted from our previous chapter [1], shows more than double the usage of antipsychotic medication for male and female LTCH residents with than without diagnosed dementia. The findings for no other form of psychotropic medication approach this level of discrepancy. Consequently, antipsychotic medication is the most frequently used psychotropic medication

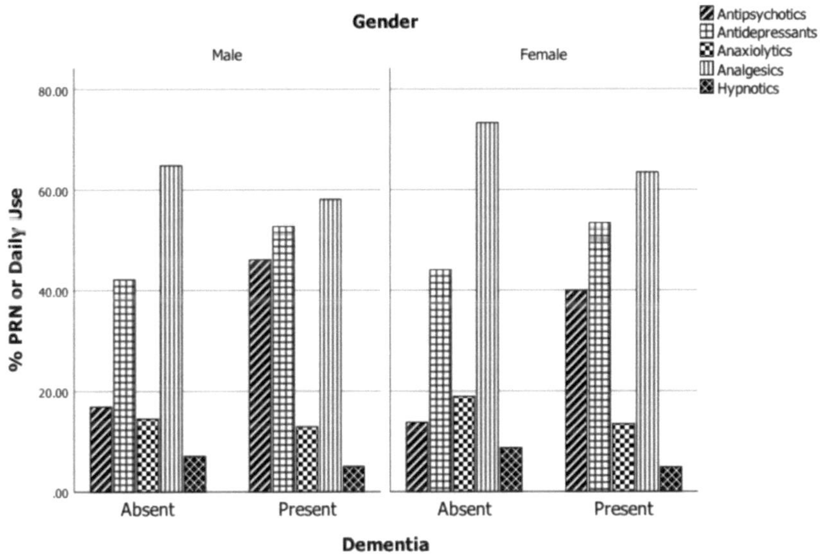

Figure 1.
Percentage of PRN or daily use of psychotropic medications for residents with or without diagnosed dementia.

specifically used with demented individuals, which is a conclusion consistent with that reported in previous publications [7].

Concerns arose early in this millennium about adverse effects associated with the use of antipsychotic medications for the management of dementia. Such effects include cardiovascular and cerebrovascular events, cardiac arrythmia, cognitive decline, extrapyramidal symptoms, falls, fractures, pneumonia and elevated mortality [8]. Levels of the preceding for people with antipsychotic prescriptions exceed those among elderly people in general, people with dementia but without antipsychotic prescriptions, and those exhibiting BPSD without antipsychotic prescriptions [9].

From 2002 onwards, manufacturers of antipsychotic medications issued warnings about health and mortality risks when prescribed for elderly people. In 2005, the USA's Federal Food and Drug Administration required "black box" warnings on packages of atypical antipsychotics, which in 2008 was extended to typical antipsychotics. This warning reads: "WARNING: Elderly patients with dementia-related psychosis treated with antipsychotic drugs are at an increased risk of death." Health authorities in other countries subsequently issued comparable warnings.

Recent meta-analysis [10] and scoping reviews [11] draw the following conclusions about mortality and antipsychotic usage in elderly people. The mortality risks are comparable between typical and atypical antipsychotics, and approximately twice that of people without such usage. The risks are comparable between individuals with or without dementia; they increase with dosage, and are highest during with first month(s) of usage. The latter suggests to authors of the scoping review [11] that factors other than antipsychotic medication may contribute to findings of elevated mortality. The authors of the meta-analytic study [10] recommend restriction and de-prescribing of antipsychotics with older people.

1.2 Methodology of retrospective studies of antipsychotic-mortality relationships

The findings discussed in our earlier chapter [1] indicate that, after control for variables that include gender, age, activities of daily living, level of cognition and mortality risk, mortality was (1) significantly elevated with PRN use for each type of psychotropic medication (2) significantly attenuated with daily use of antipsychotic and antidepressant medications, (3) significantly elevated for combinations of psychotropic medications that include PRN use and (4) significantly attenuated for combinations of psychotropic medications that include their daily use. These findings are consistent with and build upon unpublished thesis research on antipsychotic medication use by Worobetz [12]. Differences and confounds that might relate to discrepancies between our findings and previous reports of excessive mortality associated with antipsychotic medication use include the following.

First, the analyses in our chapter use generalized linear mixed modeling (GLMM) procedures. Such modeling includes a random variable that encompasses clustering of observations within that variable. This structure is appropriate for the analysis of LTCH data, with the individual homes assumed to be a random variable (i.e., the homes are independent and uncorrelated entities). In contrast, observations of residents living within a given home have commonalities because of localized admission practices, treatment preferences that differ in content and/or frequency from those in other homes, the mutual interactions of residents, etc. Traditional regression and survival analyses fail to account for such commonalities, thereby violating assumptions of independence of observations of residents, which adds to correlated error, potentially with adverse implications for the correctness of analytic outcomes. Unfortunately, it appears that the majority of studies of LTCH residents fail to address this problem. The specific form of mixed modeling used in our earlier [1] and present studies is interval censored survival (i.e., a binomial distribution with a complementary log–log link), which is appropriate for analysis of clustered observations, some of which are without a terminal event.

Second, the majority of studies of relationships between antipsychotic medication and mortality report the type and dosage of medication but not the frequency of usage [11]. Although a few studies treat PRN use as an exclusionary criterion [11], it is more likely grouped with daily use in the majority of studies. The implications of such inclusion include augmented mortality beyond that associated with daily use.

Third, our earlier study indicates augmented mortality associated with PRN use of any psychotropic but ameliorated mortality associated with daily use of certain psychotropics (e.g., antidepressants) [1]. Consequently, combinations that include PRN or daily use of other psychotropics have respective implications for increased or decreased mortality levels associated with antipsychotic use.

Fourth, compliance and adherence to medication regimens are problematic among older people with chronic illness [13]. Anyone with work experience in long-term care settings knows that "residents who put pills into their mouths do not necessarily swallow them" [1]. Some residents chose to hide those pills, others throw them away. In effect, such 'hidden' non-compliance transforms daily prescriptions to intermittent usage, potentially with adverse effects on the estimated risk of mortality.

2. The present study

The motivation that underlies the present research is to explain our earlier finding that daily use of antipsychotic medication ameliorates mortality, which contradicts conclusions reported in the majority of previous studies [9–11]. The research that follows analyzes the same database as our earlier chapter [1] to answer questions about the frequencies of concurrent combinations of antipsychotic with other psychotropic usage and their associations with subsequent mortality. As in the earlier study, the target variable is mortality within 90 days following the final RAI 2.0 assessment. The reason for this duration is that successive RAI 2.0 assessments occur at approximately 90-day intervals.

To simplify the presentation of results, we limit the control variables in analyses of mortality to the *Changes in Health, End-Stage Disease, Signs, and Symptoms Scale* (CHESS), which is an established indicator of mortality risk [14]. Although preliminary analyses also included demographic measures of age, gender and objective scales from the RAI 2.0 that include the Cognitive Performance Scale, the Activities of Daily Living Hierarchy and the Aggressive Behavior Scale (ABS), their inclusion fails to add appreciably to an interpretation of effects associated with the primary predictor variable. The latter is represented in **Table 1** by concurrent combinations of antipsychotic use and other psychotropic use.

The 1st and 2nd columns in **Table 1** represent combinations of concurrent usage of antipsychotic and other psychotropic medications. The frequencies for antipsychotics include no use, PRN use and daily use. The inclusive frequencies all other types of psychotropic are no use, PRN and daily use, only PRN use and only daily use. The 3rd, 4th, 5th and 6th columns represent possible combinations of antipsychotics with antidepressant, analgesic, anxiolytic or hypnotic medications, respectively. The possible frequencies for each of the latter are no use, PRN use and daily use.

The main hypotheses derive from our previous findings that, after control of the major risk factor for mortality, daily use of psychotropic medication ameliorates risk, whereas PRN use exacerbates risk. Consequently, we anticipate that combinations of antipsychotics with the daily use of other psychotropics ameliorate mortality to levels below that associated with absence of psychotropic use. In contrast, we predict augmented mortality associated with combinations of antipsychotic and other psychotropics that involve PRN use.

Antipsychotic prescription	Prescriptions for other psychotropics				
	All psychotropics	Antidepressant	Analgesic	Anxiolytic	Hypnotic
None	None	None	None	None	None
None	PRN & Daily	.	.	.	.
None	PRN	PRN	PRN	PRN	PRN
None	Daily	Daily	Daily	Daily	Daily
PRN	None	None	None	None	None
PRN	PRN & Daily	.	.	.	.
PRN	PRN	PRN	PRN	PRN	PRN
PRN	Daily	Daily	Daily	Daily	Daily
Daily	None	None	None	None	None
Daily	PRN & Daily	.	.	.	.
Daily	PRN	PRN	PRN	PRN	PRN
Daily	Daily	Daily	Daily	Daily	Daily

Table 1.
Antipsychotic prescription frequencies combined with frequencies for other antipsychotic medications on the final assessment.

2.1 Participants and measures

The participants are all new admissions, aged 65 years and older, to LTCHs in the Canadian province of Ontario during the financial year April 1st 2010 to March 31st 2011. They include 20,414 residents from 631 LTCHs. The distribution of men to women is 33.6% to 66.4%. The mean age of men is 83.03 years with a standard deviation of 7.37 years. The mean age of women is 85.29 years with a standard deviation of 7.19 years.

The main assessment tool used here is the RAI 2.0, which, to the authors' knowledge, (1) is used in more countries, (2) has a more thorough psychometric evaluation, and (3) is more comprehensive than any other geriatric assessment tool. The RAI 2.0 requires trained heath care professionals to score quantifiable assessment items relevant to medical diagnoses, levels of functioning, behavioral and emotional problems, forms of treatment, etc. The information is from medical records, clinical observations, and communication with residents, their family members and the facility's staff members. As already indicated, the RAI also contains objective scales that are evaluated against 'gold standard' measures from the relevant literature. The measures in the present analyses are the CHESS and items on antipsychotic, analgesic, antidepressant, anxiolytic and hypnotic medication use. The latter items record the number of days of usage during the week preceding an assessment. We report here on three usage categories: no use, PRN (i.e., intermittent) use, and daily use.

The RAI 2.0 also provides information on the mortality of residents in a LTCH. Other databases linked to the RAI 2.0 are the Discharge Abstract Database (DAD) and the National Ambulatory Care Reporting System (NACRS). The DAD reports mortality data for hospital discharges and the NACRS reports mortality in settings for emergency and ambulatory care. Consequently, our data encompasses mortality throughout the health care system. We are grateful to the Canadian Institute for Health Information (CIHI) for the provision of the data with encrypted personal and facility level identifiers.

Residents receive RAI 2.0 assessments upon admission and thereafter at quarterly intervals. The maximal follow-up period in the present study is 1-year. We report here on data from the final assessment, with mortality indexed by its absence or presence during 90 days following that assessment (i.e., a period that precedes the scheduled date of any subsequent assessment).

2.2 Statistical analyses

The statistical analyses relate to three issues. The first concerns the types of concurrent combination of usage frequencies between antipsychotics with other psychotropics. These analyses begin graphic and tabular statistics that relate to concurrent relationships between frequencies antipsychotic usage with frequencies for other types of psychotropic usage. Then follows findings from *Statistical Package for the Social Sciences* (SPSS Version 25) GLMM multinomial analysis of frequencies of antipsychotic usage (i.e., the target variable) against corresponding frequencies for each other psychotropic (i.e., the fixed effect variables). The random variable for this and every subsequent GLMM analysis are LTCHs.

The second issue concerns mortality within 90 days of the final assessment. The primary analysis is a GLMM interval censored survival model (i.e., a binomial distribution with a complementary log–log link). The CHESS (i.e., centered on its grand mean) and concurrent combinations of frequencies for antipsychotic and other psychotropic usage comprise the fixed effects. Then follows GLMM interval censored survival models that attempt to clarify implications of the preceding by analyzing summative categories that respectively relate to antipsychotic use and other psychotropic use. Next, we analyze models that examine combinations of antipsychotics with each type of psychotropic. The purpose is to ascertain the types of antipsychotic that may ameliorate of exacerbate risk of mortality at different levels of usage. All the latter models include the CHESS as a measure of mortality risk.

The final issue concerns the effects on mortality of changes in health condition and prescribing practices from the penultimate to final assessment. This GLMM analysis examines whether changes in the CHESS and PRN prescriptions have independent implications for survival. In contrast, an alternative hypothesis suggests that changes in PRN prescription are a consequence of changes in health condition, with the former having with no direct implications for survival.

2.2.1 Analyses of psychotropic combinations

The following graph and table illustrate relationships between frequencies of usage for antipsychotic medication with corresponding usage of all other psychotropic medications. **Figure 2** shows 95% confidence intervals for the totality of any other psychotropic use against no use, PRN, and daily use for antipsychotic medication. The mean use of other psychotropic medication is significantly lower with no use of antipsychotic medication than for PRN and daily use, as evidenced by non-overlapping confidence intervals. **Table 2** shows percentages of residents with a given frequency of antipsychotic medication combined with the use of 1, 2, 3 or 4 other psychotropic medications. The statistical mode (i.e., the most frequent value) within columns of this table indicates that residents without antipsychotics most frequently receive one other psychotropic, whereas those with PRN and daily antipsychotic use most frequently use two other psychotropic medications.

The following figures illustrate frequencies of use of specific psychotropics that accompany no, PRN or daily use of antipsychotics. **Figure 3** shows findings associated with antidepressant medication. The findings indicate that approximately 60% of residents with daily antipsychotics and just over 40% of those with no antipsychotics receive antidepressants on a daily basis. Of those residents with PRN use of antipsychotics, the majority show either PRN (18%) or daily (35%) use of antidepressants.

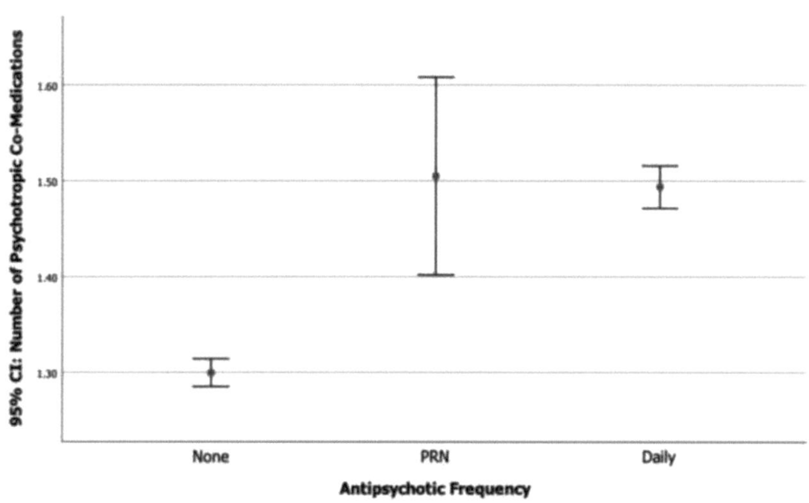

Figure 2.
95% confidence intervals for summative Co-medication frequencies for other psychotropics against frequencies for antipsychotic medication.

Number of other of psychotropics	Percentage of residents		
	Antipsychotic use		
	None	PRN	Daily
0	18.6%	13.6%	13.2%
1	41.4%	35.6%	36.6%
2	31.8%	38.6%	38.9%
3	7.7%	11.2%	10.4%
4	0.5%	1.0%	1.0%

Table 2.
Percentage of residents with No, PRN or daily use of antipsychotics 1, 2, 3 or 4 other psychotropics.

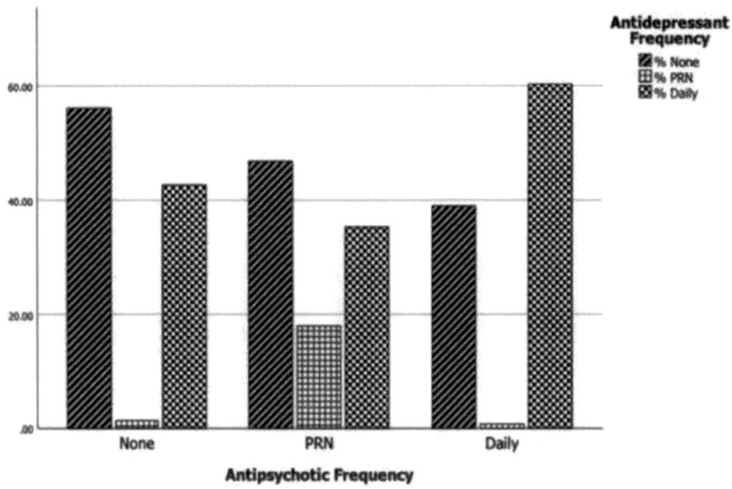

Figure 3.
Percentage antidepressant frequency against antipsychotic frequency.

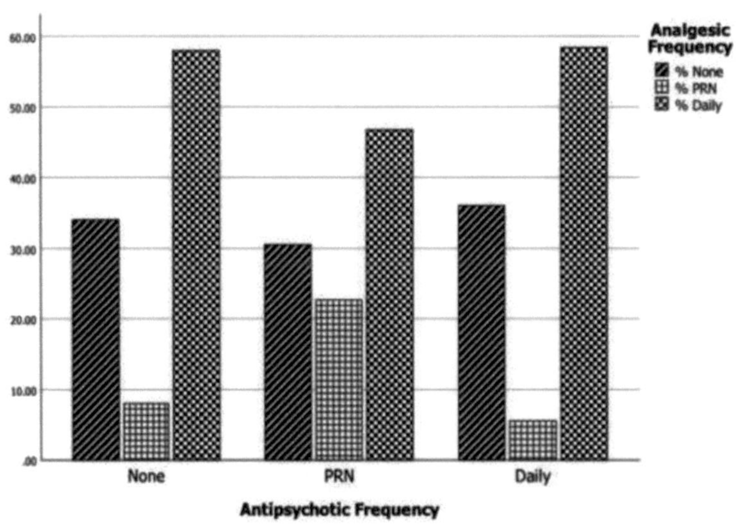

Figure 4.
Percentage analgesic frequency against antipsychotic frequency.

Levels of analgesic medication are uniformly high. **Figure 4** shows PRN or daily use among approximately 65–70% of residents regardless of frequency of usage of antipsychotic medication. Consistent with finding for antidepressants and anxiolytics (see below), the highest PRN use of analgesics corresponds with PRN use antipsychotic medication (approximately, 22%).

Figure 5 indicates a low overall use of anxiolytic medication. The levels of daily use are approximately 7–10% regardless of frequency of use for antipsychotics. However, among residents with PRN use of antipsychotics, PRN use of anxiolytics is approximately 14%, which is considerably higher than daily use for this subgroup of residents.

Figure 6 shows hypnotic use to be lower than for any of other psychotropic (i.e., approximately 6.3% of residents). The highest PRN use of hypnotics occurs

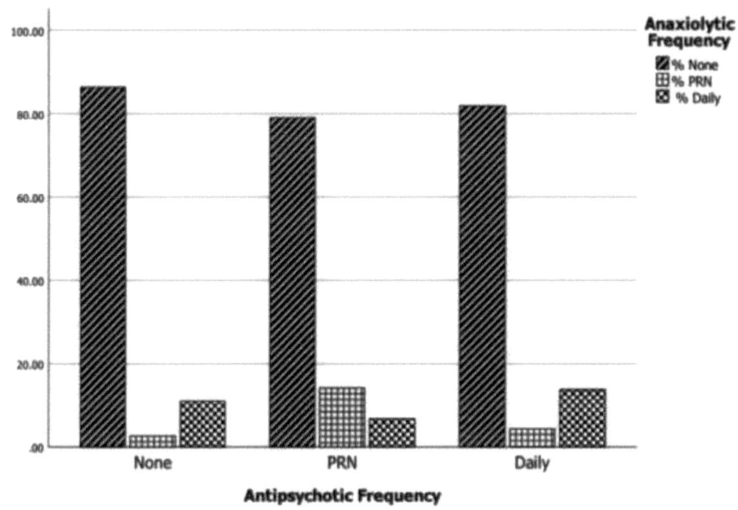

Figure 5.
Percentage Anaxiolytic frequency against antipsychotic frequency.

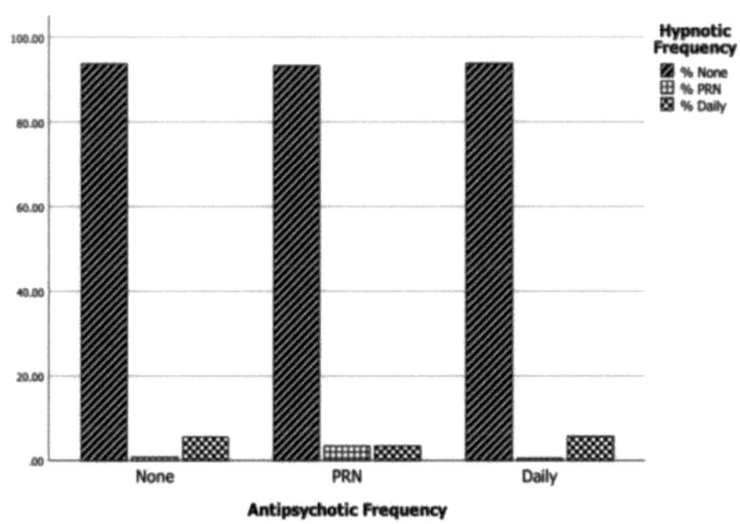

Figure 6.
Percentage hypnotic frequency against antipsychotic frequency.

Antipsych. frequency	Model term	Coefficient	Std. error	Sig.	95% confidence interval		Exponential coefficient
					Lower	Upper	
Daily	Intercept	−1.119	.0372	.000	−1.192	−1.046	.327
	Antidepress. Daily	.682	.0329	.000	.617	.746	1.977
	Antidepress. PRN	−.242	.1705	.155	−.576	.092	.785
	Antidepress. None	0	.	.	.	.	1.00
	Analgesic Daily	−.134	.0347	.000	−.201	−.066	.875
	Analgesic PRN	−.384	.0701	.000	−.521	−.246	.681
	Analgesic None	0	.	.	.	.	1.00
	Anxiolytic Daily	.207	.0484	.000	.112	.302	1.230
	Anxiolytic PRN	.561	.0863	.000	.392	.730	1.753
	Anxiolytic None	0	.	.	.	.	1.00
	Hypnotic Daily	−.033	.0694	.634	−.169	.103	.967
	Hypnotic PRN	−.302	.2145	.160	−.722	.119	.740
	Hypnotic None	0	.	.	.	.	1.00
PRN	Intercept	−4.151	.1246	.000	−4.395	−3.907	.016
	Antidepress. Daily	.054	.1330	.683	−.206	.315	1.056
	Antidepress. PRN	2.378	.1898	.000	2.006	2.750	10.788
	Antidepress. None	0	.	.	.	.	1.00
	Analgesic Daily	−.120	.1398	.389	−.394	.154	.887
	Analgesic PRN	.703	.1777	.000	.355	1.052	2.020
	Analgesic None	0	.	.	.	.	1.00
	Anxiolytic Daily	−.312	.2373	.188	−.777	.153	.732
	Anxiolytic PRN	1.399	.1907	.000	1.025	1.773	4.050
	Anxiolytic None	0	.	.	.	.	1.00
	Hypnotic Daily	−.392	.3289	.234	−1.036	.253	.676
	Hypnotic PRN	.986	.3710	.008	.259	1.713	2.680
	Hypnotic None	0	.	.	.	.	1.00

Table 3.
Fixed effects coefficients and odds ratios for prediction of antipsychotic frequency by frequencies of all other antipsychotic categories.

in combination with PRN use of antipsychotics. Daily use of hypnotics has approximately similar levels among residents with no of daily use of antipsychotic medication.

Inferences from the preceding graphs and table include the following. First, residents with PRN or daily use of antipsychotics have higher concurrent use of other psychotropic medications than those without antipsychotic use. **Table 2** shows that over 80% of residents without antipsychotic use receive at least one other psychotropic. The psychotropics that appear most frequently in these combinations are antidepressants and analgesics, which have the highest overall frequency of usage. Second, PRN use of antipsychotics combines with the highest PRN in each other psychotropic category. This finding suggests a clustering of PRN prescribing that encompasses all types of psychotropic medication.

The final analysis this section is a GLMM multinomial analysis. This analysis includes LTCHs as a random variable and fixed effect predictors that evaluate the independent contributions by other psychotropics to frequencies of antipsychotic use. The target and predictor variables are on nominal scales of no use, PRN use and daily use, respectively, with the former designated as reference category.

The findings in **Table 3** include the regression coefficients, standard errors, levels of statistical significance and 95% confidence intervals. **Table 3** also includes derivative exponential coefficient for readers that prefer odds ratios over regression coefficients. Positive or negative regression coefficients respectively indicate mean values above or below those associated with the reference category, with odds ratios greater or less than unity having comparable meaning. The overall findings for the model include significant random effects of LTCHs at $p < .001$. Findings for the fixed effect terms are as follows.

Daily antidepressants, daily anxiolytics and PRN anxiolytics are all positive predictors of daily antipsychotic use (all $p < .001$). Daily analgesics and PRN analgesics are negative predictors (both $p < .001$). These findings suggest that psychotropics purportedly relevant to mood improvement and anxiety reduction are likely to accompany daily antipsychotic use, whereas medications purportedly relevant to pain relief are less likely to occur in combination with daily antipsychotic medication.

PRN use of antidepressants ($p < .001$), anxiolytics ($p < .001$), analgesics ($p < .001$) and hypnotics ($p < .001$) are positive predictors of PRN use of antipsychotics. There are no significant relationships between daily use of other psychotropics and PRN use of antipsychotics. These findings indicate a clustering of PRN prescribing.

2.2.2 Survival analyses

Mortality during the 1-year follow-up period of data collection is 18.1% overall. The mortality rates for men and women are 21.1% and 16.3% respectively. The distribution of mortality across assessments indicates that 45% of residents died within 90 days of the admission assessment, with a decreasing proportion of deaths at each subsequent assessment.

The primary interval censored survival analysis shows a significant random effect for LTCHs $p < .001$. Because the same level of significance is present in all subsequent GLMM analyses, we need not report them henceforth. **Table 4** shows findings for the fixed effects. Unsurprisingly, the positive coefficient for the CHESS indicates higher mortality for residents at greater risk of mortality. The reference category for combinations of medications is the daily use of both antipsychotics and other psychotropics, which numerically is associated with the lowest level of mortality. This combination has significantly lower mortality ($p < .005$ or beyond) than any other combination except for those that combine no antipsychotics with daily psychotropics and PRN use of antipsychotics with daily psychotropics.

Fixed effects	Coefficient	Std. error	Sig.	95% Confidence interval		Exponential coefficient
				Lower	Upper	
Intercept	−1.938	.0412	.000	−2.019	−1.858	.14
CHESS	.569	.0136	.000	.543	.596	1.77
AP, None: PT, None	.366	.0600	.000	.248	.483	1.44
AP, None: PT, Mixed	.552	.0776	.000	.400	.704	1.74
AP, None: PT, PRN	.643	.0782	.000	.490	.797	1.90
AP, None: PT, Daily	.084	.0459	.066	−.005	.174	1.09
AP, PRN: PT, None	.999	.2851	.000	.441	1.558	2.72
AP, PRN: PT, Mixed	.818	.2480	.001	.332	1.304	2.27
AP, PRN: PT, PRN	.910	.1978	.000	.522	1.298	2.48
AP, PRN: PT, Daily	.346	.1739	.047	.005	.687	1.41
AP, Daily: PT, None	.273	.0944	.004	.088	.458	1.31
AP, Daily: PT, Mixed	.421	.1036	.000	.218	.624	1.52
AP, Daily: PT, PRN	.549	.1537	.000	.248	.850	1.73
AP, Daily: PT, Daily	0	.	.	.	.	1.00

Table 4.
Fixed effect coefficients for the CHESS and combinations of antipsychotic (AP) and other psychotropic (PT) frequencies in prediction of mortality.

Fixed effects	Coefficient	Std. error	Sig.	95% Confidence interval		Exponential coefficient
				Lower	Upper	
Intercept	−1.846	.0355	.000	−1.915	−1.776	.16
CHESS	.577	.0134	.000	.550	.603	1.78
No Antipsychotics	.113	.0380	.003	.039	.188	1.12
PRN Antipsychotics	.566	.1095	.000	.352	.781	1.76
Daily Antipsychotics	0	.	.	.	.	1.00

Table 5.
Fixed effect coefficients for combined categories of antipsychotic frequencies with other psychotropic medications.

An implication is that daily use of psychotropics ameliorates mortality associated with antipsychotics to levels below that associated with no use of the latter.

A Bonferroni multiple comparison with the combination that includes neither antipsychotic nor any other psychotropic provides further support for this inference. The only other combination with significantly lower mortality than zero use of any psychotropic is that of no antipsychotics but daily use of other psychotropics ($p < .001$). Consequently, the latter ameliorates mortality below the level associated with zero psychotropic medications.

The next two analyses condense the preceding array of combinations into those associated with antipsychotic use (i.e., none, PRN and daily) and other psychotropic use, respectively (i.e., none, mixed, PRN and daily). Both analyses include the CHESS, with daily use as the reference category for the combinational variable.

Fixed effects	Coefficient	Std. error	Sig.	95% Confidence interval		Exponential coefficient
				Lower	Upper	
Intercept	−1.879	.0262	.000	−1.930	−1.827	.15
CHESS	.572	.0135	.000	.546	.598	1.77
No Psychotropics	.294	.0455	.000	.205	.383	1.34
Mixed Psychotropics	.457	.0578	.000	.344	.570	1.58
PRN Psychotropics	.589	.0626	.000	.466	.712	1.80
Daily Psychotropics	0	.	.	.	.	1.00

Table 6.
Fixed effect coefficients for combined categories of other psychotropic medication use with antipsychotic use.

The findings in **Table 5** show the findings from the analysis of psychotropic use. In addition to significance for the CHESS, daily use of antipsychotics is associated with significantly lower mortality than no use or PRN use ($p < .005$ or beyond). Moreover, a Bonferroni multiple comparison shows that no use has a significantly lower level of mortality than PRN use. These findings replicate the trends for antipsychotic use reported in our earlier publication [1].

Table 6 shows findings from the analysis of the use of other psychotropics. With daily use as the reference category, no use, mixed use and PRN use are associated with higher levels of mortality ($p < .005$ or beyond). Sequential Bonferroni multiple comparisons of no, mixed and PRN use reveal higher mortality for PRN than no use ($p < .001$), with no comparison that involves mixed use significant at $p < .01$ level. These findings suggest that daily use of other psychotropics has ameliorative effects on mortality. **Figure 7** provides a graphic portrayal of the combined finding from last two analyses, indicating inverted-V or inverted-U structures corresponding to frequencies of no, mixed, PRN and daily use, with lowest frequencies associated with daily use of other psychotropics.

Fixed effects	Coefficient	Std. error	Sig.	95% Confidence interval		Exponential coefficient
				Lower	Upper	
Intercept	−1.984	.0464	.000	−2.075	−1.893	.14
CHESS	.575	.0135	.000	.549	.601	1.78
AP, None: AD, None	.370	.0510	.000	.270	.470	1.45
AP, None: AD, PRN	.718	.1374	.000	.448	.987	2.05
AP, None, AD, Daily	.069	.0547	.207	−.038	.176	1.07
AP, PRN: AD, None	.819	.1541	.000	.517	1.121	2.27
AP, PRN: AD, PRN	1.040	.2203	.000	.608	1.472	2.83
AP, PRN, AD, Daily	.301	.2127	.157	−.116	.718	1.35
AP, Daily: AD, None	.320	.0647	.000	.193	.447	1.38
AP, Daily: AD, PRN	.625	.2955	.034	.046	1.204	1.87
AP, Daily, AD, Daily	0	.	.	.	.	1.00

Table 7.
Fixed effect coefficients for the CHESS and combinations of antipsychotic (AP) and antidepressant (AD) use in prediction of mortality.

Fixed Effects	Coefficient	Std. Error	Sig.	95% Confidence Interval		Exponential Coefficient
				Lower	Upper	
Intercept	−1.891	.0450	.000	−1.979	−1.803	.15
CHESS	.573	.0136	.000	.546	.599	1.77
AP, None: AN, None	.225	.0551	.000	.117	.333	1.25
AP, None: AN, PRN	.566	.0714	.000	.426	.706	1.76
AP, None, AN, Daily	.055	.0501	.276	−.044	.153	1.06
AP, PRN: AN, None	.701	.2015	.001	.306	1.096	2.02
AP, PRN: AN, PRN	.721	.2139	.001	.302	1.140	2.06
AP, PRN, AN, Daily	.510	.1579	.001	.200	.819	1.67
AP, Daily: AN, None	.012	.0705	.860	−.126	.151	1.01
AP, Daily: AN, PRN	.546	.1117	.000	.327	.764	1.73
AP, Daily, AN, Daily	0	.	.	.	.	1.00

Table 8.
Fixed effect coefficients for the CHESS and combinations of antipsychotic (AP) and analgesic (AN) use in prediction of mortality.

Fixed effects	Coefficient	Std. error	Sig.	95% Confidence interval		Exponential coefficient
				Lower	Upper	
Intercept	−1.925	.0886	.000	−2.099	−1.751	.15
CHESS	.574	.0134	.000	.548	.601	1.78
AP, None: AX, None	.199	.0898	.027	.023	.375	1.22
AP, None: AX, PRN	.537	.1322	.000	.278	.797	1.71
AP, None, AX, Daily	.042	.1078	.695	−.169	.254	1.04
AP, PRN: AX, None	.546	.1503	.000	.251	.840	1.73
AP, PRN: AX, PRN	1.143	.2503	.000	.652	1.633	3.14
AP, PRN, AX, Daily	.649	.4058	.110	−.146	1.444	1.91
AP, Daily: AX, None	.081	.0941	.390	−.104	.265	1.08
AP, Daily: AX, PRN	.302	.1580	.056	−.007	.612	1.35
AP, Daily, AX, Daily	0	.	.	.	.	1.00

Table 9.
Fixed effect coefficients for the CHESS and combinations of antipsychotic (AP) and anxiolytic (AX) use in prediction of mortality.

The following GLMM interval censored survival analyses examine combinations of antipsychotic with separate types of other psychotropic. These combinations correspond to frequencies of usage outlined in last four columns of **Table 1**. All these analyses include the CHESS among the fixed effects, with daily usage of both

Fixed effects	Coefficient	Std. error	Sig.	95% Confidence interval		Exponential coefficient
				Lower	Upper	
Intercept	−1.707	.1230	.000	−1.948	−1.466	.18
CHESS	.576	.0134	.000	.550	.602	1.78
AP, None: HY, None	−.027	.1237	.828	−.269	.216	.97
AP, None: HY, PRN	.657	.2081	.002	.249	1.065	1.93
AP, None, HY, Daily	−.123	.1495	.411	−.416	.170	.88
AP, PRN: HY, None	.450	.1633	.006	.130	.770	1.57
AP, PRN: HY, PRN	.001	.5223	.999	−1.023	1.025	1.00
AP, PRN, HY, Daily	.350	.5583	.531	−.744	1.444	1.42
AP, Daily: HY, None	−.149	.1264	.239	−.397	.099	.86
AP, Daily: HY, PRN	−.009	.4182	.982	−.829	.810	.99
AP, Daily, HY, Daily	0	.	.	.	.	1.00

Table 10.
Fixed effect coefficients for the CHESS and combinations of antipsychotic (AP) and hypnotic (HY) use in prediction of mortality.

an antipsychotic and the other specified psychotropic as the reference category for combinations.

Tables 7–10 show fixed effect findings for combinations that include antidepressants, analgesics, anxiolytics and hypnotics respectively. **Tables 7** and **8** show coefficients for the combinations that include the most frequently used psychotropics. **Table 7** shows significantly lower mortality for a combination of daily antipsychotic with antidepressant use than for two of three combinations without antipsychotics ($p < .001$); the exception being a combination of no antipsychotics with daily antidepressants. **Table 8** shows comparable findings for the combination of daily antipsychotics with analgesic use. Also, every combination that includes PRN use of an antipsychotic and/or another psychotropic has significantly higher mortality than the reference category.

Tables 9 and **10** show findings for combinations of antipsychotic use with anxiolytic and hypnotic use, respectively. Neither psychotropic has a high prevalence of usage in LTCHs. The findings mainly indicate non-significant differences in mortality against the reference category. The significant differences include higher mortality than for the reference category for combinations that include PRN use of antipsychotic or another psychotropic ($p < .001$).

A final analysis in this section relates mortality to the duration of residence in a LTCH. Because previous reviews indicate higher mortality during the beginning phase of antipsychotic use, we would be remiss not to examine such effects [10, 11]. We report at the beginning of this section that nearly half the deaths occurred within 90 days of the admission assessment. Consequently, the following GLMM multinomial analysis uses as the target variable categories of (1) death after the admission assessment, (2) death after subsequent assessments, with (3) absence of mortality as the reference category. Findings in **Table 11** for death after the initial assessment indicate significantly lower mortality for the daily antipsychotic with other psychotropic use combination than for any other combination ($p < .005$ and beyond). Bonferroni multiple comparison also shows that the no antipsychotic but other daily psychotropic use combination has lower mortality than the combination with neither antipsychotic nor other

Assessment	Model term	Coefficient	Std. error	Sig	95% Confidence interval		Exponential coefficient
					Lower	Upper	
Initial	Intercept	−2.932	.0717	.000	−3.072	−2.791	.053
	CHESS	.557	.0230	.000	.512	.602	1.745
	AP, None: PT, None	.906	.0961	.000	.717	1.094	2.474
	AP, None: PT, Mixed	1.211	.1223	.000	.971	1.450	3.356
	AP, None: PT, PRN	1.423	.1187	.000	1.190	1.655	4.148
	AP, None: PT, Daily	.420	.0802	.000	.263	.577	1.522
	AP, PRN: PT, None	2.079	.3858	.000	1.323	2.835	7.995
	AP, PRN: PT, Mixed	1.605	.4089	.000	.803	2.406	4.977
	AP, PRN: PT, PRN	1.714	.3130	.000	1.100	2.327	5.549
	AP, PRN: PT, Daily	.819	.2808	.004	.268	1.369	2.268
	AP, Daily: PT, None	.688	.1474	.000	.399	.977	1.991
	AP, Daily: PT, Mixed	.839	.1701	.000	.506	1.172	2.314
	AP, Daily: PT, PRN	.768	.2735	.005	.232	1.304	2.156
	AP, Daily: PT, Daily	0	.	.	.	.	1.00
Subsequent	Intercept	−2.315	.0558	.000	−2.424	−2.206	.099
	CHESS	.773	.0214	.000	.731	.815	2.166
	AP, None: PT, None	.006	.0908	.949	−.172	.184	1.006
	AP, None: PT, Mixed	.152	.1253	.225	−.094	.397	1.164
	AP, None: PT, PRN	.015	.1361	.912	−.252	.282	1.015
	AP, None: PT, Daily	−.140	.0636	.028	−.265	−.015	.869
	AP, PRN: PT, None	.206	.5757	.720	−.922	1.334	1.229
	AP, PRN: PT, Mixed	.626	.4299	.145	−.216	1.469	1.871
	AP, PRN: PT, PRN	.882	.3216	.006	.252	1.513	2.416
	AP, PRN: PT, Daily	.058	.2753	.834	−.482	.597	1.059
	AP, Daily: PT, None	.075	.1397	.589	−.198	.349	1.078
	AP, Daily: PT, Mixed	.331	.1522	.030	.033	.629	1.392
	AP, Daily: PT, PRN	.483	.2271	.033	.038	.928	1.621
	AP, Daily: PT, Daily	0	.	.	.	.	1.00

Table 11.
Fixed effect coefficients for the CHESS and combinations of antipsychotic (AP) and other psychotropic (PT) frequencies in the prediction of mortality after the first and later assessments.

psychotropic use ($p < .001$). These findings are comparable to those reported for mortality over the full range of assessments. However, the findings for mortality after the admission assessment show no significant effects. We conclude, therefore, that effects associated with the medicinal combinations are stronger for mortality that occurs shortly after the admission assessment.

2.2.3 Survival analysis against measures of change

The preceding analyses relate mortality to CHESS scores and prescription profiles on the final assessment. Questions raised in our preceding chapter concern issues about causality with respect to relationships between health and medicinal

Model term	Coefficient	Std. error	Sig	95% Confidence interval		Exponential coefficient
				Lower	Upper	
Intercept	−2.249	.0308	.000	−2.309	−2.188	.053
CHESS Preceding, High	1.958	.2346	.000	1.499	2.418	1.745
CHESS Preceding, Low	0	.	.	.	.	2.474
CHESS Change, Worse	2.015	.0756	.000	1.867	2.163	3.356
CHESS Change, Better	−1.052	.2904	.000	−1.621	−.482	4.148
CHESS Change, None	0	.	.	.	.	1.522
PRN Preceding, Present	.349	.1005	.001	.152	.545	7.995
PRN Preceding, Absent	0	.	.	.	.	4.977
PRN Change, Increase	.648	.0731	.000	.505	.791	5.549
PRN Change, Decrease	−.123	.1247	.325	−.367	.122	2.268
PRN Change, None	0	.	.	.	.	1.00

Table 12.
Fixed effect coefficients for the CHESS and PRN levels on penultimate assessment and their changes from the penultimate to final assessments in the prediction of mortality after the final assessment.

prescriptions, with potential implications for subsequent mortality [1]. One hypothesis is that changes toward higher PRN prescribing explains both worsening in health condition and subsequent mortality.

A second hypothesis is that worsening of health condition results in higher PRN prescribing and subsequent mortality, such that any relationship between PRN and mortality is artifactual rather than actual. A third hypothesis is that changes toward higher PRN prescribing and changes in health conditions make independent contributes to levels of mortality.

The following GLMM analysis tests these hypotheses with the data necessarily restricted to the penultimate and final assessments among residents with two or more assessments. With mortality as the target variable, the fixed effects include binary scores of (1) high-risk scores *versus* low risk on the CHESS (i.e., high risk scores are 4 or 5 on a 5-point scale) (2) the presence or absence of any PRN prescription on the penultimate assessment; and (3) changes in the CHESS index and (4) the PRN index from the penultimate to final assessment. **Table 12** shows the findings.

Levels of mortality are significantly higher for high risk scores on the CHESS and the presence of PRN prescription. Changes on the CHESS toward worsening health are associated with significantly higher mortality, whereas changes toward lower risk scores are associated with significantly lower mortality, when compared an absence of change on the CHESS index. Compared to no change on the PRN index, an increased frequency of PRN prescription is associated with significantly increased mortality. Consequently, the findings indicate that detrimental levels and detrimental changes on the CHESS and PRN indexes contribute independently to higher levels of mortality.

2.3 Discussion

Our previous research with this database [1] includes a number of resident-level and facility-level control variables from the RAI 2.0. The analyses reported here simplify the presentation of results by inclusion of only the CHESS as a control variable. The justification is that unreported analyses, which included a wider range of fixed effect predictors of mortality, did not substantially alter the present findings. We should also mention findings from unreported analyses with Cox regression, which is a common form of survival analysis that takes no account for correlated error in SPSS 25. Despite this limitation, the findings with Cox regression are otherwise comparable to those reported here.

The present findings indicate that approximately 30% of residents are in receipt of antipsychotic medication, with more than 99% of those residents in receipt of at least one other psychotropic medication. The most frequently used among the latter are antidepressants and analgesics. The GLMM analysis in **Table 3** indicates that psychotropics with positive effects on mood and anxiety are frequently combined with daily use of antipsychotics, whereas analgesics are more frequent in residents without antipsychotic usage. PRN use of other types of psychotropic significantly predicts PRN use of antipsychotics, which indicates that residents typically receive PRN prescription for multiple types of psychotropic medication.

To our knowledge, the study presented here is the first to examine how concurrent prescriptions of other psychotropics can affect elevated mortality among the elderly, which is attributed in many previous studies to the use of antipsychotics. Although limitations in present data includes absence of information on the types and dosages of psychotropics, a limitation common to previous studies is an absence of information on the frequencies of usage. Although prior evidence indicates the good overall quality of RAI 2.0 data [2], a limitation for present purposes is an absence of information about medicinal use prior to admission. A consequence is uncertainty about whether high mortality shortly after admission reflects effects associated with short-term antipsychotic use, relocation to a LTCH, or other unknown effects. However, the findings reported in **Table 12** on residents with at least two RAI 2.0 assessments indicate that changes in prescribing practices do have effects on mortality beyond those associated with changes in high risk health conditions measured by the CHESS. Consequently, we conclude that the relationship between PRN usage and mortality is one of primary determination, rather than secondary to the relationship between declining health and mortality.

The overall findings on mortality support our hypotheses that daily use of other psychotropics may ameliorate mortality levels associated with antipsychotic use, whereas PRN use of other psychotropics augments that mortality. **Figure 7** provides a cogent illustration of the supportive findings. The specific psychotropics that support amelioration with daily use are antidepressants and analgesics, whereas concurrent PRN use of analgesics, anxiolytics and hypnotics are associated with augmented mortality. However, despite the high percentage of death among LTCH residents with PRN prescriptions on the final assessment, it must be remembered that only 12.9% are in receipt of such prescription.

Implications of the findings are that retrospective studies may incorrectly estimate the mortality associated with antipsychotic prescriptions by failure to take account of the deleterious effects of PRN usage and the beneficial effects of daily usage of other psychotropics. We reasoned in our previous chapter that the clinical rationale for psychotropic prescription is to renormalize disturbances to a resident's equilibrium (e.g., aggression, depression, pain, anxiety, insomnia), with

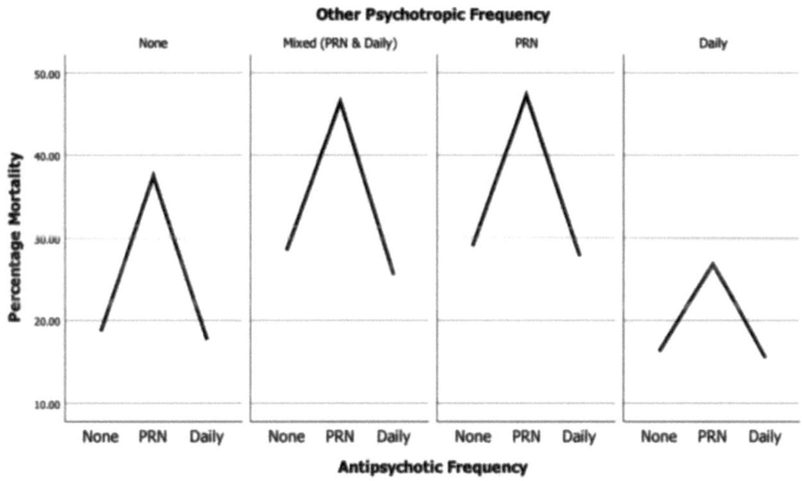

Figure 7.
Percentage mortality for frequency combinations of antipsychotic with other psychotropic medication.

such disequilibrium considered a risk to wellbeing and mortality [1]. Successful treatment is associated with regained equilibrium after adaptation to regular prescription of the requisite medication. However, intermittent medication usage is antagonistic to adaptation, may exacerbate disequilibrium, with an elevation of mortality risk. Consequently, implications for caregiving of residents with BPSD may include daily antipsychotic and other daily psychotropic usage if non-pharmaceutical intervention fails to bring relief, but should avoid PRN usage of any form of psychotropic medication.

3. Conclusions

Behavioral disturbance is common among residents with dementia in LTCH. Such disturbance is associated with poor quality of life, caregiver burden and adverse health care outcomes. Although non-pharmacological procedures are recommended as the first line of treatment [15], the usual treatment in LTCHs includes the use of antipsychotics despite limited evidence for effectiveness and health outcomes reported to include elevated mortality. The research described here suggests that daily use of antipsychotics with daily use of other psychotropics (particularly antidepressants and analgesics) attenuate mortality whereas concurrent combinations that include PRN usage exacerbate mortality. The implications for caregiving include avoidance of PRN prescriptions of psychotropic medications.

Acknowledgements

All the authors contributed to the research and manuscript preparation, and verified their authorship of this chapter. The authors wish to thank the editors, Robert Reynolds and Steven Day, for very helpful comments on an earlier draft.

Conflict of interest

No author has any conflict of interest.

Author details

Michael John Stones[1*], Jason Randle[2] and Peter Brink[1]

1 Lakehead University, Thunder Bay, Ontario, Canada

2 University of Waterloo, Waterloo, Ontario, Canada

*Address all correspondence to: mstones@lakeheadu.ca

References

[1] Stones MJ, Worobetz S, Randle J, Marchese C, Fossum S, Ostrom D, et al. Psychotropic medication use and mortality in long-term care residents. In Reynolds, R.J., *Aging – Life Span and Life Expectancy*. London: IntechOpen. . DOI: 10.5572/intechopen.89571 https://www.intechopen.com/online-first/psychotropic-medication-use-and-mortality-in-long-term-care-residents

[2] Hirdes J, Poss JW, Caldarelli H, Fries BE, Morris JN, Teare GF, et al. An evaluation of data quality in Canada's continuing care reporting system (CCRS): Secondary analyses of Ontario data submitted between 1996 and 2011. BMC Medical Informatics and Decision Making. 2013; 13:27. Available from: http://www.biomedcentral.com/1472-6947/13/27

[3] Barlas S. Medicare adds new long-term-care pharmacy rules: Agency passes again on pharmacist independence requirements. Pharmacy and Therapeutics. 2016;**41**(12):762-764

[4] Kozman MN, Wattis J, Curran S. Pharmacological management of behavioural and psychological disturbance in dementia. Human Psychopharmacology: Clinical and Experimental. 2006;**21**(1):1-2. DOI: 10.1002/hup.745

[5] Cerejeira J, Lagarto L, Mukaetova-Ladinska E. Behavioral and psychological symptoms of dementia. Frontiers in Neurology. 2012;**3**:73. DOI: 10.3389/fneur.2012.00073

[6] Kapur S, Mamo D. Half a century of antipsychotics and still a central role for dopamine D2 receptors. Progress in Neuro-Psychopharmacology and Biological Psychiatry. 2003;**27**(7):1081-1090. DOI: 10.1016/j.pnpbp.2003.09.004

[7] Madhusoodanan S, Shah P, Brenner R, Gupta S. Pharmacological treatment of psychosis of Alzheimer's disease: What is the best approach? CNS Drugs. 2007;**21**:101-115 http://dx.doi.org/10.2165/00023210-200721020-00002

[8] Prakash S, Masand MD. Side effects of antipsychotics in the elderly. The Journal of Clinical Psychiatry. 2000;**61**:43-49

[9] Banerjee S. The Use of Antipsychotic Medication for People with Dementia: Time for Action. London: Department of Health, UK Government; 2009 Available from: http://psychrights.org/research/digest/nlps/banerjeereportongeriatric

[10] Ralph SJ, Espinet AJ. Increased all-cause mortality by antipsychotic drugs: Updated review and meta-analysis in dementia and general mental health care. Journal of Alzheimer's Disease Reports. 2018;**2**(1):287-312. DOI: 10.3233/ADR-170042

[11] Randle JM, Heckman G, Oremus M, Ho J. Intermittent antipsychotic medication, and mortality in institutionalized older adults: A scoping review. International Journal of Geriatric Psychiatry. 2019 Jul;**34**(7):906-920. DOI: 10.1002/gps.5106

[12] Worobetz S. Effects of Antipsychotic Medications on Older Adults with Dementia in Canadian Complex and Long-Term Care Facilities [Doctoral Thesis]. Thunder Bay: Lakehead University; 2014

[13] Meyer L. Improving medication adherence. Today's geriatric. Medicine. 2015;**8**(1) https://www.todaysgeriatricmedicine.com/archive/0115p12.shtml

[14] Hirdes JP, Poss JW, Mitchell L, Korngut L, Heckman G.

Use of the interRAI CHESS scale to predict mortality among persons with neurological conditions in three care settings. PLoS One. 2014;**9**(6):e99066. DOI: 10.1371/journal.pone.0099066

[15] Gerlach, LB & Kayles, HC Managing Behavioral and Psychological Symptoms of Dementia. Psychiatric Clinics North America 2018 41: 127 139 https://doi.org/10.1016/j.psc.2017.10.010

Chapter 13

Depression: A Challenge during Palliative Care

Manish Shandilya, Soumya Sharma, Prabhu Prasad Das and Sonika Charak

Abstract

Depression is a serious concern among patients and their family members undergoing treatment for acute and chronic illnesses. The quality of palliative care has great significance in improving the mental health of patients. The patient usually undergoes various stages of treatment before reaching the palliative care stage. Therefore, the tendency of denying treatment at later stages of illness increases. Depression could arise either early or at later stages of treatment. Most doctors feel restrained to prescribe antidepressants to the patient, as antidepressants could have a serious side effect on the physiology of the patient. Antidepressants only work for a smaller group of patients. A proper diagnostics and structured interview with extensive checks of reliability and viability could be used for assessment. Various factors like sociodemographic, gender, age, support health groups have a drastic effect on the mental health of the patient. Palliative care to the patients with social health support groups psychotherapy, relaxation meditation yoga, along with the appropriate pharmacological approach, works wonders for some patients. Continued efforts should be made to treat and deal with depression in palliative care.

Keywords: depression, palliative care, acute, chronic illness, assessment, antidepressants

1. Introduction

Depression is thought to be one of the most serious and common mental disorders that could arise in palliative care settings. The term depressed is widely misunderstood among a large section of people. Often depressed is misused by the word "feeling sad". Many physical symptoms like fatigue, weight loss, sleep cycle, weakness, lack of interest are common in advanced illness. There should be proper monitoring of symptoms in depression. A survey was done by Lauren Rayner and team [1] that determined the pervasiveness of depression in patients receiving palliative care, after the initial assessment by clinicals, nurses 300 patients were interviewed. According to the survey, 58 patients met the criteria for MDD (major depressive disorder) while 109 met the criteria for any depressive disorder. Males were more prone to MDD. Depression could not be only identified by somatic symptoms, but a proper psychological assessment and support are also needed. A study done by Franca Warmenhoven and team suggested that [2] many physicians failed to distinguish between the normal and abnormal sadness, patients receiving palliative care, the therapeutic and diagnostic processes for depression is a continuous and overlapping process. There is high non-specificity in diagnostic methods for depression in palliative care settings. The occurrence of depression also depends upon the past life of the patients and their relationship with their family members. A study conducted by Moira o Connor, Kate white RN and team upon patients with cancer in Western Australia and new south wales [3], has shown that depression is more prevalent in patients with a family history of anxiety. Many patients battling life-threatening illnesses have gone through a lot of pain, trauma, diagnostic measures by the time they approach palliative care. Each of the phases they have gone through has a psychological impact on the patient. Depending upon the diagnostic criteria used the rates of depression could range from 3–69% [4]. Gender, age, demographics widely influence the personality and mental status of patients. Participants diagnosed with mental disorders were significantly younger than the other participants and have a smaller social network. Women are significantly likely to be more depressed than men (P = 0.082) [5]. Patients receiving palliative care with moderate to severe depression could be benefited from an intense narrative intervention as the score reduced on PHQ-9 [patient health questionnaire, it is a multiple-choice questionnaire that is used for screening for depression]. Healthcare workers who understand the background of patients thoroughly with practitioners could deliver the intervention. Intervention is a partially structured narrative that is performed by experienced scientists with research trainers who had background knowledge of patients with advanced illness [6]. Patients are more prone to depression in advanced stages of illness (**Figure 1**). Helping patients with support groups in the initial stages of disease could prove effective. Taking care of patients suffering from idiopathic pulmonary fibrosis is very challenging because at that time no medication could prove its efficacy that could improve the quality of patient's life, but many therapies could reduce symptoms in patients. However, a placebo effect could have improved the outcome, when introduced to the support groups and palliative care have increased the quality of life [7]. A comorbid condition for the patient in palliative care could be very challenging to treat. A study suggested that psychotherapy when given to patients with advanced and serious illness in palliative care can reduce symptoms of depression and tends to improve the quality of life [8]. Cognitive-behavioral therapy helps the patients to accept the condition and treat emotional distress, intervention narrated by health professionals also has significant effects [8]. Detection of depression in palliative care screening could be an effective way as it excludes the non-depressed patients from the depressed ones, but one disadvantage is that it could not detect the degree to which a diagnostic criterion is applied to the patient. Comprehensive clinical evaluation should not be substituted by screening but supplement it. Mostly the detected cases rarely take into account the duration of symptoms. The ability to detect and treat depressive symptoms should be an initial priority to treat depression in palliative care [9, 10]. To achieve quality palliative care, an acceptable or good amount of psychological care is a must.

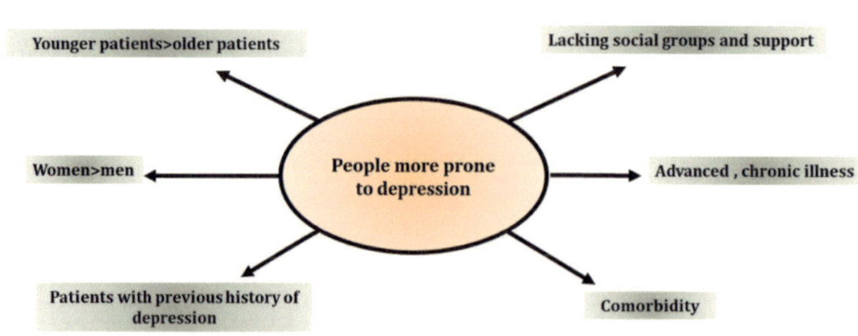

Figure 1.
Factors responsible for depression in patients.

Most patients face a stigma from seeking help from medical professionals, thus it should be dealt with and solved. Members of the medical and research team should arm themselves with interactive communication skills. Unconsciously or unknowingly the healthcare workers should be very vigilant not to portray hopelessness or any negative thought in respect to the disease diagnosis or treatment to the patient. They should be compassionate and empathetic towards the patient. In the advanced stages of the disease, the intensity and frequency of physical symptoms can vary. Screening for mood disorders and depression should be done in patients expressing the significantly high intensity of physical symptoms to provide treatment to the condition [11]. Lack of support system from friends and family at the time of palliative care is certainly a risk factor for non-remission. A strong correlation was found between remission of depression and improvement of physical symptoms [12]. An additional amount of psychological care could benefit depressed patients in palliative care with low support groups for their treatment [12]. Psychological therapies including cognitive behavior therapy showed some positive results in the treatment procedure. Some interventions like antidepressants and psychostimulants remain challenging, requiring a wide level of clinical trials. Pharma logical approach when combined with psychotherapy, support group therapy, an aromatherapy massage could be proven very effective in treating depression [13]. A study performed in cancer patients to detect depression states that no method has been completely accurate for definitive screening. Detailed tests combined with simple questions could be considered as a method. Work carried out in future generation should be beyond screening for psychopathy alone, there is a wide variety of psychological distress that also require medical help [14].

2. Assessment and diagnosis

The first step is the assessment and is one of the most important and crucial steps in the diagnosis of depression. This step could itself be very challenging in the environment. In a study, a structured interview was constructed for assessing the symptoms of patients in the advanced cancer stage receiving palliative care. Visual analogue scales (VAS) were also completed by the participants along with the interview. Impressive interrater reliability was shown by interview items (interclass correlations were > 0.9). Structured interview for symptoms and concerns was found to be sensitive between each participant of the subgroup. Thus, a structured interview method of assessment could be proven reliable and valid way in determining depression during palliative care [15]. To treat a disease, the first step is to identify it. Undetected depression in patients receiving palliative care could lead to severe consequences. Often physicians find it difficult to distinguish between sadness and depression in patients with advanced illness at the end of their life so there should be a different diagnostic mechanism for determining depression in terminally ill patients. Correlation between subscale of depression and HADS (hospital anxiety and depression scale) of the 25 patients that were admitted to a hospice correlated with 100 mm linear Visual analogue scale (VAS). VAS thus was thought to be an effective screening tool for patients who were suffering from depression in advanced disease [16]. Hospital anxiety and depression scale (HADS) could be used in yielding numerical scores and is quite acceptable to the patients. The person who deals with this scale should have proper knowledge and time to deal with psychological and emotional stress generated by its use. There comes a time when patients tend to have consistent high HADS scores, a proper review should be maintained in that situation. Earlier detection could be made possible by regular screening from the referral time and thus could be followed by treatment protocols [17].

Psychological distress comes in many ways and forms. Its proper assessment makes it a big task. Psychiatric questionnaires when routinely assessed by the clinical staff could produce proper results. Awareness could be raised in non-psychiatric staff by educational programs, screening for the disease could be most effective when it coupled with informative and educational seminars in the presence of responsible psychiatric input. The attention of psychologists and researchers is often attracted by unidimensional scales like distress thermometers because they are easy to use, but there is always a question on their validity in complex psychological constructs. The scale with a length of 6–30 items is multidimensional scales that focuses on a wide variety of distress like somatic, behavioral. The large size of the questionnaire poses one disadvantage. Identifying the causes of depression, distressing symptoms, mood swings that co-exist with other illnesses in the patient could be detected through the HADS anxiety subscale. To improve the clinical issue, screening for psychological issues should be the priority. To gain as many benefits as possible from screening it should be accompanied by validation of treatment. There is a minute difference between assessment and screening for a disorder that is assessment is a more complex process that involves various steps like identification of the problem, a good therapeutic relationship followed by management strategies, whereas screening involves only identification of the psychological distress that eventually leads to assessment in the identified patients [18]. Patients suffering from advanced stages of cancer often face mood disorders and various psychiatric problems which are often underdiagnosed or overlapped with the symptoms of the disease. This may be led to severe difficulties and the patient could lead to poor quality of life. A comparison was bought in the screening procedure between Edmonton Symptom Assessment System (ESAS) for depression with Hospital Anxiety and Depression Scale (HADS). The study suggested that a sample of 216 patients were analyzed using ESAS and the score for depression was found to be 2(0–10) and 6(0–16) using HADS. The sensitivity using ESAS was found out to be 77% and 83% and specificity was found out to be 55% and 47% for moderate to severe depression. The cut-off point that was analyzed using ESAS for the screening of depression in palliative care was 2 out of 10 [19]. Interviewing for psychiatric illness in the palliative care setting is very important. There was a comparison between formal psychiatric interview compared with two-item screening interview which determined the specificity and sensitivity of two item screening interview was the main objective in the study to identify the depressed patients in palliative care study. The sensitivity and specificity of the two-item questionnaire were found out to be 90.7% and 67.7%. The false-positive and false-negative results were 32.3% and 9.3%. The study concluded that the two-question screening tool has high sensitivity and low false-negative results. There was also an easy detection and the patients tend to respond positively to the two-item questionnaire who previously had some experience of depression in the earlier stage than the patients with no prior history of depression [20]. One in four palliative care patients tends to show symptoms of depression, so the screening tool therefore must be very accurate. A comparison was drawn out between three screening tools. The initial was the verbally rating mood on the scale of 0–10, responding to the question that was asked to the patients "Are you Depressed?" in either yes or no format, and last was the completion of the Edinburg depression scale. Using DSM IV criteria, a semi-structured interview was also performed. When determined the sensitivity and specificity of the "yes" answer it was found to be 55% and 74%. The sensitivity and specificity of verbally rating mood on the scale were found to be 80% and 43% and at last, the Edinburg depression scale was found to be highly accurate with the sensitivity of 70% and specificity of 80%. In comparison to these three scales, the Edinburg depression scale was found to be highly reliable in detecting depression in patients in palliative care [21]. In medical oncology and palliative care settings patients are prone to depression. The rapid screening for depression could be validated by BCD (Brief Case find for Depression). A comparison was drawn out to carry the validation of BCD in a palliative care setting with Primary Care Evaluation of Medical Disorders (PRIME -MD), HADS and beck depression inventory (BDI). Validity was constructed by comparing depressed patients and non-depressed patients relating to symptoms, pain, performance status by using these methods the prevalence of depression was found to be 34%, 12%, 19% and 14% respectively of BCD, PRIME MD, BDI and HADS. BCD was found to be much sensitive than other instruments as it detected a higher rate of depression as compared to other methods. BCD when compared to PRIME MD could recognize both major and minor depression whereas PRIME MD could be used for detection for major depression among patients. The validity of BCD could also be proved by patients having a high BDI score, HADS depression score with probable depression on BCD compared to those without probable depression. A comparison was also drawn between depressed patients according to BCD and non-depressed patients significantly showed scores on the higher side on PRIME MD. The administration of BCD is not very complicated, could be a part of a routine clinical interview. The results could be obtained immediately. Depression and anxiety are often thought to be the same, distinction was obtained between these two by using BCD that supports its discriminatory validity. Thus, BCD could be introduced in standard clinical practices [22].

3. Diagnostic challenges

Patients with severely ill conditions receiving palliative care are prone to depression and other psychiatric illnesses but assessing these psychiatric conditions could be very challenging by the medical staff. Multiple somatic symptoms are expressed in the patients with advanced cancer which could overlap with symptoms of depression, thus depression assessment could be very challenging. The study found out the occurrence of depression was significantly related to poor performance status and more pain. One could not exclude somatic symptoms in the assessment of depression which could have a direct or indirect relation with it. Comorbid depression characterization was increasing pain, poorer physical condition than expected normally [23]. There should be no omission of somatic symptoms when as they remain influential in the diagnosis of depression. All somatic symptoms were present in any depressive disorder (ADD) like insomnia or sleeping too much, poor appetite, lack of concentration, etc., whereas major depressive disorder includes both somatic and non-somatic symptoms. Defining depression with HADS score the symptoms were psychologically followed up by somatic symptoms. Thus, in a palliative care setting symptoms like poor appetite, feeling tired overpowered symptoms like feeling bad or speaking slowly. There should be proper symptom diagnosis to determine the broad or narrow concept of depression [24]. Many clinical find these steps challenging as to differentiate between the symptoms (**Figure 2**). Mood disorders symptoms can be the effect of physiological impairment in the body. Pancreatic cancer is highly malignant, and it is very hard to treat. Patients are often feared for it because of its deadly reputation. Patients that develop psychological conditions like mood disorders, depression is likely the outcome of disruptive physiological conditions of the pancreas like impaired secretion of hormones, digestive enzymes or neurotransmitters. Thus, here the reason for psychological symptoms was impaired physiological processes of the patients [25]. Depression prevalent among cancer patients could range from 3.8–58%. 25% patients suffer from depression who have

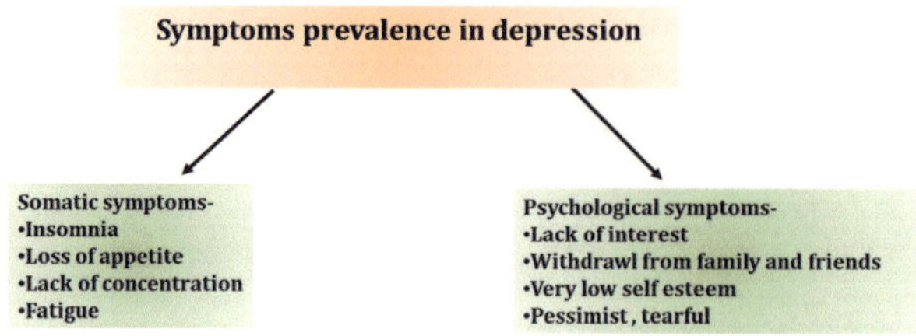

Figure 2.
Differentiating between symptoms of depressions.

been hospitalized with a significant level of physical impairment [26]. Barriers in assessment could form if there arises confusion about depression with some different sources of sadness among cancer patients. The consequence of depression could lead to suicidal or self-harm tendencies if not assessed properly. It is unclear that patients having a comorbid condition like having cancer with depression could be worse than patients only having depression without underlying disease. There is an uncertainty in identifying symptoms of depression in patients with severe diseases because the symptoms tend to overlap with the disease. The cases of depression are often missed. Physicians and nurses were capable of identifying only half of the cases and half of the cases were left undetected [27, 28]. A study was conducted that determined the accuracy of physicians to detect depressive symptoms among patients. A survey was performed on 1,109 subjects who were treated by 12 oncologists by 25 ambulatory oncology clinics that were affiliated with community cancer care Indiana [29]. Subjects had to complete ZSDS (Zung Self-Rating Depression Scale) and physicians rated their patients based on depressive symptoms, pain, anxiety. To detect depression physicians, tend to rate their patients based on how the patient endorses on the ZSDS scale (**Figure 3**). The rating of the physician was also influenced by the medical correlation of the patient. The patient's mood symptoms like sadness, hopelessness also affected the rating. Physicians tend to be affected by symptoms like crying mood, depressive mood, but this could not be labeled as the reliable indicator of depression [29]. In the UK, a study was done to assess the ability of 143 doctors in 34 cancer centers and hospitals [31]. It was found out that the misclassification of psychiatric morbidity in 34.7% of 797 patients and wrong assessment was made. There was a lack of proper communication skills between doctors and the patients. There should be a need in the improvement of skills during the consultation [31]. Many patients from rural background who are not economically capable of affording a psychiatrist are often left undetected. In physically ill patients, the diagnosis of depression is often complicated because of pervasive somatic symptoms that could be or could not be due to primary disease. In confounding somatic symptoms many options have been proposed. Symptoms that are directly caused by medical conditions are excluded according to DSM IV. The distinction between the symptoms practically could be very challenging.

Zung self rating depression scale

Score range	Interpretation
25-49	Normal
50-59	Mild depression
60-69	Moderate depression
70 and above	Severe depression

Figure 3.
Zung self rating depression scale (ZSDS standard scale) [30].

For the diagnosis of major depressive disorder, 5 out of 9 symptoms should be present when all the symptoms were excluded. This is highly standardized that could only identify severely depressed patients [32, 33]. When the false-negative results are greater, there is a failure to treat depression, or false-positive results the risk of initiating unnecessary therapy. Cassem suggests that clinicals should include on the side of caution the somatic symptoms in diagnosing medically ill patients [34]. However, when the approach suggested by Cassem is used there could be a possibility of prevalence of an exaggerated number of patients with the depressive disorder [15, 34].

4. Treatment and therapies

When depression is identified in patients with terminal illness requires various measures to treat it. Treatment procedures could include pharmacological treatment, psychological treatment or the combination of both of these. A study was conducted to prove the efficacy of antidepressants in patients with depression in palliative care. It was found out the administration of antidepressants in these patients was found to be more effective than the placebo effect, and it was more apparent within 4–5 weeks and increased with its continuous use [35]. Patients showing depressive symptoms or depressed anxiety mixed symptoms were daily given oral doses of ketamine hydrochloride. In this 28-day trial, there was found to be a significant improvement in both depressive and anxiety symptoms in patients, the improvement was significant and gradual for 28 days with some rare side effects like diarrhea, insomnia, trouble sitting [36]. There is a slight misconception that the psychotherapeutic approach is not beneficial in severely depressed patients but in a study done by Driessen, et al., it was found that psycho-therapeutic approaches could be beneficial in both mild and severe depression [37].

5. Psychotherapy

Depressive symptoms that diminish with psychological interventions can also be provided by medical caregivers apart from the specialist in psychological oncology. When the relation of health care workers with the patients is perceived as supportive then the patients with cancer tend to show less traumatic stress. Patients with leukemia significantly show stress symptoms which are associated with physical symptoms, psychological intervention could prevent traumatic stress in the patients. A study of breast cancer patients identified that women who don't have emotional support from family and friends have difficulty in interacting with nurses and physicians [38, 39]. For both undergraduate and postgraduate medical training, there is deterioration in clinical empathy [40].

Several types of psychological therapies are being performed depending upon the severity of depressive symptoms (**Figure 4**) stage of the disease, the interest of the patient and motivation to participate in psychological therapy. Cancer patients who were diagnosed with mild to moderate depression could be benefitted from cognitive behavioral therapy, methods of relaxation, approaches to problem-solving [40–42]. Supportive expressive therapy could be beneficial for the patients who have more advanced disease that targets the fear related with death and existential concerns. Many psychotherapies have been developed like meaning-centred group therapy which is beneficial spiritual and emotional wellbeing [43], dignity therapy which empowers meaning to life [44], mindfulness-based meditation therapy, effective in cancer patients [45], and managing cancer and living peacefully [46].

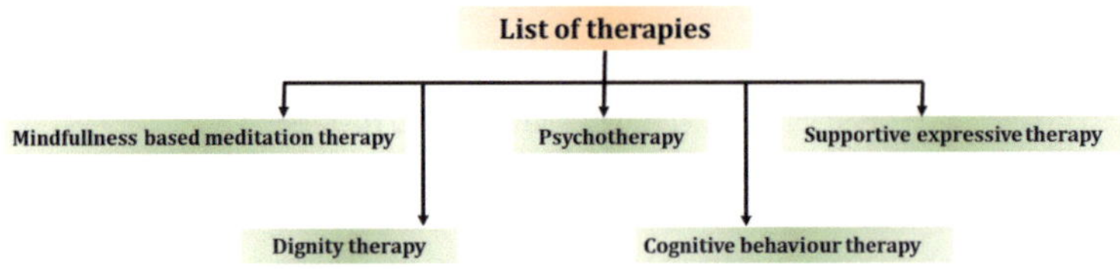

Figure 4.
Therapies performed to treat depression.

6. Pharmacological approaches

Administration of antidepressants in physically healthy patients has shown improvement in treating depression, but when it comes to treating physically ill patients there has been a serious doubt in using it. Tricyclic antidepressants (TCA) and selective serotonin reuptake inhibitors (SSRI) are two classes of antidepressants that showed effective results than the placebo effect. But patients stopped taking them after 6–8 weeks of treatment because they experienced serious side effects like sexual dysfunction and dry mouth [47]. There is an inhibition of cytochrome P450 by SSRI drug–drug interaction. Citalopram is well tolerated as it has the fewest drug interaction compared to fluvoxamine which is a potent inhibitor of CYP1A2 and CYP2C19. The assessment of SSRI drug combination should be administered on an individual basis [48]. Drugs such as quetiapine and olanzapine are some antipsychotic medications that have been proposed for symptom palliation because they are thought to improve insomnia, appetite changes, nausea related to chemotherapy with some additional effects on depression, but rather than cancer population its efficacy is derived from general psychiatric [49]. Fatigue and symptoms of depression are very common in terminally ill older patients with advanced illnesses. Administration of methylphenidate showed possible effectiveness towards depressive symptoms and fatigue because of its rapid onset of action [50]. Patients that develop depression in palliative care were restricted and not allowed to use psychostimulants according to European guidelines [51]. Physicians prescribing drugs should be well aware of their toxicity and interactions with other drugs. When antidepressants were administered to the patient's suicidal tendencies increased mostly between young adults and adolescents [52]. It is important to study drug interaction because patients with cancer when administered antidepressants can alter the pharmacokinetics of the other drugs that were prescribed to the patient for its illness. For example, women who received tamoxifen for the treatment of breast cancer when administered with antidepressants can significantly decrease the survival chances. Paroxetine which is a potent irreversible inhibitor of CYP2D6 which is an antidepressant when administered with tamoxifen increases the risk of death in breast cancer patients [53]. Antidepressants to the patient should be provided following its symptoms of depression and physical illness. In a study done by Mehmet et al., it was found that when low doses of mirtazapine were administered for the treatment of depression in cancer patients, it was significantly safe until 24 weeks period of time, which reduced depressive symptoms [54].

7. Age, demographics gender

Depression is common in patients with serious illness in palliative care. Age factor could also contribute to its prevalence. A study was conducted in determining the prevalence of depression in heart failure patients [55]. In the total of patients, it

Age scale

Age range	Depression severity in percentage
19-29	5%
30-44	7.5%
65 and above	1.4%

Figure 5.
Prevalence of depression in different age groups [55].

was found out 48% of the patients were depressed [55]. Younger patients tend to be more depressed when compared to non-depressed patients. The age group between 19 and 29 had a 5% depression rate, 30–44 years had a 7.5% prevalence of depression and those over 65 years had the least depression rate that is 1.4% (**Figure 5**). When compared between men and women (64%) of women are likely to be more depressed than men (44%) [55].

8. Social support and support groups

Support groups for the patients suffering from depression in palliative care could be beneficial as it is associated with the gradual improvement of depressive symptoms and helps in improving the patient's emotional stress and quality of life of the patient. Cancer patients when participated in these support groups had a positive impact [56]. Patients with ostomy when participated in ostomy support group functioned at much more advanced levels than they were in any other previous support group. They experience a willingness to live and tried making new friends [57]. The efficiency of support groups increases when there is additional social support provided by friends and family members. A study done on breast cancer patients analyzed that how women cope with stress and anxiety [58]. It was found out that women who received social support from family showed an effective way of coping with stress. For effective stress management, it was determined that social support was very necessary [58]. Apart from family and friends nurses also play a crucial role in providing social support to the patients. In the medical staff nurses are the ones that are closest to the patient when they need anything. The connection between patients and healthcare is built by nurses themselves, so they need to understand the whole social support system and the nurses should be trained in providing counseling to the patients who are unable to get social support. In a study done on breast cancer patients, there was found to be a direct relationship between psychiatric morbidity and social [59]. For patients suffering from different types of cancer, one year after diagnosis for psychological disorder it was found out that 31.8% of the patients were diagnosed with depression who had low social support scores [59, 60]. A study conducted on different types of cancer, breast cancer, other cancer and mixed cancer by Bina Nausheen and team, results collectively suggested that there is a relationship between cancer progression and social support is strong for breast cancer [61].

Depression is treatable in palliative care patients if one identifies it at the right time. Delayed diagnosis will always lead to delayed treatment which in order will worsen the situation. In the assessment procedure VAS (Visual analogue scale) is very effective for screening depression that correlated well with HADS [16]. Another sensitive diagnostic method is BCD (Brief Case find for Depression) which is very simple to administer which could detect both major and minor depression. PRIME MD (Primary Care Evaluation of Medical Disorders) has a certain limitation that it could identify only major depressive disorders [22]. For the assessment to be smooth and functioning, there should be well-equipped hospitals with improvised mechanisms and techniques and well-trained staff. When patients were openly asked about feeling depressed the responses recorded from most of the patients were less sensitive and showed false results because the patients tend to hide their illness because of them being stigmatized. The stigma of depression should be eradicated as it hampers the testing problem. To eradicate this stigmatization one must preach to everyone in the family and hospital staff, should organize some seminars and conduct workshops. Many of the medical staff and even doctors treating patients are not well aware of depression as a psychological illness. For the patients to be comfortable with the doctors and staff, there should be good interpersonal communication skills between both doctors and the patients, which could be established by a non-judgemental and emphatic behavior of doctors towards patients [31]. The mental and emotional support from friends and family to the patient at the time of illness could also help the patient to recover more likely than those who do not have it. In the hospital where nurses play a vital role and act as a bridge between doctors and patients, they need to be well trained and highly professional. Untrained staff and nurses in the hospital could be a major reason for prolonged and untreated depression in the patients. Once the depression is assessed, treatment methods could be both psychological and pharmacological. The major limitation of pharmacological drugs is it has certain side effects in some patients apart from treating depression [35, 47, 49, 51]. Patients who experience side effects from antidepressants or psychostimulants should be treated in combination with psychotherapy, yoga and meditation are also effective in the treatment process which helps the patient to achieve peace of mind.

9. Conclusion

Depression is very common in patients with terminal or life-threatening illnesses in a palliative care setting. It is therefore important to diagnose it at a right time. Diagnosing it at a right time will result in effective treatment and could improve the symptoms. There could be many hurdles for the physician to diagnose it because of the overlapping with physical symptoms of the illness. The medical staff should be trained to give counseling to the patients. Many patients tend to resist their treatment because of a lack of social support from family and friends. Psychotherapy which includes various therapies like cognitive behavior therapy was found to be effective in the treatment procedure. Antidepressants when given to patients with depression but with no illness could be very effective but when given to patients with some advanced illness had severe side effects. Doctors must resist the use of drugs that tend to interact with other drugs because it could hamper the treatment of the patients. Social support from family and friends plays a crucial role in combatting depression as it increases the quality of life and gives meaning to live a life, lack of a support system could also be a reason for depression. When it comes to gender, women are the ones who tend to be more depressed than men. Young adolescents and adults when compared to people on the older side are more depressed. There is a lack of hope, suicidal tendencies in the patient with depression. Thus, depression could be a serious challenge in the palliative care settings due to various reasons and we need to deal with it in a more precise way.

Author details

Manish Shandilya[1], Soumya Sharma[1], Prabhu Prasad Das[2] and Sonika Charak[3]*

1 Amity School of Applied Sciences, Amity University Haryana, Gurugram, Haryana, India

2 ACOAST, Amity University Haryana, Gurugram, Haryana, India

3 National Brain Research Centre, Gurugram, Haryana, India

*Address all correspondence to: sonu.mbhu@gmail.com

References

[1] Rayner, L., et al., *The clinical epidemiology of depression in palliative care and the predictive value of somatic symptoms: cross-sectional survey with four-week follow-up.* 2011. **25**(3): p. 229-241.

[2] Warmenhoven, F., et al., *How family physicians address diagnosis and management of depression in palliative care patients.* 2012. **10**(4): p. 330-336.

[3] O'Connor, M., et al., *The prevalence of anxiety and depression in palliative care patients with cancer in Western Australia and New South Wales.* 2010. **193**: p. S44-S47.

[4] Payne, S.J.I.J.o.P.N., *Depression in palliative care patients: a literature review.* 1998. **4**(4): p. 184-191.

[5] Wilson, K.G., et al., *Depression and anxiety disorders in palliative cancer care.* 2007. **33**(2): p. 118-129.

[6] Lloyd-Williams, M., et al., *Pilot randomised controlled trial of focused narrative intervention for moderate to severe depression in palliative care patients: DISCERN trial.* 2018. **32**(1): p. 206-215.

[7] Danoff, S.K. and E.H.J.C.o.i.p.m. Schonhoft, *Role of support measures and palliative care.* 2013. **19**(5): p. 480-484.

[8] Fulton, J.J., et al., *Psychotherapy targeting depression and anxiety for use in palliative care: a meta-analysis.* 2018. **21**(7): p. 1024-1037.

[9] Rayner, L., et al., *The detection of depression in palliative care.* 2009. **3**(1): p. 55-60.

[10] Onyeka, T.C.J.I.j.o.p.c., *Psychosocial issues in palliative care: A review of five cases.* 2010. **16**(3): p. 123.

[11] Delgado-Guay, M., et al., *Symptom distress in advanced cancer patients with anxiety and depression in the palliative care setting.* 2009. **17**(5): p. 573-579.

[12] Goodwin, L., et al., *Predictors of non-remission of depression in a palliative care population.* 2012. **26**(5): p. 683-695.

[13] Price, A., M.J.C.o.i.s. Hotopf, and p. care, *The treatment of depression in patients with advanced cancer undergoing palliative care.* 2009. **3**(1): p. 61-66.

[14] Mitchell, A.J., et al., *Prevalence of depression, anxiety, and adjustment disorder in oncological, haematological, and palliative-care settings: a meta-analysis of 94 interview-based studies.* 2011. **12**(2): p. 160-174.

[15] Wilson, K.G., et al., *Diagnosis and management of depression in palliative care.* 2000: p. 25-49.

[16] Lees, N. and M.J.E.j.o.c.c. Lloyd-Williams, *Assessing depression in palliative care patients using the visual analogue scale: a pilot study.* 1999. **8**(4): p. 220-223.

[17] Holtom, N. and J.J.P.M. Barraclough, *Is the Hospital Anxiety and Depression Scale (HADS) useful in assessing depression in palliative care?* 2000. **14**(3): p. 219.

[18] Thekkumpurath, P., et al., *Screening for psychological distress in palliative care: a systematic review.* 2008. **36**(5): p. 520-528.

[19] Vignaroli, E., et al., *The Edmonton Symptom Assessment System as a screening tool for depression and anxiety.* 2006. **9**(2): p. 296-303.

[20] Payne, A., et al., *Sensitivity and specificity of a two-question screening tool for depression in a specialist palliative care unit.* 2007. **21**(3): p. 193-198.

[21] Lloyd-Williams, M., M. Dennis, and F.J.G.h.p. Taylor, *A prospective study to compare three depression screening tools in patients who are terminally ill.* 2004. **26**(5): p. 384-389.

[22] Jefford, M., et al., *Rapid screening for depression–validation of the Brief Case-Find for Depression (BCD) in medical oncology and palliative care patients.* 2004. **91**(5): p. 900-906.

[23] Lie, H., et al., *Depression in advanced cancer–assessment challenges and associations with disease load.* 2015. **173**: p. 176-184.

[24] Mitchell, A.J., K. Lord, and P.J.J.o.a.d. Symonds, *Which symptoms are indicative of DSMIV depression in cancer settings? An analysis of the diagnostic significance of somatic and non-somatic symptoms.* 2012. **138**(1-2): p. 137-148.

[25] Passik, S.D. and W.S. Breitbart, *Depression in patients with pancreatic carcinoma: Diagnostic and treatment issues.* 1996. **78**(S3): p. 615-626.

[26] Lynch, M.E., *The Assessment and Prevalence of Affective Disorders in Advanced Cancer.* 1995. **11**(1): p. 10-18.

[27] Greenberg, D.B., *Barriers to the Treatment of Depression in Cancer Patients.* JNCI Monographs, 2004. **2004**(32): p. 127-135.

[28] Hardman, A., P. Maguire, and D. Crowther, *The recognition of psychiatric morbidity on a medical oncology ward.* Journal of Psychosomatic Research, 1989. **33**(2): p. 235-239.

[29] Passik, S.D., et al., *Oncologists' recognition of depression in their patients with cancer.* Journal of Clinical Oncology, 1998. **16**(4): p. 1594-1600.

[30] Kirkby, R., Saif, A.A., & Mohamed, G. (2005). Validation of an Arabic translation of the Zung Self-Rating Depression Scale. *Annals of Saudi Medicine, 25*, 205 - 208.

[31] Fallowfield, L., et al., *Psychiatric morbidity and its recognition by doctors in patients with cancer.* British Journal of Cancer, 2001. **84**(8): p. 1011-1015.

[32] Cohen-Cole, S.A. and A. Stoudemire, *Major Depression and Physical Illiness: Special Considerations in Diagnosis and Biologic Treatment.* Psychiatric Clinics of North America, 1987. **10**(1): p. 1-17.

[33] Endicott, J., *Measurement of Depression in Patients With Cancer.* 1984. **53**(S10): p. 2243-2248.

[34] Cassem, E.H., *Depression and Anxiety Secondary to Medical Illness.* Psychiatric Clinics of North America, 1990. **13**(4): p. 597-612.

[35] Rayner, L., et al., *Antidepressants for the treatment of depression in palliative care: systematic review and meta-analysis.* 2011. **25**(1): p. 36-51.

[36] Irwin, S.A., et al., *Daily oral ketamine for the treatment of depression and anxiety in patients receiving hospice care: a 28-day open-label proof-of-concept trial.* 2013. **16**(8): p. 958-965.

[37] Driessen, E., et al., *Does pretreatment severity moderate the efficacy of psychological treatment of adult outpatient depression? A meta-analysis.* 2010. **78**(5): p. 668.

[38] Rodin, G., et al., *Traumatic stress in acute leukemia.* 2013. **22**(2): p. 299-307.

[39] Han, W.T., et al., *Breast cancer and problems with medical interactions: relationships with traumatic stress, emotional self-efficacy, and social support.* 2005. **14**(4): p. 318-330.

[40] Li, M., P. Fitzgerald, and G.J.J.C.O. Rodin, *Evidence-based treatment of depression in patients with cancer.* 2012. **30**(11): p. 1187-1196.

[41] Strong, V., et al., *Management of depression for people with cancer (SMaRT oncology 1): a randomised trial.* The Lancet, 2008. **372**(9632): p. 40-48.

[42] Ell, K., et al., *Improving treatment of depression among low-income patients*

with cancer: the design of the ADAPt-C study. General Hospital Psychiatry, 2007. **29**(3): p. 223-231.

[43] Breitbart, W., et al., *Meaning-centered group psychotherapy for patients with advanced cancer: a pilot randomized controlled trial.* 2010. **19**(1): p. 21-28.

[44] Chochinov, H.M., et al., *Dignity therapy: a novel psychotherapeutic intervention for patients near the end of life.* 2005. **23**(24): p. 5520-5525.

[45] Michiyo Ando, T.M., Tatsuo Akechi, Sayoko Ito, Masaya Tanaka, Yuka Ifuku, and Toshimichi Nakayama, *The Efficacy of Mindfulness-Based Meditation Therapy on Anxiety, Depression, and Spirituality in Japanese Patients with Cancer.* 2009. **12**(12): p. 1091-1094.

[46] Nissim, R., et al., *Managing Cancer and Living Meaningfully (CALM): a qualitative study of a brief individual psychotherapy for individuals with advanced cancer.* 2012. **26**(5): p. 713-721.

[47] Rayner, L., et al., *Antidepressants for depression in physically ill people.* 2010(3).

[48] Hemeryck, A. and F.M.J.C.d.m. Belpaire, *Selective serotonin reuptake inhibitors and cytochrome P-450 mediated drug-drug interactions: an update.* 2002. **3**(1): p. 13-37.

[49] Komossa, K., et al., *Second-generation antipsychotics for major depressive disorder and dysthymia.* 2010(12).

[50] Hardy, S.E.J.T.A.j.o.g.p., *Methylphenidate for the treatment of depressive symptoms, including fatigue and apathy, in medically ill older adults and terminally ill adults.* 2009. **7**(1): p. 34-59.

[51] Rayner, L., et al., *The development of evidence-based European guidelines on the management of depression in palliative cancer care.* 2011. **47**(5): p. 702-712.

[52] Stone, M., et al., *Risk of suicidality in clinical trials of antidepressants in adults: analysis of proprietary data submitted to US Food and Drug Administration.* 2009. **339**: p. b2880.

[53] Kelly, C.M., et al., *Selective serotonin reuptake inhibitors and breast cancer mortality in women receiving tamoxifen: a population based cohort study.* 2010. **340**: p. c693.

[54] Ersoy, M.A., A.M. Noyan, and H.J.C.d.i. Elbi, *An open-label long-term naturalistic study of mirtazapine treatment for depression in cancer patients.* 2008. **28**(2): p. 113-120.

[55] Gottlieb, S.S., et al., *The influence of age, gender, and race on the prevalence of depression in heart failure patients.* 2004. **43**(9): p. 1542-1549.

[56] Zabalegui, A., et al., *Nursing and cancer support groups.* 2005. **51**(4): p. 369-381.

[57] Byfield, D.J.J.o.W., Ostomy and C. Nursing, *The Lived Experiences of Persons With Ostomies Attending a Support Group: A Qualitative Study.* 2020. **47**(5): p. 489-495.

[58] Ozdemir, D. and F.J.P.o. Tas Arslan, *An investigation of the relationship between social support and coping with stress in women with breast cancer.* 2018. **27**(9): p. 2214-2219.

[59] Simpson, J.S.A., et al., *Effects of a brief intervention on social support and psychiatric morbidity in breast cancer patients.* 2002. **11**(4): p. 282-294.

[60] Usta, Y.Y.J.A.P.J.o.C.P., *Importance of social support in cancer patients.* 2012. **13**(8): p. 3569-3572.

[61] Nausheen, B., et al., *Social support and cancer progression: a systematic review.* 2009. **67**(5): p. 403-415.

Chapter 14

Multimodal Pain Management in the Setting of Palliative Care

Marija V. Sholjakova and Vesna M. Durnev

Abstract

Pain as an integral part of palliative care (PC) is often present at the end of the life. Today, many different analgesics from opioids and non- opioids origin are in use. The integration of their use is the most effective method for pain relief. The aim of this chapter is to discuss different therapeutic approaches to pain management in palliative care. Palliative care is being confronted between the expectations and the possibilities to provide an efficient relief from the symptoms, the pain and the stress. The possibility to use opioids for pain management, with all side effects, and non-addictive drugs as additional treatment, improves the quality and the duration of life for the patients in palliative care. Since the origin of the pain is different, the use of analgesic therapy should be individualized and adapted to the real need of every person. Finally, only a good organization and institutionalization of palliative care in the society could allow for better prevention of suffering at the end of the life.

Keywords: pain in palliative setting, multimodal analgesia, non-opioids, opioids, non-pharmacological therapy

1. Introduction

Pain is an integral part of palliative care (PC) and it is often present at the end of the life. Nowadays the understanding of "palliative care" has changed. The new approach in palliative care services integrates the latest knowledge and developments in medicine [1], providing care by specialized team of doctors for pain treatment, surgery, interventions' radiology, oncology, intern medicines and others. This integration of the knowledge from different specialties, offers in "hospices" a very high-quality care for the patients at the end of their life, where pain is managed by specialized professional teams [2]. This care is enriched with support in daily living, with psychological and spiritual care for patients and their families [3].

The philosophy of palliative care is to provide advanced care planning and support which helps the patient live an active, pain-free life, and the pain treatment is one of the most important curative methods during their habitation in a Hospice. Difficulties with impairments, such as sense of hearing, sight, and speech, often represent barriers in communication. Since the patients in palliative care are elderly persons, they are also burdened with the presence of some neurological diseases such as Alzheimer's disease, dementia, or cognitive impairment, which is an additional problem in this context. Additionally, in patients with cardio-circulatory, respiratory or kidney disorders, symptoms of fatigue, insomnia, and shortness of breath dominate.

Pain is very often present at the end of the life, but unfortunately the presence of pain in palliative care is underestimated. The reasons for that are multi-factorial. One of the reasons is a lack of communication and difficulties between the patients and the palliative care providers; the second is unrecognized and misunderstood presence of pain; the third is the mixture of different symptoms or other reasons [4]. Due to these reasons, it is necessary to improve the knowledge about the pathogenesis of pain and the modern approaches to the management of pain relief.

2. Pain

According to the last guidelines by the International Association for the Study of Pain (IASP), pain is defined as unpleasant sensory and emotional experience associated with or resembling that of actual or potential tissue damage [5].

The presence of pain in patients at PC is associated with actual or potential tissue damage which has implications on their daily physical activities, produces debilitation and mental destabilization and has social consequences. In general, pain is a special medical condition which pathophysiology is complex and originates from different causes [6].

Many stimulations arising from injuries or destroyed tissues, commonly associated with prime pathological event in the body, produce noxious stimuli. Peripheral painful stimuli are detected by nociceptors, which are free nerve endings located in tissues and organs. Following complex mechanisms, the noxious stimuli are transformed and recognized by the brain as pain [7].

The released neurotransmitters and neuropeptides enable the pain stimuli to ascend to the thalamus and midbrain through two main tracts, the spinothalamic tract and the spinoreticular tract (involved in descending inhibition of the pain) and through the spinomesencephalic tract. They go from the spinal cord, are synapsing in the periaqueductal gray meter in the midbrain and are involved in the modulation of the pain [8]. Descending pathways descend in the dorso-lateral fasciculus and synapse in the dorsal horn inhibitory tracts; they are coming mainly from areas (periaqueductal gray matter, the raphe nuclei, and the locus ceruleus) in the brainstem tracts.

Modulation of the pain is a process of inhibition or amplification of the pain signals [9]. It happens along its ascending pathways on several levels, at segmental level (the primary afferent neuron and dorsal horn), supra-segmental level (midbrain) and cortical, or through the descending pathways. In this process the following excitatory substances are included: excitatory amino acids (EAA), acetylcholine (Ach), glycine, substance P (sP), Oxytocin, central corticotropin releasing hormone (CRH), and the inhibitory substances as serotonin, noradrenalin (NE), and gamma-amino butyric acid (GABA) including endorphins (eg, enkephalin) [10].

Many drugs are acting as modulators of pain. They are acting at segmental level (local anesthetics), supra segmental (opioids, non-opioids, and adjuvants), and central or cortical levels (opioids). The endogens opioids endorphins and enkephalins are acting via the descending system and are responsible for the analgesia induced by stress.

Modulation and perception are the component of the plasticity of the pain. Pain plasticity is a result of the possibility of the nervous system to modify its function under different conditions [9]. For the perception of the noxious stimuli and the formation of the memory of the pain, the middle and higher levels of the brain are responsible. The subconscious pain information's are ended in sub cortical level at hypothalamus, thalamus, amygdale, and hippocampus. They are transferred to the cortical centers where they are recognized as pain in somato sensory cortex, insula, and anterior cingulate cortex [10].

In general, pain can be acute (physiological) and chronic (pathological). Some authors make a distinction between physiological and pathological pain, classify it as Nociceptive (somatic, visceral), and Neurophatic (burning along the nerves, dysesthesia, allodynia, Hyperalgesia) [11]. Under certain conditions, acute pain can become maladaptive and non-protective and turn to pathological, dysfunctional pain - chronic pain.

The evidence concerning pain among patients in PC show that during the care phase, pain is present in one moment in approximately 70–90% of the patients [9]. Pain is seen in many end stage diseases. The prevalence of pain is most common in cancer; 70–90% in latter stages of the illness and 33–70% in patients receiving treatment [12]. Comparatively, the prevalence of chronic pain in the general adult population ranges from 2% to 40%. It is known that back pain alone affects "up to 84%" of adults.

Many conditions in palliative settings could provoke the pain. Mainly they are caused by the primary diseases, disorders, and conditions. An accidental situation such as trauma, blunt trauma, broken bone, burning, electrical injury, eye injury, heart attacks or postoperative state (amputation, removal of a part of an organ) needs corresponding analgesia. In chronic illnesses from circulatory, infectious, or malignant origins, the pain is expressed as neural compression or malignant infiltration, bone metastasis, obstructions, and infiltration of the soft tissues. Many degenerative processes produce inflammation and are reason for pain.

Resulting from the type of the pain, the feeling pain is different. The pain is reported as dull, achy, stabbing, shooting, burning, severe, or pins-and-needles sensations.

The patients on PC fear pain because of its physical, emotional, and psychological components [3]. Unrelieved or undertreated pain with all its effects to the body systems, may transit to chronic pain. The pain experience is unique for each individual and the way everyone perceives pain, and its severity is different, leading to changes in the personality that has social implications. If the pain is with chronic persistence, it disturbs the sleep and appetite, lowers the tolerance to stress and is often the reason for depression. There are evidences that pain contributes to the development of some cognitive dysfunctions. It impairs attention, memory, concentration, and content of thought [13].

The reaction to pain and thresholds to pain are complex and individual and depend to the individual experiences to pain. The intensity of the pain is in the proportion of the extent of the tissue damage, the severity of the illness and the degree of the patients' discomfort [14]. The after-effects of persistent pain are multiple due to stress-reaction with the involvement of the adreno-cortical axis and hyperactivity in many organs and systems. Increased heart rate with low cardiac output, presence of fear, increase respiration rate, cold vasoconstricted skin, neurological dysfunctions and other impairments in homeostasis are often seen as associated symptoms to the pain [15]. Patients with chronic pain may have low levels of endorphins in their spinal fluid [16].

Modifications of the quality of the pain are product of different physiological and psychological phenomena. The protective function of the pain has function to restore the homeostasis at both levels (autonomic and psychological). The intensity of pain can be modulated by psychological factors where emotions have an important role in the perception of pain. The memory of pain episodes, the patients' reactivity to pain, families and friends supports, religion, personal defense skills, and therapeutic strategies are the most frequent reasons for these modifications [8]. The levels of education, culture and tradition have an important part in the formation of the pain experience. Severe pain produces mental and physical torture of the body [17]. The person is exhausted, fatigued and without energy. Fatigue is one of the leading symptoms of terminal states and often concomitant symptom of the malignancy, producing a poor quality of life.

3. New approaches of pain treatment

Pain is a common symptom in many advanced illnesses [18]. Nowadays, the treatment of pain is approached from neurobiological, clinical, and behavioral perspective.

The main goals of the pain management are early recognition, early proper pain relief, monitoring and documentation. New approaches to the management of pain in palliative care integrate the standard pain relief methods with complementary health techniques [19]. The expectations of the patients at a Hospice are to have an active, pain-free life. The potential to reach these expectations is though the patients tailored analgesia and the integrations of alternatives with medical treatment in multimodal analgesic approach. A multimodal flexible approach to pain relief therapy for palliative care provides the best results. It consists of the use of more therapeutic abilities at the same time frame, at different time intervals. The main characteristic of this therapy is a continuum of analgesic management [20]. The last advancement in pain management treatment is multimodal analgesia with individual tailoring of the therapy to the real needs [21].

3.1 The multimodal approach to pain management

The multimodal approach to pain management which was introduced in 1993 by Kehlet and Dahl as an analgesic model for postoperative pain is already well established [22]. The fact that nearly 10–30% of patients with cancer pain were not satisfied with the standard pain relief treatment (use of systemic analgesics alone) [23] commanded research for new analgesic approaches for more severe pain. The complex mechanism of pain in which physical and psychological disorders are involved need corresponding therapeutic approaches; complex and focused on pain relief, improvement of mental status, psychological treatment, education, and socialization. It seems that multimodal approach in pain management can reach all those necessities providing less use of opioids for 10–20% sparing effect [24].

The multimodal analgesia (MMA) and its opioids sparing effect, provides a significant efficacy in pain treatment and takes an important place for curing acute or chronic pain in palliative medicine. It involves multiple combinations of drugs (opioids, non-opioids, and sedatives), non-pharmacological therapies and some specialized techniques to provide better analgesia.A variety of fixed combinations of analgesic drugs are available on the market. In those combinations, the paracetamol, and non-steroidal anti-inflammatory drugs (NSAIDS) play important part of the multimodal approach to analgesia. Used in palliative setting the multimodal approach may meet the individual patient needs of altered nociception and the variety of experiencing pain [25, 26].

The main goal of this therapeutic approach is the treatment of pain by targeting different physiological causes of the pain.

Data about genetic polymorphism speaks about the necessity to tailor the pain management according to the real patients' need [27]. According to the ladder algorithm, selection of non-opioid, opioid, and adjuvant analgesic therapy should be adapted to the intensity of the pain [28]. Identification of opioid receptor gene regulation, its transcription factors and post-transcriptional events are considered as alternative variations in mRNA stability and translation efficiency.

Additionally, the development of genes that increase or decrease pain opens a new dimension in the treatment of pain [29]. Perhaps the genomic profile of every person will be key to more efficient pain control. The choice of certain pain strategy and adequate medications are key principles for effective pain management.

3.2 Assessment of the pain

The assessment of the pain is the most important part of pain treatment. It is an initial step in the evaluation of the level of pain and continues during all pain relief episodes, as constant reevaluation of the effects of pain management. An effective relief of pain depends mainly on a comprehensive assessment to identify the different physical, psychological, social, and spiritual aspects. The oral description of the presence of pain is insufficient to express the real patients' suffering. It is more visible by other objective, autonomic and behavioral sights that are expressed through mimics, sweating, tears, or with changes in vital parameters in the person [4].

The subjective feeling of pain is difficult to be measured, but its effects on vital parameters may be measured. Based on this, the evaluation of the pain is being based. Generally, there are two main principles: objective (Type I) and subjective (Type II) method for pain evaluation. The difference between those two methods is the opportunity to present the individual feelings of pain in measurable values. The objective evaluation is measurable by the detection of the changes in physiological, neuropharmacological, and neurological parameters. In the Type II evaluation approach, the subjective patients' feelings of pain, measured by self-evaluation, are presented in measurable values- scores. In practice, for PC use, more applicable are the less invasive methods, which are present in Type II evaluation [30].

Taking anamnesis is the first step which helps enormously, where the patient must describe the pain in detail. It is necessary to provide information about the severity of the pain, the history – when, where, how the pain appeared, examine the location of pain, and to investigate the state of the other systems (imaging, organ function). To assign the appropriate management, it is important to discover: the origin of the pain, the states in which the pain is more intensive, the quality of the pain, the route of propagation of the pain, and the degree and the intensity of the pain. In assessing the symptoms, one can use the OPQRSTUV mnemonic (O- Onset, P- Position, Q- Quality, R- Radiation, S- Severity, T- Timing, A- Associated features, A- Aggravating Factors, A- Alleviating Factors) [19].

The received information helps in understanding the pathophysiology and in classification of the pain as nociceptive or neuropathic. An objective evaluation of the pain during palliative care is difficult; it is caused by the lack of communication with the patients so the use of conventional scales for measurement of pain is almost impossible [31]. For this reason, for patients in palliative care and in children, a multidimensional approach is accepted worldwide [4]. It works by using subjective explanations or common methods for self-evaluation of the level of pain, and objective signs from behavior and other vital parameters. Subjective feelings of the pain are measured with self-evaluation using several scales that help in the evaluation of the severity of the pain or pain questionnaires useful for children and older people (**Table 1**). In multidimensional approach the subjective methods in Type II evaluation are supplemented with the objective reports of the medical staff, relatives, parents, guardian, and others involved in the palliative care [32].

Type I – PAIN EVALUATION	Type II – PAIN EVALUATION
PHYSIOLOGICAL CHANGES	**ONE DIMENSIONAL METHODS**
Increased Plasma Cortisol	Categorical Scale
Increased Plasma Catecholamine's	Numerical Scale
Cardio-Circulatory Changes (Pulse, BP, CVP)	Visual Analog Scale
Respiratory Changes (RR, VC, FEV, TV)	
Tears, Facial grimacing	
NEUROPHARMACOLOGICAL	**MULTI DIMENSIONAL METHODS**
Inverse Correlation with Plasma Beta Endorphins	
Changes in Dermal Temperature	
	Mc GILL Questionnaire
NEUROLOGICAL	Dartmaut' Questionnaire
Changes in Nervous Conductance Velocity	List of West Haven-Yale
Evoked potential (neurologic dysfunctions)	Pain perception profile
Micro- neurographics	Behavior observation
	Pain Diary
	Pain Scoring
	Prevocational Test
	Rehabilitation Test
Legend: BP-blood pressure; CVP-central venous pressure; RR-respiratory rate; VC-vital capacity. FEV-forcefully expired volume; TV-tidal volume.	

Table 1.
The evaluation of pain [4].

A simple observation can discover any kind of discomfort, lack of interest, anxiety, crying, tears, abnormal position or movement, or changes in vital parameters as high blood pressure, tachycardia, sweating, impairment in dieresis and other [30].

3.3 Treatment plan

In the *preparation of the treatment plan,* it must be considered that pain is a syndrome with neuropathic, nociceptive, emotional, and psycho-social overlays and it can be used to guide an individually tailored treatment plan because of its subjective nature. To improve outcomes, it is necessary to integrate the PC with other settings [33]. Patient / family must be involved in the planning of the pain treatment. The common problems in planning appear from the conservative believes and myths about pain. The existence of the pain is inevitable at the end of the life; the patient/family has fears about the use of opioids because of addiction and side effects. For this reason, is necessary to discuss the management strategy for pain relief. All parties must be very well informed about the multimodal approach and the incorporation of the interdisciplinary team in pain management that comprises integration of the use of medicines, physical therapy, music, meditation, hypnotherapy, and others alternative methods. Additionally, the personal abilities of the patient/family regarding the terminal stage, culture, religion, and other socio-economic factor must be taken in consideration.

3.4 Pain services

The pain services as special teams working on pain treatment takes place in or out of the Hospices. They could practice pain treatment as "patronage services", visiting the homes of persons at the end of their life or patients with cancer pain. The goal of such services is to achieve the best care and to improve the life for patients and their families.

4. Pharmacotherapy in pain management in palliative setting

In normal conditions, the primary analgesic management in palliative care starts with *oral administration of the medicines.* The WHO in 1986, for nociception pain, proposed a "step by step" approach which understands escalation of the drugs from non-opioid to opioid analgesics [34].

Primarily the ladder approach was used for cancer pain, but today it is widely used for any kind of pain. In 2010, Vargas-Schaffer G. suggested a re-adapted four steps ladder [35] (**Figure 1**), which in 2012 was revised by Leung, who advised pain treatment in a tridimensional multimodal platform [36], and at list, in 2019 Cuomo introduced the trolley model for multimodal tailored therapy [37].

The administration of drugs in palliative care is recommended to be less invasive. When possible, the most appropriate method is oral administration. Also, among less invasive methods well accepted by the patients are rectal or transdermal (patches) application. When it is necessary to apply the invasive parenteral routes, intra venous (IV), intramuscular (IM), subcutaneous (SC), can be considered. Dosing is different and varies depending on the type of the pain from around-the-clock dosing, "as-needed dosing" to "patient-controlled analgesia (PCA)".

4.1 Non-opioids

Non –opioids are a group of medications consisting of anti-inflammatory and non-steroidal anti-inflammatory drugs. They have antipyretic, anti-inflammatory, and anti-platelet effects. Their use in palliative care takes an eminent place because most of the etiological factors of the pain are related to inflammation. Traditionally they include anti-inflammatory drugs such as salicylic acid, paracetamol, and non-steroidal anti-inflammatory drugs (NSAIDs), which remain the major players for the treatment of pain in PC [38]. They have an opioid sparing effect when used in multimodal therapeutic approach (see below).

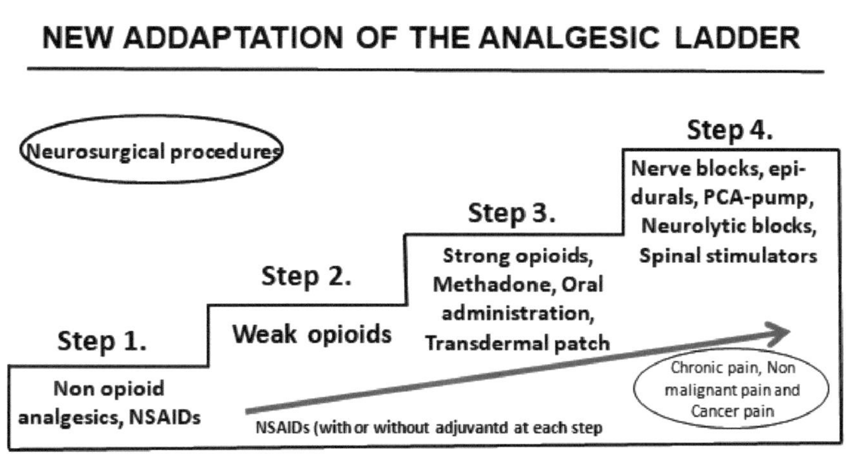

Figure 1.
Readapted WHO ladder for analgesic management [22]. (legend: NSAIDs- non-steroidal anti-inflammatory drugs; PCA- patient control analgesia).

4.1.1 Anti-inflammatory drugs

Acetaminophen (paracetamol) chemically belongs to para-aminophenol derivatives; it is an active metabolite of phenacetin with an analgesic-antipyretic property and weak anti-inflammatory activity. It is recommended as a first step analgesic for mild to moderate pain [39]. Its mechanism of action is based to inhibition of central prostaglandin synthesis in the central nervous system and possible increases of noradrenaline in CNS and peripheral beta-endorphins [40]. It describes its analgesic and antipyretic activity without any effects on inflammation. Its use in PC is crucial on its formulations in form of tablets, coated tablets, or ampoules; therefore, it can be administered orally or IV. The onset of action for oral form is slow (15 min), so the use of intravenous application is the more appropriate. The maximum recommended therapeutic dose is 4000 mg/24 h, or 80/kg BW/24 h. According to a Meta analyses made from Schüchen RH et al. (2018), it was shown that there was no conclusive evidence that Acetaminophen in treatment of cancer pain produces satisfactory pain relief [41], but often it is used in combinations with opioids and it shows a decrease of the need for opioids (spearing effect). Its metabolites contribute to the toxic effects, so doses over its maximum dosage provoke liver damage. Therefore, it must be used with precaution in patients with liver diseases.

Aspirin (acetylsalicylic acid) chemically belongs to the group of salicylates [42]. It is the most widely used drug for the treatment of mild to moderate pain. Aspirin has an analgesic-antipyretic, anti-inflammatory effect and prevents clotting. It is usually used for pain relief with low intensity. Its mode of action is through the decreased production of prostaglandins and thromboxane A2 by an irreversible inactivation of the ciclooxygenase enzymes (COX). It is an important additional medicine for patients with severe inflammatory pain (rheumatoid arthritis and similar). It is suitable for long-term use, because it is safe, with lower toxicity than paracetamol or opioids. In PC it can be safety used for pain control of acute pain, such as headache, toothache, minor back pain, for prophylaxis of myocardial infarction due to its well-established anti-platelet action. Its formulation is prepared in tablets and suppositories (100 mg, 300 mg, and 500 mg). Its use is 4–6 times per day, with maximum dose of 3000 mg/24 h. Among its side effects, the most important are appearance of peptic ulcer, allergy to salicylates and development of Reye's syndrome, if it is used in children younger than 16 years old. Overdosed, aspirin can cause cardiovascular instability, exacerbate underlying renal insufficiency, and even lead to coma with renal failure, metabolic acidosis, and respiratory arrest [42].

4.1.2 Non-steroidal anti-inflammatory drugs

Non-steroidal anti-inflammatory drugs (NSAIDs) are a group of potent analgesics, antipyretics, and anti-inflammatory agents which are efficient in reliving of moderate to severe pain from musculoskeletal origin. They are widely in use at the institutions of palliative care as mono or combined therapy. The list of NSAID medicines is long and, in this document, only the most often used drugs will be mentioned. The NSAIDs mode of action is through peripheral and central inhibition of prostaglandin production from arachidonic acid through acetylating of two cyklooxygenase isoenzymes (COX-1 and/or COX-2). The non-selective NSAIDs inhibit the activity of both cyklooxygenase - COX-1 and COX-2. The most often used non-selective NSAIDs are ibuprofen, ketonal, diclophenac, naproxen, etc. [43].

On the other side, the selective inhibitors to isoenzyme COX-2 (celecoxib, valdecoxib and rofecoxib) have the same analgesic effects as the non-selective NSAIDs, but with a reduced risk for gastrointestinal tract (GIT) and platelets that makes those acceptable for pain management [44]. Unfortunately, the COX-2 inhibitors in 2001–2010 failed to be adopted because of cardiovascular side effects [45]. Some authors described the development of acute myocardial infarction and sudden cardiac death, and in 2004 rofecoxib was withdrawn from the market. However, some additional studies show that inhibitors to isoenzyme COX-2 are powerful agents for control of intractable pain. They also have antitumor effects and are suitable for treatment of patients with bone metastasis what is due to inhibition of the production of cytokine and prostaglandin responsible for solid tumors and bone pain [46].

4.1.3 Recommended non-conventional non-steroidal anti-inflammatory drugs

They are used in palliative medicine for the treatment of moderate and severe chronic pain, alone or in combination, including cancer pain:

Metamizole or dipyrone is an old non-opioid drug patented in 1922 in Germany. It has analgesic, antipyretic, spasmolytic, and fewer anti-inflammatory effects. The possibility to provoke a life-threatening agranulocytosis after long use made metamizole for a long time to be under scrutiny. It was restricted in many countries in the world, but today after relevant clinical studies, the evidence has changed. Now, metamizole is recommended as an effective pain reliever in treatment of acute pain, particularly for renal colic and acute pancreatitis. It is found in form of tablets, suppositories, and injections for IM use [47].

Ketorolac is the most widely used non-steroidal, anti-inflammatory drug for treatment of moderate to severe pain in adults. Its mode of action is by blocking both cyklooxygenase (COX1 and COX2) and decreasing the prostaglandin production. Its' medical use dates to 1989, predominantly for postoperative pain relief. It is found in form of tablets, nose spray, injection for IM and IV use, as well as eye drops. Its use shows many benefits. It is an efficient analgesic, an opioid sparing NSAID drug, and improves the bowel motility what makes it suitable for postoperative analgesia in abdominal and obstetric surgery. Its adverse effects limit its use up to 6 days [48].

4.1.4 Toxicity of NSAIDs

In general, the use of non-steroidal and NSDAIDs in recommended therapeutic doses is well tolerated, but they contribute in various degrees to gastrointestinal (GI), renal and cardiovascular (CV) toxicity. In 2003 Schung SA and all [49] studied the efficacy and potential toxicity of opioids and non-opioids. They concluded that paracetamol used in therapeutic doses is safe, but an overdose is fatal, requiring specific treatment. The inhibition of the activity of COX-1 provokes impairment of gastric mucosa, renal parenchyma, and platelet function, manifesting several life-threatening side effects. The most important are the development of gastrointestinal bleeding, asthma, renal dysfunction, hepatotoxicity, cardiotoxicity, and others.

There are general recommendations for the choice of NSAIDs in palliative medicine based on individual risk of GI or CV toxicity [50]. With the aim to avoid any GI risks, all patients on regular NSAIDs/COX-2 inhibitors -therapy, must receive proton pump inhibitors (**Table 2**).

NSAIDs used alone may not achieve its satisfactory effects; the combination of NSAIDs and step III opioids showed beneficial effect [38]. The essential drugs for palliative care are drugs that are effective for the treatment of common symptoms in palliative medicine, easily available, and are affordable, and are ones that correspond with the use of non-opioid drugs [51].

Drugs	*Only GI problems*	*CV problems/±GI*	*CV/GI problems*	*No CV/GI problems*
NSAIDs	*Avoid if possible, if is essential:* Celecoxib 200 mg/24 h	*Avoid as possible or:* naproxen –1 g/24 h or ibuprofen 1.2 g/24 h	*Alternative therapy*	naproxen, ibuprofen, diclofenac

Legend: GI-gastrointestinal; CV-cardiovascular; CV/GI – bough (gastrointestinal and cardiovascular).

Table 2.
Recommended NSAIDs therapy in patients with risks [32].

4.2 Opioids

They are particularly important medicines in PC for treatment and control of moderate to severe, acute, or chronic pain. Opioids are a group of medical agents that have opium or morphine –like properties with analgesic and many other pharmacological effects. In the past, their use was limited by the clinicians as undesirable drugs, especially in high doses, because of its possibility for addiction and appearance of several side effects, including respiratory depression.

Nowadays, as the population ages, with an increased prevalence of chronic pain, it has been agreed that this concern was unfounded. The new multimodal approach for pain control, the development of safer opioids analgesics and the use of opioids sparing agents, promise more regular prescription [42]. Cancer's intractable pain remains the most horrific condition where opioids take an eminent place in the treatment [43]. Concerning the ladder algorithm for severe pain, patients tailored therapy to its need, provides the right choice of opioids, non-opioids and adjuvant leading to more satisfactory pain relief [52].

Today it is accepted that opioids act on an endogenous opioidergic system which controls the nociception, and participates in modulation of other functions as autonomic, GI, endocrine or cognition. Exogenous opioids administered in the body have the affinity to bind with several distinct types of receptors for opioids. These receptors are the previously known G-protein-coupled receptors: "delta", "kappa" and "mu", which were named according to the exogenous ligand or tissue where they were isolated. By a recommendation from the International Union of Pharmacology (IUPHAR), in 2000 the opioid receptors were renamed to DOP, KOP and MOP [53].

The identification of the MOP receptors and the isolation of its protein helped in more profound study of the structure and pharmacological properties of morphine. The opioid receptors are found in peripheral and central nervous system including spinal cord (PNS & CNS). They are found also within vas deferens, GIT, heart, immune system, and knee joint. The endogenous opioids peptides, active ligands to the receptors, were identified in the brain extract, having analgesic properties similar as morphine, and known as "endogenous opioids". Endogenous opioids in CNS are derived from their precursors: pro-enkephalin, pro-opiomelanocortin, pro-dynorphin, and pre-pro-N/OFQ (pp-noc), and function as neurotransmitters important in control of hormone secretion, thermoregulation, and cardiovascular system [54]. The opioids' receptors are presented at **Table 3**.

The main event is in the CNS where, by the opioids activated MOP receptors, the descending inhibitory neurons producing opioids are activated –induced analgesia.

Opioids are divided upon its pharmaco-chemical origin in naturally occurring, semi-synthetic and synthetic compounds. According to their activity at opioids receptor, they are divided to agonists, partial agonists, and antagonists.

DOI: http://dx.doi.org/10.5772/intechopen.96579

Receptor& Precursor of endogenous ligand	Peptide-endogenous ligand	Effects	Clinical drugs		
			Agonists	Partial agonists	Antagonists
MOP (POMC Unknown)	β-Endorphin Endomorphin-1/2	Analgesia, sedation, nausea, vomiting, reduction of gastric motylity	Morphine Meperidine Diamorphine Fentanyl/ Remifentanyl	Pentazocine Buprenorphine Butorphanol	Naloxone Butorphanol Nalbuphine
DOP Pro-enkephalin	[Met]-enkephalin [Leu]-enkephalin	Spinal/supraspinal analgesia, reduced gastric motility	Low Affinity; Fent/remifen– no affinity	Weak affinity Buprenorphine	Low Affinity;
KOP Pro-dynorphin	Dynorphin A/B	Spinal analgesia, dieresis, dysphoria	Low Affinity;	Butorphanol	Buprenorphine Low Affinity;
NOP Pre-pronociceptin	N/OFQ	Spinally–analgesia, hyperalgesia&allodynia; Intracerabrovasular antianalgesic effect	**X** No Affinity;	**X** No Affinity	**X** No Affinity

Table 3.
Opioid receptors, endogenous ligands, and clinical drugs.

Agonists are all opioid drugs which by binding to the receptors produce complete response morphine-like. Antagonists binding to the receptor have functional response and prevent binding of an agonist (naloxone). Partial agonists provide only partial functional response which is not corresponding to the amount of the drug [55].

According to the ladder algorithm, which is in use in palliative care centers, the opioids are divided upon their power in weak and strong opioids. In the following text, this classification will be taken in consideration.

4.2.1 Weak opioids

4.2.1.1 Tramadol

It is centrally acting non-opiate analgesic with low affinity for MOP receptors and is effective in the treatment of moderate to severe pain. It has modest affinity to MOR and has weak interaction with DOR and KOR receptors. Because of its non-opioid properties, it is included in bouts group as weak non opioid agent with centrally acting analgesic effect and is favorable for PC use. As it possesses MOR agonist properties, it also, through the activation of monoaminergic spinal inhibition of pain, acts in inhibition of the reuptake of serotonin and norepinephrine, which synergistically enhances its weak opioid mechanism of action [56].

Chemically tramadol is present in two isomers which separately (one or other) inhibit the reuptake of noradrenalin or serotonin. The activity of tramadol depends on its metabolic activation which differs among the patients. Its' use is convenient for treatment of acute and chronic pain, moderate and severe, from cancer and non–cancer origin, as diabetic neuropathy, and fibromyalgia as well.

Tramadol is found as tramadol hydrochloride in form of tablets or capsules (50 mg, and 100 mg) for oral use 4–6 times per day, and in injections of 2 ml (50 or 100 mg/ml) for IV, SC, IM and via spinal routes. The maximal daily dose is 400 mg which could be exceeded only in special clinical circumstances. Clinically used for moderate pain, can provoke some adverse reactions as, dizziness, nausea, sedation, dry mouth, sweating and gastrointestinal dysfunctions. It is an extremely popular drug used for pain relief in PC in musculoskeletal injuries and as postoperative analgesic drug.

4.2.1.2 Codeine

It is used as a weak opioid. It is a naturally occurring substance derived from opium (opiate) and is a pro-drug of morphine. Codeine is metabolized in the liver and is excreted through the urine. About 10% of codeine by demethylation is converted to morphine [57]. Codeine has incredibly low affinity to opioid receptors - 200 times lower than morphine; its analgesic property is due to converted morphine. Its dominant use is orally, in the form of tablets or suspensions, for control of mild to moderate pain, coughing and diarrhea. It is a drug with reliable effects, and particularly useful in PC for pain relief. It can be used alone or as a combination with some non-opioid drugs, which increases its analgesic profile. The onset of its effect is after 30 minutes, with maximum effect at two hours and its offset about four to six hours. It comes in form of tablets (15 mg, 30 mg and 60 mg), a liquid (25 mg/5 ml spoon) to swallow, and syrup (15 mg/5 ml) or as an injection-codeine phosphate - of 2 ml (60 mg/ml). The dose is repeated every 4 hours and should not exceed more than 4 times per day. The adverse effects of codeine are like all opioids: constipation, nausea, vomiting, drowsiness, lightheadedness, confusion, euphoria, vertigo, dry mouth, headaches, pruritus.

The safe treatment of codeine understands titration of the doses of codeine (starts with a small dose of the drug and gradually increases it, until a satisfied result of complete analgesia is obtained). Symptoms of overdoses of codeine are also like those of morphine and other opiate analgesics. They are miosis, sweating, cold skin, respiratory depression, bradycardia, hypotension, skeletal muscles flaccidity and other which need an emergent resuscitation.

Hydrocodone is a more potent synthetic opioid, hydrogenated ketone derivative of codeine. It is selective full agonists to MOP receptors. It is used for control of moderate to severe pain. It comes in form of tablets (5 mg and 10 mg) for oral use. Its duration of action is 4–5 h, and plasma half-life of 4 h. It is typically available in combination with acetaminophen or ibuprofen, which is very well suited for the treatment of mild to moderate pain syndromes in multimodal analgesia. In the past, hydrocodone has been used as a cough suppressant. For the treatment of severe chronic cancer pain, it has found a wide use with prolonged duration and the more potent metabolite hydromorphone [58]. As an agonist it poses all adverse reactions described above.

4.2.2 Strong opioids

4.2.2.1 Morphine

Morphine is a strong naturally occurring opiate, isolated in 1805 from the poppy straw. Morphine is a "gold standard" among the opioids, against which the other drugs are measured in equal-analgesic doses. Morphine is a full MOP agonist with appreciable affinity to DOP and KOP. Its major effects are apperceived on parts of the CNS (posterior amygdala, hypothalamus, thalamus, nuscleus caudatus, putamen, and some cortical areas), producing drowsiness, analgesia, changes in the mood. MOP agonists further inhibit gastrointestinal tract (GIT) secretions and peristalsis; often causing constipation, also present is decreased bowel motility, vomit, nausea, and other sensations. MOP opioids also have effects on the cardiovascular system, thermoregulation, hormone secretion and immune function [59].

Morphine in PC is primarily used to treat acute and chronic severe pain and is a drug of first choice in PC for treatment of moderate to severe cancer pain. The oral formulation is easy for administration and especially useful for long treatment. It comes in form of tablets (30 mg, 60 mg, 100 mg), sub-lingual pastilles (60 mg), or as solution/suspensions (10 mg/5 ml). It is also valuable as injections (for IV, IM, SC, or PCA), rectal and spinal applications. In some countries extended-release capsules are present and extended-release tablets which are prescribed 1–2 times in 24 h. They are suitable for patients who are long time on morphine treatment. The onset of analgesic activity appears in 30 minutes, reaching the peak effect at 60–90 minutes. The average plasma half-life is 3 hours with offset of 6 h. The rest of morphine in plasma is present up to 15 hours [49]. The best way of the application of morphine is titrating of the doses. As it has no roof of its effect, the cure starts with small dose which may be increased by 30–50% every 12–24 hours until the optimal control of the pain. The titration continues to maximum tolerability, before moving on to another opiate [60].

Proper dosing of morphine is especially important for elderly patients in PC institutions. They may be overly sensitive to the effects of morphine and a continuous monitoring of the respiration, blood pressure (BP) and the level of consciousness is necessary to be performed.

The clinical use must be corresponding to the current recommendations at national or institutional levels. In most of the recommendations it has been shown that starting with a low-dose oral morphine (eg ≤30 mg/day) gives better pain relief than using weak opioids. National Institute for Heath and Care Excellence, UK, (NICE) [61] in its Guidelines recommends that morphine should be used as first-line oral opioid for relief of cancer pain. It is also recommended for children with cancer pain; in the guidelines of the Royal Children's Hospital Melbourne, it is advised the use of oral morphine for children over six months with start dose of 0.2–0.5 mg/kg/dose, every 4-6 h orally [32].

The adverse effects of morphine include sedation, cognitive impairment, nausea and vomiting which are frequently seen. Also seen are respiratory depression, etching, circulatory disturbances, hormonal imbalance with hypogonadism, immunodeficiency, changes in the mood with hallucinations and depression. Constipation is seen with chronic therapy; patients do not develop tolerance to it and typically require preemptive treatment with laxatives. Also seen are tolerance or intolerance to morphine and addiction. The genetic approach confirms that those effects of morphine are result of the action at the MOP receptor and N/OFQ–NOP system [62, 53].

Many opioids are made by the modification of the morphine molecule, as Apomorphine, Oxycodone, Hydromorphone. They have similar properties as morphine and only the specificity of their use in PC will be mentioned.

Oxycodone–is a synthetic opioid, with high selective affinity to MOP and low affinity to DOP and KOP receptors, working as typical agonist. It is used for treatment of moderate to severe pain, is metabolized hepatically to the active oxymorphone [63]. It comes in form of tablets with immediate and controlled release of action or in injection. The onset of the analgesic effect starts within 15 minutes and it is used widely as analgesics especially for postoperative pain. One study compared the controlled-release oxycodone and morphine tablets in 45 cancer patients and was found that both were transformed in liver to the active oxymorphone. Oxycodone was the most often used drug in USA in the last two decades and was responsible for the "opioid crisis" due to – "too much free use" of this drug [64]. It is a particularly good pain killer and because of its oral application it is recommended for patients at PC. It develops the same side effects as other morphine like drugs.

Hydromorphone- is a water-soluble opioid that is several times more potent than morphine allowing for smaller dosage. It is found in parenteral, rectal, subcutaneous, and oral formulations. It is also used for epidural and intrathecal administration for postoperative pain relief or when other ways are not appropriate [65]. It was shown more effective pain relief properties for continuous dull pain and provides superior analgesia when is mixed with epinephrine.

Meperidine- is a synthetic analgesic drug indicated for the treatment of moderate to severe pain. It is delivered as hydrochloride salt found in form of tablets (50 and 100 mg), emulsion, or injections. It is predominantly a MOP agonist with main action on CNS and the bowel. Its analgesic effects exceed after 15 minutes and the peak effect after 45 minutes. The effectiveness of parenteral application is the same as that of morphine. The adverse reactions are like those of other agonists [63].

Methadone- is synthetic opioid, MOP agonist, which is used for pain relief in PC. Its pharmacological profile is like that of morphine, but it has a very long half-life with considerably longer duration of action. It is also an antagonist of the N-methyl-D-aspartic acid (NMDA) receptor [64]. Methadone is without any active metabolites but is found as racemic mixture of 2 enantiomers; the R- methadone is responsible for analgesic effects, while S-methadone is a NMDA antagonist. It has little tendency to induce tolerance in patients, which makes it suitable drug for treatment of opioid dependence. It has unique properties that make it useful in treating pain which is poorly controlled by other opioids. Its dosing is flexible, although it can be used in neuropathic and somatic pain relief. It is safe for patients with renal impairment and is only long-acting liquid opioid. As a result of the lack of knowledge of its metabolic changes, it has possible interactions with other drugs, and its' long half-life made, methadone is seen to be an incriminated drug [59].

Fentanyl-is a synthetic powerful opioid, related to phenyl piperidine family that includes sufentanil, alfentanyl and remifentanil, with similar properties to the other opioids, selective MOP agonists. It is a powerful analgesic, lipophylic opioid, quick acting drug which is 70 to 100 times more potent than IV morphine.

Fentanyl is used for treatment of severe acute and chronic pain, as a medicine for anesthesia, for postoperative pain relief and in the treatment of intractable cancer pain in PC. It is available in parenteral, transmucosal, and transdermal formulations. Intravenous fentanyl has very rapid onset of action 5 minutes to peak analgesia, with offset of two hours. Fentanyl and its forms administered in intrathecal and epidural space provide prolonged postoperative analgesia up to 8 hours [50].

Because of the variety of forms, fentanyl has become the most widely used drug in palliative medicine. It is found in form of fentanyl buccal soluble film (FBSF), fentanyl buccal tablets (FBT), fentanyl pectin nasal spray (FPNS), oral transmucosal fentanyl citrate (OTFC), intranasal fentanyl spray (INFS), sublingual fentanyl and transdermal patches (FTP) [66]. Most of those forms are extremely valuable for analgesia of patients whose oral access is compromised, or with existence of profuse nausea and vomiting, limiting the swallowing of the required dose of opioid. The lowest transdermal dose of patch currently available is 2.5 mg which delivers 25 mcg/h of transdermal fentanyl. Due to its quick effect, Fentanyl is the drug of choice in control of breakthrough cancer pain (BTcP) [67].

Buprenorphine - is a semi-synthetic highly lipophilic opioid. It has partial MOP agonist properties and has been in clinical use for over 25 years for treatment of acute and chronic pain [63]. Recent studies have confirmed that buprenorphine binds with high affinity to MOP and KOP opioid receptors, and with relatively lower affinity to DOP receptors. It is found in several formulations for parenteral, sublingual, and transdermal use. It is also used as supplement to anesthesia and for psychiatric disorders (treatment of opioid addiction). Now Buprenorphine is widely used for cancer pain management. There is still debate about the potential damage of the transdermal patch and most of the authors think that because of this reason it is not suitable for PC [68]. As an opioid, a respiratory depression could occur, but it does not response to naloxone. The lowest patch strength of buprenorphine (5 mcg/h) is suitable for opioid naive patients.

Tapentadol is a new, centrally acting analgesic agent approved in Europe in 2010, used for treatment of acute and chronic, moderate to severe pain. Its molecular structure is chemically like tramadol. It has a dual mode of action, as a MOP agonist and a norepinephrine reuptake inhibitor. This metabolic change makes it a more potent opioid.

Its potency is somewhere between tramadol and morphine, like hydrocodone, oxycodone, and meperidine with more tolerable side effects profile [58–60]. Its formulation is in a form of tablets and solutions; tablets for immediate release (IR) of 50 mg, 75 mg, and 100 mg, are indicated for treatment of acute to moderate pain, with maximum toxic dose of 700 mg/day. For treatment of chronic pain, it is advised to use tablets with extended release (50 mg, 100 mg, 150 mg, 200 mg, and 250 mg). This formulation for long-release, with once-daily dosing of Tapentadol is especially acceptable for treatment in PC of chronic severe pain because of its simple use and more powerful effect [69]. The daily dose must not exceed 500 mg/24 h.

Clinical studies show that tapentadol is efficient pain reliever in various pain settings including PC setting. In a Clinical trial (NCT01500317) where the adverse effects of tapentadol with the equivalent doses of oxycodon were compared, tapentadol reported significantly lower incidence of GI side effects [70]. Its characteristics offer an improvement in pain therapy, and easier coping with severe pain for PC patients.

The described side effects are like those of other opioids- such as development of allergy, nausea, vomiting, and loss of appetite; dizziness, worsening tiredness or weakness may be seen in some consumers. Overdose, addicting, and abstention syndrome are also present with an inappropriate use of the drug.

"*Breakthrough cancer pain*" (BTcP) - is a state of chronic pain with adequate analgesia where a temporal intensive peak pain occurs, interrupting the state of controlled pain. Traditionally the patients with cancer pain were treated with oral opioids, but for the treatment of BTcP it is recommended the fast-realizing forms of fentanyl (FPNS or INFS). Some authors reported good response to short-acting immediate-release (IR) oral opioid in advanced cancer, supporting the use of these opioids in clinical practice [67]. In this context, the National Institute for Health and Care Excellence guidelines do not recommend transdermal opioids as a first-line treatment, when oral opioids are appropriate, specifically fentanyl formulations, are now the gold standard for BTcP due to rapid action and high efficacy.

4.2.2.2 Side effects of the use of morphine and morphine like opioids

The development of constipation, nausea and vomiting; delirium, hallucinations, sedation, myoclonus, hyperalgesia, seizures, headaches, euphoria, or dysphoria are often seen as adverse reaction to morphine like opioids. Respiratory depression or non-cardiogenic pulmonary edema can appear. Pruritus, urinary retention and altered renal function may be seen also, and signs from CV system as bradycardia and hypotension as well, hypogonadism, sexual dysfunction, osteoporosis and impairment in the immune system, physical dependence, and the tolerance to the drugs [71].

In most of the Guidelines for PC is emphasized that during the pain management at the end of life, addiction should not be an issue [61, 72, 73]. It is also reported that development of life-threatening overdoses of morphine and morphine like opioids in palliative setting is exceedingly rare. In 2005, the American Assembly of Nurses referred that overdoses may be avoided with rational prescribing of opioids, proper conversion to other drugs, titration and use of adjuvant analgesics [74, 75]. The proper titration of opioids and multimodal approach with the use of other techniques such as radiotherapy, bisphosphonates, and other medicines in [76] Ca pain management, or increased dose of current analgesics, and adding adjuvants analgesic for neuropathic pain, may help patients in PC to easier cope with severe pain without a danger for overdoses.

At the commencement of therapy with opioids, sedation and drowsiness appeared, which are common side effects of opioids. The use of light stimulants such as caffeine, or methylphemidate [32] may be helpful. Other mental dysfunctions such as euphoria, dysphoria or nightmares need some additional treatment.

The main sign of overdose with morphine and morphine like opioids, besides drowsiness, is the appearance of respiratory depression (respiratory rate - RR < 8/min, SpO2 < 90% and cyanosis). Because of the progression of the main disease, the respiration at the end of the life could be slow, shallow, and noisy, what may be misunderstood as a respiratory depression. The recommendations proposed by the North East London Cancer Network (NHS)-2018, did not advise immediate use of antagonist naloxone for treatment of respiratory depression. The reason for that is the ability of naloxone to break the optimal analgesia and produce a "pain crisis" which is distressing for the patient and the family [77].

It is advised to use a conservative protocol for such events, which is as follows:

If the patient with slow RR (8/min) is not dying, has no cyanosis and is rousable, the measure “wait and observe” must be performed. If the RR decreases (<8/min), the patient is unconscious, cyanotic with SpO2 < 90% and tachycardia, opioids should be stopped and an oxygenation via mask should be administered. The treatment compromises of emergent resuscitation and application of MOP antagonist, naloxone. Naloxone (0.4 mg/ml) is given as a diluted solution of 0.04 mg/ml. The start of the application is with 0.5 ml of diluted solution (0.02 mg), and this dose is repeated until higher responsiveness is obtained [65]. If the patient is not treated, the respiratory depression can cross to respiratory arrest, with hypoxia, cyanosis, hemodynamic instability, hypotension until shock and death [63].

4.3 Adjuvant analgesics

They are drugs with indications different than analgesia. Today is known that adjuvants in combination with some analgesic drugs produce efficient analgesia. In use are several groups of medicines: antidepressants, antiepileptic drugs, corticosteroids, NMDA receptor antagonists and others [78].

The *tricyclic antidepressants* (TCA) adjuvant agents are very well accepted by patients with cancer pain due to their positive effects on the mood and sleep. Amitriptyline 1–2 mg/kg oral is a useful agent for treatment of children with nocturnal pain, neuropathic pain or sleeping difficulties. Amitriptyline, imipramine, doxepin, and clomipramine are also useful and attractive drugs for MMA of the patients in PC and for treatment of neuropathic pain. Because of common side effects of TCA, is advised the use of *Nontricyclic* compounds as safer [79]. Some authors suggest that the use of secondary amines desipramine and nortriptyline, are less anticholinergic and could be better tolerated than tertiary amines [80]. It has been also shown that trazadone, a nontricyclic antidepressant, has the same effectiveness as amitriptyline [81].

Antiepileptic drugs (AED) can offer a remarkably effective treatment strategy in combination with opioids and non-opioids in MMA. It has been proposed that pregabalin and gabapentin, which are effective in neuropathic pain, target accessory $\alpha 2\delta$ subunits of Ca^{2+} channels. An alternative mechanism of action has also been suggested - that additionally gabapentin blocks spine morphogenesis [82]. The initial daily dose of 100–300 mg of gabapentin can be increased every 3 days. The usual maximum dose is 3600 mg daily. It was reported that carbamazepine, lamotrigine, levetiracetam have been efficacious in alleviating different neuropathic pain syndromes and cancer pain. Precautions must be taken at liver function and bone marrow: suppression is possible to develop.

Corticosteroids are frequently used in PC as an adjuvant therapy for cancer related pain syndromes, which include bone pain, neuropathic pain from infiltration or metastatic compression of neural structures, headache due to increased intracranial pressure, or if the pain is from inflammatory origin (nerve, bone). If the pain is aggravated by tension or muscle spasms, the use of muscle relaxants can play an important role in relieving the pain [83], sedation and anti-cholinergic are present as side effects.

*Bisphosphonates*as adjuvant can help control the pain in certain situations such as: cancer-related neuropathic pain [84], in prevention of fractures in people whose cancer has spread to the bone, in metastatic bone pain, bone pain, breast cancer, bone fractures, osteoporosis with past fracture, etc.

NMDA antagonists has been shown that play an important place and are efficient modulators of the pain in postoperative allodynia and hyperalgesia. A representative of this group is *Ketamine,* a dissociative anesthetic which is used for analgesia as well. It produces, sedation, amnesia, and as an adjuvant sufficient analgesia.

It is used for treatment of severe acute and chronic pain. Its mechanism of action is complex but acts mainly as an antagonist of the NMDA receptor.

Ketamine is given through IV, IM, SC, oral, rectal, nasal, transdermal, epidural, and intrathecal way. It is a safe drug, without effects on respiration at analgesic doses, and less nausea and vomiting compared to opioids [85]. It is used with success in treatment of postoperative pain, refractory neuropathic pain syndromes, and severe Hyperalgesia as well. Its use in PC is controversial and is based on few un-homogeny studies and with a variety of obtained results. Recent study examining refractory cancer pain showed that ketamine used at moderate doses provides efficient analgesia [86].

Canabis still is with limited evidence of its use. The recent controlled trials and studies are unable to answer to the questions about its analgesic efficacy [87].

5. Invasive analgesic techniques

When the pain is refractory to pharmacological treatment, it is advised the use of *invasive analgesic techniques*. The use of local anesthetics provides a novel therapeutic approach in the treatment of pain. It is now established that neuraxial administration of drugs and use of neurolytic blocks are efficient in reduction of intractable cancer pain [88].

The analgesic effect of local anesthetics (procaine, bupivacaine, and lidocaine) is enabled by blocking the voltage sensitive Na^+ channels, preventing the generation and conduction of nerve impulses. It has been also shown that chemical neuromodulation produces effective pain relief. For this purpose, intrathecally can be administered as local anesthetic, opioids, and adjuvant medications (alpha-adrenergic agonists, eg, clonidine), baclofen, and ziconotide. Baclofen is a GABA-B agonist who intrathecally inhibits both monosynaptic and postsynaptic reflexes at the spinal level producing muscle relaxation useful in some neuropathic pain syndromes [89]. Neuroaxial blocks as the epidural/intrathecal application of opioids (in low-dose) and non-opioids drugs (low concentration local anesthetic 0.125–0.25% levo-bupivacaine) increases the analgesic effects with few side effects [90].

Also, directly to the area of pain intrathecal pumps for small doses of medication can be used. The peripheral nerve blocks techniques, catheterization, and tumor infiltration prevent and reduce the bad memories of pain. The quality, duration, and safety of epidurally applied opioids have been intensively studied and compared [91]. It was suggested that sufentanil is a drug with the most promising profile [92]. Agents may be delivered via variety of catheters and ports. The implantation of a self-contained pump delivers medication at a specific rate into the subarachnoid space by a subcutaneously tunneled intrathecal catheter.

Neurolytic blocks or neurolysis of peripheral nerves or plexuses (celiac plexus or superior hypogastric plexus blocks), with phenol or alcohol, can be used for treatment of neoplasm pain, refractory to pharmacological treatment [93].

6. Non-pharmacological therapy

In recent years, due to the advancement of medical techniques and technology, other forms of treatment such as vertebroplasty, spinal cord stimulation, and prolo therapy are being used. The integration of the use of *interventional* medical and rehabilitative techniques improves the patients' lifestyle and helps reduce the pain. The use of surgical procedures is very rare for treatment of pain. There are some cases where surgery was used for relieving a nerve from compression, or at the disseminated metastatic cancer, a kyphoplasty was used at painful vertebral compression fractures [94].

The other alternative forms of nonpharmacological therapy such as chiropractic therapy, acupuncture, music, movement therapies or yoga in integration with the standard analgesic techniques also provide effective pain relief [95].

Transcutaneous electrical nerve stimulation (TENS) therapy involves the use of low-voltage electric currents to treat pain. This small device delivers the current at or near nerves producing electro neuromodulation. It is widely used for treatment of intractable neuropathic and central pain but not for cancer pain and is advised in PC [96].

In CONCLUSION, pain management is an especially important part of improving the quality of life in terminal patients. Because of the complexity of pain, the treatment must be multidisciplinary. Aggregation of PC with other settings, the use of MMA, could only permit better prevention of suffering at the end of the life. In the conclusion the next message will be greatly beneficial: undertreated or untreated pain at the end of the life may be cause patients' discomfort, stress, and suffering, which is a message to the clinicians to increase their awareness for pain control during the terminal phase of the life with a liberal use of opioids and non-opioids.

Acknowledgements

We would like to express our gratitude for the long collaboration with the ex- Director of the Hospice "Sue Rider"in Skopje, Dr. Mira Adzic, who helped us with experiencing and empathy with the real problems of patients in a palliative care institution.

Conflict of interest

The authors declare no conflict of interest.

Notes/thanks/other declarations

We would like tank to Ms. Magdalena Mishkovska and the design studio "Magna –Scan" for their technical support.

Author details

Marija V. Sholjakova[1*] and Vesna M. Durnev[2]

1 The University "Ss. Cyril and Methodius" Medical School, Skopje, Republic of North Macedonia

2 University Clinic of Anesthesiology, Campus Mother Theresa Skopje, University "Ss. Cyril and Methodius" Medical school, Skopje, Republic of North Macedonia

*Address all correspondence to: msoljakova@yahoo.com

References

[1] Greer S., Joseph M: Palliative Care, a Holistic Discipline. Integr Cancer Ther. 2016; 15(1):5-9. doi.org/10.1177/1534735415617015.

[2] Clinical Quality and Patient Safety Unit, Queensland Ambulance Service: Palliative Care. 2016; :321-322.

[3] Rizk D: Palliative care managements. Hospital Medicine. 2017.

[4] Sholjakova M, Durnev V, Kartalov A, Kuzmanovska B: Pain relief as an integral part of the palliative care, OA MJMS 2018; 6(40:739-741 doi:10.3889/oamjms.2018.163

[5] International Association for the Study of Pain: Pain terms: a current list with definitions and notes on usage. Available at www.iasp-pain.org/ (Accessed January 2020).

[6] Bywater J, et al: In 'Green Book', Pain, Wessex Palliative Physicians, 1st Ed. 2014; :4-24

[7] Schug SA, Daly HCS, Stannard KJD: Pathophysiology of pain. In Fitridge R, Thompson M: Mechanisms of vascular disease: a reference book for vascular specialists [Internet]. Adelaide (AU). University of Adelaide Press.2011

[8] Vriens J, Nilius B, Voets T: Peripheral thermosensation in mammals. Nature Reviews. Neuroscience. 2014; 15 (9): 573-589. doi: 10.1038/nrn3784.

[9] Go R: Pathophysiology of pain. Columbia University Medical Center 2017.doi 20171114

[10] Yam MF, Loh YC, Tan CS at al: General pathways of pain sensation and the major neurotransmitters involved in pain regulation. Int. J. Mol. Sci. 2018; 19:2164. doi:10.3390/ijms19082164

[11] Watson JA: An overview of pain. In Merck manual, 2020. www.merckmanuals.com

[12] Dinakar P, Stillman AM: Pathogenesis of pain. Seminars in Pediatric neurology. 2016; 23(3):201-208 doi.org/10.1016/j.spen.2016.10.003

[13] Deer TD, Navalgund YA: Chronic pain, Elsevier.2019; Continuing Medical Education, 2019

[14] Gangadharan V, Kuner R: Pain hypersensitivity mechanisms at a glance. Dis Model Mech.2013; 6(4):889-895

[15] Blanco PT, Rodriguez MR, Vadivelu N.Pathophysiology of Pain and Pain Pathways. In Reach 's J, Yue JJ, Narayan D at al.Perioperative Pain Management for Orthopedic and Spine Surgery. Oxford University Press 2018; DOI: 10.1093/med/9780190626761.001.0001

[16] Dinakar P, Stillman AM. Pathogenesis of pain. Seminars in Pediatric neurology. 2016; 23(3):201-208 doi.org/10.1016/j.spen.2016.10.003

[17] Fong A, Schug S. Pathophysiology of pain. Plastic and reconstructive surgery 2014; 134 (4S-2):8S–14S

[18] Zhi WI, Smith TJ: Early integration of palliative care into oncology: evidence, challenges and barriers, APM, 2015 (7) :1-12 doi: 10.3978/j.issn.2224-5820. 2015.07.03

[19] Parker G: Assessing and managing patients' pain in palliative care, WWW paliative care 2013 :3-5

[20] Proger J at al: cancer pain continuum: a flexible approach. Clin J Pain. 201; 17:206-214

[21] Manworren RC: Multimodal pain management and the future of a

personalized medicine approach to pain, AORN 2015; 101(3):308-314

[22] Kehlet H, Dahl JB. The value of "multimodal" or "balanced analgesia" in postoperative pain treatment. Anesthesia and Analgesia. 1993;77(5):1048-1056

[23] Joseph M. The Challenge of Cancer Induced Neuropathic Pain. J Palliat Care Pediatr. 2016;1(1):5-8

[24] Martinez V, Beloeil H, Marett E, at al. Non-opioid analgesics in adults after major surgery: systematic review with network meta-analysis of randomized trials. British Journal of Anaesthesia. 2017;118 (1): 22-31 doi: 10.1093/bja/aew391

[25] Cascella M: Introductory Chapter: The Rationale for a Multimodal Approach to Pain Treatment. In:From Conventional to Innovative Approaches for Pain Treatment. Intech. 2019; p:1-10 dx.doi.org/10.5772/intechopen.85864

[26] Bujedo BM, Santos SG, Azpiazu AU: Multimodal Analgesia for the Management of Postoperative Pain. In: Pain and treatment, Chapter 4. Intech. 2015:131-172 dx.doi.org/10.5772/57401

[27] Trescot AM, Feynboym S:A Review of the Role of Genetic Testing in Pain Medicine. Pain Physician 2014; 17: 425-445 • ISSN 1533-3159

[28] Singh A, Zai C, Mohiuddin AG at al. The pharmacogenetics of opioid treatment for pain management. Journal of Psychopharmacology .2020; 34(11) :1200-1209 DOI: 10.1177/0269881120944162

[29] Kapur BM, Lala PK, Shaw JLV. Pharmacogenetics of chronic pain management. Clin Biochem. 2014;47(13-14):1169-1187. doi: 10.1016/j.clinbiochem.2014.05.065.

[30] Pain severity assessment tools practical Pain Management. List of clinically tested and validated pain scales. Retrieved from https://www practicalpainmanagement com / resource centers/opioid prescribing monitoring/ on 07/16/18).

[31] Rogers SK, Gomez CF, Carpenter P et al: Quality of Life for Children with Life-Limiting and Life-Threatening Illnesses: Description and Evaluation of a Regional, Collaborative Model for Pediatric Palliative Care. American Journal of hospice & Palliative Medicine. 2011;28(3):161-170

[32] The Royal children's Hospital Melbourne. Pain in palliative care. RCHM 2020

[33] AHRO: The integration of palliative care with chronic disease management in ambulatory care. Advanced excellence in health care. 2019; (3) :1-2

[34] World HealthOrganization: Traitement de la douleur cancéreuse. Geneva, Switz: World Health Organization; 1997.

[35] Vargas-Schaffer G: Is the WHO analgesic ladder still valid? Twenty-four years of experience. Can Fam Physician. 2010; 56(6): 514-517.

[36] Leung L: From ladder to platform: A new concept for pain management. Journal of Primary Health Care. 2012;4(3):254-258

[37] Cuomo A,Bimonte S, Forte CA at al:Multimodal approaches and tailored therapies for pain management: the trolley analgesic model.J Pain Res. 2019; 12: 711-714. doi:10.2147/JPR.S178910

[38] PaezBorda A, Charnay-Sonnek F, Fonteyne V at al: Guidelines on Pain Management & Palliative Care. European Association of Urology.2013; :15-25

[39] Care search-palliative care knowledge: Non-opioids. Source Internet. *Last updated 06 November 2019*; www.caresearch.com.au

[40] Remy C, Marret E, Bonnet F. Effects of acetaminophen on morphine side effects and consumption after major surgery: meta-analysis of randomized controlled trials. British Journal of Anaesthesia 2005; 94(4) :505-513

[41] Schüchen RH, Mücke M, Marinova M at al: Systematic review and meta-analysis on non-opioid analgesics in palliative medicine. J Cachexia Sarcopenia Muscle. 2018;9(7):1235-1254. doi: 10.1002/jcsm.12352. Epub 2018 Oct 29.

[42] Pathan SA, Mitra B, Cameron PA: A systematic review and meta-analysis comparing the efficacy of non-steroidal anti-inflammatory drugs, opioids, and paracetamol in the treatment of acute renal colic. Eur Urol 2018; 73:583-595.

[43] Clark GT, Dionne RA: Orofacial Pain. A guide to medications and management. Wiley-Blackwell Ed I. Oxford 2012; :3-405

[44] Carter JA, Black LK, Sharma Dat al: Efficacy of Non-opioid Analgesics to Control Postoperative Pain. BMC Anesthesiol. 2020;20(272)

[45] Mukherjee D, Nissen SE, Topol EJ: Risk of cardiovascular events associated with selective COX-2 inhibitors. JAMA 2001; 286:954-959

[46] Rouff G, Lema M: Strategies in pain management: new and potential indications for COX-2 specific inhibitors, J Pain Symptom Manage. 2003 Feb;25(2 Suppl):S21–S31.doi: 10.1016/s0885-3924(02)00628-0.

[47] Gonnert FA, Meissner W: Case report - metamizole-induced agranulocytosis. Anasthesiol Intensivmed Notfallmed Schmerzther 2018; 53:388-94.

[48] Maslin B, Lipana L, Roth B at al. Safety considerations in the use of Ketorolac for postoperative pain.Curr Drug Saf. 2017;12(1):67-73. doi: 10.2174/1574886311666 1607 19154420.

[49] Schung SA, Garett WR, Gillespie G: Opioids and non-opioids analgesics. Best Pract Res Clin Anaesthesiol. 2003;17(1):91-110. doi: 10.1053/bean.2003.0267.

[50] O'Neil Ch K. Pain Management. In Chisholm-Burns' AM at al: Pharmacotherapy principals and practice, Section 5, Chapter 34. McGrow-Hill Medical Ed.2019

[51] Williams K. Evidence on NSAID use in soft tissue injuries. Nurs Times 2012; 108:12-14.

[52] Pathan H, Williams J: Basic opioids pharmacology: an update. Br J Pain.2012; 6(1):11-16

[53] Law PY. Opioid receptor signal transduction mechanisms. In: Pasternak GW, Ed. The opiate receptors. New York: Humana Press 2011; :195-238.

[54] Spetea M, Asim MF, WolberG, Schmidhammer G. The opioid receptor and ligands acting at the μ opioid receptor, as therapeutics and potential therapeutics. Current Pharmaceutical Design. 2013; 19:7415-7434

[55] Wood H, Dickman A, Star A, Boland JW: Updates in palliative care – overview and recent advancements in the pharmacological management of cancer pain. Clinical Medicine. 2018; 18(1) : 17-22

[56] Russell IJ, Kamin M, Benn RM: Efficacy of Tramodol in Treatment of Pain in Fibromylagia. Journal of Clinical Rheumatology, Practical Reports on Rheumatic & Musculoskeletal Diseases

November 2000; 6(5):250-257 DOI: 10.1097/00124743-200010000-00003

[57] Prommer E: Role of codeine in palliative care. Journal of Opioid Management. 2010; 7 (5): 401-406. doi:10.5055/jom.2011.0081.

[58] Hydrocodone: MedlinePlus Drug Information. *medlineplus.gov*. Retrieved 15 April 2019.

[59] Eldahah B: Seeking new approaches to pain management, DGCG 2019; :1-13

[60] Wiffen PJ, Derry S, Moore RA: Impact of morphine, fentanyl, oxycodone or codeine on patient consciousness, appetite and thirst when used to treat cancer pain. Cochrane Database of Systematic Reviews. 2014; 5: CD011056. doi.org/10.1002/14651858. CD011056

[61] National Institute for Heath and Care Excellence: Osteoarthritis: care and management: NICE Guideline (CG177). NICE, 2014. Nice.org. uk/guidance/ gc177 [27 November 2017].

[62] Ebenau A, Dijkstra B, terHuurne C. et al: Palliative care for patients with substance use disorder and multiple problems: a qualitative study of experiences of healthcare professionals, volunteers and experts-by-experience. BMC Palliat Care 2020; 19 (8). doi: org/10.1186/ s12904-019-0502-x

[63] Sharma V, Dutt S, Kumar R, at al: Opioid Pharmacology: A Review. IJSRST 2015; 1(5):1-11 ISSN: 2395-6011 | Online ISSN: 2395-602X

[64] Cardiff (UK): National Collaborating Centre for Cancer (UK). Opioids in Palliative Care: Safe and Effective Prescribing of Strong Opioids for Pain in Palliative Care of Adults. 2012; Bookshelf ID: NBK115257 PMID: 23285502

[65] Maharaj R: Pain management in palliative care. 50th Annual scientific meeting Florida ACP. 2018.

[66] Vallejo R, Barkin RL, Wang VC: Pharmacology of opioids in the treatment of chronic pain Syndromes. Pain Physician. 2011; 14: E343-E360. ISSN 2150-1149

[67] Madescape org: CMA. Stewardship in breakthrough cancer pain management. The right treatment in right dose. Madescape. 2020; November

[68] Guniona MV, MarchionneaAM, Andersona CTM: Use of the mixed agonist—antagonist nalbuphine in opioid based analgesia. Acute Pain. 2004; 6: 29-39 doi:10.1016/j.ac pain.2004.02.002

[69] Singh DR, Nag K, Shetti AN at al: Tapentadol hydrochloride: A novel analgesic. Saudi Journal of Anaesthesia.2013; 7 (3): 322-326. doi:10.4103/1658-354X.115319.

[70] Camilleri M: Comparison of the Effects of Tapentadol and Oxycodone on Gastrointestinal and Colonic Transit in Humans (tap-oxy). Clinical Trials. gov Mayo clinic 2012; Identifier: NCT01500317

[71] Bywater J, et al. In 'Green Book', Pain, Wessex Palliative Physicians, 1st Ed. 2014; :4-24

[72] Hariharan U, Garg R: Update on opioid addiction for perioperative and Critical Unit Care: Anesthesiologists perspective. J Addict Med Ther Sci 2015; 1(1): 027-030

[73] Nord of England Cancer network: Palliative and end of life care Guidelines. Ed 3. NHS 2008:7-9

[74] ArnsteinP: Multimodal approaches to pain management. Nursing 2011. 2011; 41(3) :60-61 doi:10.1097/01. NURSE.0000394384.65192.3c

[75] Anand KJS, Willson DF, Berger J, at al. Tolerance and Withdrawal from Prolonged Opioid Use in Critically Ill Children. Pediatrics. 2010; 125(5): 1208-1225. doi:10.1542/peds.2009-0489.

[76] Torrance N, Smith BH, Bennett MI, Lee AJ. The epidemiology of chronic pain of predominantly neuropathic origin. Results from a general population survey. The Journal of Pain. 2006;7(4):281-289

[77] MMG021: Guidance on the use of Naloxone in the management of opioid-induced respiratory depression. NHS 2018. https://www.nhft.nhs.uk/

[78] Shim JH:Multimodal analgesia or balanced analgesia: the better choice?Korean Journal of Anesthesiology 2020;73(5):361-362. doi:10.4097/kja.20505

[79] Arbuck D: The Use of Antidepressants in Multimodal Pain Management. PPM 2021;21(1):1-7

[80] Prakash S. Masand& Sanjay Gupta (1999) Selective Serotonin-Reuptake Inhibitors: An Update, Harvard Review of Psychiatry, 7:2, 69-84. doi: 10.3109. hrp. 7.2.69

[81] Piedad MA, Carmen Ma RL, Barea RM at al: Trazodone for the treatment of fibromyalgia: an open-label, 12-week study. BMC MusculoskeletDisord. 2010; 11: 204. doi: 10.1186/1471-2474-11-204

[82] Ratini M: Pain Medications for Palliative Care. WebMD Medical Reference.2017 Pmid:28874624.

[83] Shim JH:Multimodal analgesia or balanced analgesia: the better choice?Korean Journal of Anesthesiology 2020;73(5):361-362. doi:10.4097/kja.20505

[84] Joseph M: The Challenge of Cancer Induced Neuropathic Pain. J Palliat Care Pediatr. 2016;1(1):5-8

[85] Urban MK, YaDeau JT, Wukovits B at al: Ketamine as an adjunct to post-operative pain management in opioid tolerant patients after spinal fusions: A prospective randomized trial.HSSJ. 2008; 4: 62-65 DOI:10.1007/s11420-007-9069-9

[86] Hocking G, Cousins MJ: Ketamine in chronic pain management: an evidence-based review. AnesthAnalg. 2003;97(6):1730-1739. doi: 10.1213/01.ane.0000086618.28845.9b.

[87] Bettinger JJ, Chu R: Analgesics of the Future: The Potential of the Endo-cannabinoid System. PPM 2019; 19, (3):56-62

[88] Johnson Q, Borsheski RR, Reeves-Viets JL: Pain management mini-series. Part I. A review of management of acute pain. Mo Med. 2013; 110(1):74-79. PMID: 23457757; PMCID: PMC6179627.

[89] Obs& Gynae Clinical Guidelines Co-ordinator: Clinical practice guidelines Palliative Care: Intrathecal administration of medications, WNHS, May 2017, Part. :1-3

[90] Salins NS, Crawford GB: Intrathecal Analgesia and Palliative Care: A Case Study. Indian J Paliat Care. 2010;16(1):44-47. doi.org/10.4103/0973-1075.63134

[91] Sholjakova M, Kuzmanovska B, Durnev V, Kartalov A, Isjanovska R: Epidural analgesia for intractable cancer pain - An old story used until now. Arch Pub Health 2020; 12 (2): 15-24 (English)

[92] Chambers WA: Nerve blocks in palliative care. British Journal of Anesthesia. 2008; 101 (1):95-100. doi.org/10.1093/bja/aen105.

[93] Smith TJ, TeminS, Erin R et al: American Society of Clinical Oncology Provisional Clinical Opinion: The Integration of Palliative Care into Standard Oncology Care. Feb 26,

2012. Accessed from www.asco.org March 2012.

[94] Fourney DR, Schomer DF, Nade R at al: Percutaneous vertebroplasty and kyphoplasty for painful vertebral body fractures in cancer patients. J Neurosurg. 2003; 98(1 Suppl):21-30. doi: 10.3171/spi.2003.98.1.0021.

[95] O'Brien T, Kane CM:Pain services and palliative medicine- an integrated approach to pain management in cancer care patients, Br J Pain. 2014; 8(4): 163-171. doi:10.1177/204 9463714548768

[96] National health Servis UK Last review 10 August 2018 (TENS) www.nhs.uk

Section 5

Ethics, Organization and Policy Issues

Chapter 15

Holistic/Palliative Management of Patient's Health Care and Home Situation in a Depressed Economy

Akon Emmanuel Ndiok, Emilia Oyira and Busisiwe Ncama

Abstract

In most middle and low economic nations, problem in the active management of health complaints is patients defaulting on follow-up appointments, attributable to financial constraints and cost of health services due to economic recession. This increases the danger of aggravation and deterioration of the condition and leads to re-hospitalisation. Most terminally ill patients and elderly prefer to be cared for at home by family caregivers or paid health professionals towards the end of their life. Holistic/palliative care is a key component of home health care. Current structure of health and social care services shows that the home is gradually becoming a significant location of long-term care. Holistic care as advocated by Florence Nightingale and others takes cognizance of the care of total human being looking at the spiritual, physical, social and psychosocial care of individual. Quality care for patients and their families can be achieved by establishing principles of holistic/palliative care as an integral part of daily practice both in the hospital and home care, as advocated by the WHO. Challenges in seeking to do this can be overcome if adequate funding is allocated for palliative care activities and setting up machineries for training of families on home care.

Keywords: depressed economy, holistic/palliative care, home care, management

1. Introduction

The economic recession in developing countries especially in sub-Saharan region has affected various sectors of the economy. This includes the health sector, leading to low productivity, poor service delivery and poor health outcome [1]. In some of these countries, home services are not available. The health sector is still trying to deliver basic health care services with the collective efforts of government but efforts to accomplish this seem not achievable due to the present state of the economy. Holistic health care is good, both ethically and practically but it is hard to find as any obvious expression of what holistic health care is or any plain explanation of its realistic usefulness especially in terminally ill patients in need of palliative care, which may require home care.

In most developing countries, patients generally report late to health facility due to a sequence response to event: improper health-seeking behaviour, economy and ignorance of the disease, treatment by unqualified and unorthodox medication, non-availability of personnel, equipment, culture/belief and family decisions [2].

Terminal diseases have often been linked with having one of the worst effects on the quality of life among affected patients and their families.

This chapter, therefore, considers what holism is and then what a holistic approach to illness might be, and how this might improve health care at home in a depressed economy.

1.1 Learning outcomes

By the end of this chapter you should be able to:

- review holistic care and identify its principles
- understand palliative care and its principles
- recognise the relevance of spirituality in health care
- assess the impact of economic depression on health
- assess the home care situation in a depressed economy
- discuss the integration of palliative/holistic care in clinical and home-based care in terminally ill patients and the elderly.

2. What is holistic care?

Holistic care means reflection of the whole person, physically, psychologically, socially and spiritually, in the care and prevention of disease. These different conditions can be similarly important. They should be managed together so that a person is cared for as a whole. A holistic approach means that the health care providers are well versed with a patient's whole life situation. Maintaining one's health requires continuous effort to attain a balance of all aspects of life. To accomplish this balance, an amount of consistent factors must be considered when providing health care to patients/clients. Such factors include age, sex, family relationship, cultural influences and economic status. This broad approach to health care is recognised as holistic health care [3]. In order to have a good understanding of holistic nursing, Katie Eriksson, who is a nurse, came up with the theory of Caritative care that helps distinguish the relationship between a nurse and a patient and the concept of caring principles, which guide the nurses in decision-making. The theory of Caritative care comprises love, which is known as caritas. It shows the significance of regarding the self-esteem of a human being and holiness [4].

Almost all health care professionals would assert to put into practice holistic health care. It is obvious that; no one would declare or have the same opinion that their individual, professional or organisational practice was not holistic. Consequently, few if any of these professions, people or organisations make it apparent what they mean by 'being holistic'. They do not provide any explanation, or examples of how they manifest their holism. It is difficult to discover any criteria against which their success at being holistic could be measured. I doubt that many of the people, professions or organisations have any comprehensible conceptual understanding of what they mean by 'being holistic'.

The word holism has its foundation in two Greek words, both of which denote 'whole'. This first 'holos' is the base for holism and the second 'hale' is the base for healing and health [5]. Health in general is believed to be concerned with the state of a person's mind and body, commonly meaning free from illness, injury or pain. Healing is the process of re-establishing health to a diseased, injured or damaged individual. Mariano defines healing as the consolidation of total human being in body, mind, feeling and spirit [6]. Therefore, it is an associate to holism.

'Holism' in health care is a philosophy that emanates from Florence Nightingale who advocated care that centred on unity, wellness and the interrelationship among human beings, events and the environment [6]. She discerned the importance of such components as the environment, sense of touch, light, smells, music and silent expression in the treatment process [7], hence, reaching patients in fashions that went beyond rendering just physical care. The philosophy behind holistic care is founded on the thought of holism, which stresses that for human beings the whole is greater than the sum of its parts and that mind and spirit affect the body [8]. Holistic nursing has a higher cognizance of self, others, nature and spirit. This is the same approach Florence Nightingale integrated as the first holistic nurse, which centred on harmony, wellness and interrelatedness of human beings, likewise their surroundings. Holistic nurses also have the same self-care and self-awareness of body, mind and spirit as part of their belief structure (**Figure 1**). Through caring for themselves, it is believed it gives a holistic nurse the capability to have that same consciousness for the care of others [7]. Florence Nightingale once expressed the role of nurses as 'to put the patient in the best condition for nature to act upon him' [9]. She thought that touch, kindness and other measures of comfort, provided within the setting of treatment environment, are essential for nursing care. These assumptions are applied nowadays. Even these days, nurses are educated to deal with the environment and use touch, knead, eye contact, voice and other measures to make patients more relaxed. These nursing actions, known as 'the art of nursing', constitute the basis of professional nursing [10]. Currently, different fields, such as physics, mathematics, science, philosophy, sociology, medicine, nursing, etc. endorse the opinion that the honesty of an individual is much more complicated and greater than the sum of their individual parts [10].

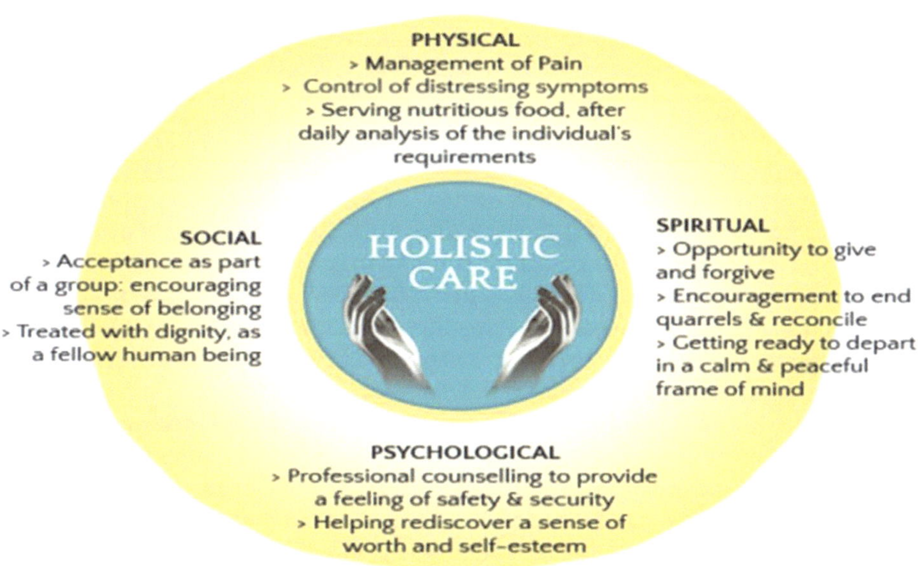
PHYSICAL
› Management of Pain
› Control of distressing symptoms
› Serving nutritious food, after daily analysis of the individual's requirements
SOCIAL
› Acceptance as part of a group: encouraging sense of belonging
› Treated with dignity, as a fellow human being
HOLISTIC CARE
SPIRITUAL
› Opportunity to give and forgive
› Encouragement to end quarrels & reconcile
› Getting ready to depart in a calm & peaceful frame of mind
PSYCHOLOGICAL
› Professional counselling to provide a feeling of safety & security
› Helping rediscover a sense of worth and self-esteem

Figure 1.
Diagrammatic presentation of the components of holistic care.

2.1 Principles of a holistic approach

- All people have natural healing powers;
- The patient is a person, not just a disease;
- Suitable healing therapy needs a team approach;
- Patient and health care professionals are collaborators in the healing process;
- Treatment comprises fixing the cause of the illness, not just reliving the symptoms [5].

3. Palliative care and its principles

The World Health Assembly approved the resolution to integrate hospice and palliative care services into national health services [11]. The body recognises these important health services as an important component of health systems worldwide and therefore calls on national authorities to make sure they be given the awareness they deserve. This is the first time that the World Health Assembly has considered a declaration on palliative care. It endorses that all countries need to take palliative care seriously [11]. The main recommendations to all member states of WHO as seen in the resolution are to integrate palliative care into health care systems, to make sure that palliative care is incorporated into the introductory and continuing education and training for all health care personnel and to make sure that appropriate medications, as well as strong pain medications, are accessible to patients [11].

Many individuals, organisations and bodies including the WHO have suggested different definitions of palliative care. WHO revised the meaning of palliative care to be 'an approach that improves the quality of life of patients and their families facing the problem associated with life-threatening illness, through the prevention and relief of suffering by means of early identification and impeccable assessment and treatment of pain and other problems, physical, psychosocial and spiritual' [12]. WHO further listed the following features of palliative care: 'provides relief from pain and other distressing symptoms; affirms life and regards dying as a normal process; intends neither to hasten nor postpone death; integrates the psychological and spiritual aspects of patient care; offers a support system to help patients live as actively as possible until death; offers a support system to help the family cope during the patients illness and in their own bereavement; uses a team approach to address the needs of patients and their families, including bereavement counselling, if indicated; will enhance quality of life, and may also absolutely influence the progression of illness; is applicable early in the course of illness, in conjunction with other treatments that are aimed to prolong life, such as chemotherapy or radiation therapy, and includes those examinations needed to better understand and manage distressing clinical complications' [12].

Boltz defined palliative care 'as expert curative care of patients with severe disorders, and it emphases providing patients with relief from symptoms, discomfort and worry of serious illness, irrespective of the diagnosis' [13]. She further explained that the word 'palliative' has its origin in the Latin word meaning to 'cloak or cover'. And upheld that, Viewpoint of how cancer, which is one of the terminal diseases is observed and not properly diagnosed, is suitable description because most cancers progress without warning signs for an extensive period before the individual tries to seek help. The National Consensus Project (NCP) and National

Quality Forum (NQF) jointly formulated the concept of palliative care so as to separate it from other types of care [14]. And so they came up with eight domains of palliative care: 'structure and processes of care; physical aspects of care; psycho-social and psychiatric aspects of care; social aspect of care; spiritual, religious, and existential aspects of care; cultural aspects of care; care of the imminently dying patient and ethical and legal aspect of care' [14].

Palliative care is often misidentified as being the same as care given to the patient approaching death where no cure is expected to be achieved [15]. It is focused on the relief of distress during the advancement of patient's illness. Even though hospice and palliative care is extensively used in the western world, many patients are seen to register in hospice very close to death, which limits the advantage these services would have obtained.

Rosser and Walsh cited WHO's principles of palliative care as follows:

- "provides relief from pain and other distressing symptoms;
- intends neither to hasten nor postpone death;
- integrates the psychological and spiritual aspects of patient care;
- offers a support system to help patients live as actively as possible until death;
- offers a support system to help the family cope during the patient's illness and in
- their own bereavement;
- uses a team approach to address the needs of patients and their families, including
- bereavement counselling, if indicated;
- is applicable early in the course of illness, in conjunction with other therapies that
- are intended to prolong life, such as chemotherapy or radiation therapy, and includes complications" [5].

These principles according to Rosser and Walsh focus on a whole, humanistic method of caring for the total being during the course of their illness, instead of concentrating on the ailment or situation [5]. Palliative care answers to the altering wishes of the patient and family, identifying that the illness development and the related involvements are distinctive to each individual. Rosser and Walsh opined that palliative care is seen as supportive care [5]. They see it as care delivered to patients, friends and family during the course of their illness; this includes the period before diagnosis has been made, as soon as patients start undergoing series of examinations, treatment and home care. The purpose of supportive care is to assist the patients and their families to be able to handle their illness and management at home.

Becker also penned principles that are relevant to providing palliative care. These include the following:

- Follow-up of all patients diagnosed with terminal illness at any stage of the disease

- Competence at putting patients at ease
- Listening and attention skills
- Questioning techniques [16].

These principles will put humanity back into the care offered by nurses. After physicians, nurses are the most important members of the palliative care team in the sense that they spend 24 hours with the patients and should be able to display the principles [16]. Skill is an important characteristic for ensuring quality, safety and cost-effective health care. The term competence according to the Royal College of Nursing "(RCN) comprises the skills, knowledge, practices, qualities and manners essential for an individual" so as to execute the work successfully [16]. A nurse is said to be competent when she has the skills and talents vital for lawful, safe and effective professional practice without direct guidance [17]. Competence can be said to be basic features of persons that result in effective performance. They can be described as a mixture of knowledge, skills, purposes and personal character traits. It can also be seen as the way someone behaves or acts.

Areas of competency include verbal message, written communication, enquiring skills and team skills [17]. Nurses are expected to communicate efficiently, generating talking and listening skills. Nurses should be able to use their knowledge and skills to promote open and honest communication skills to support open and honest interaction that recognises the needs of patients, and also creates a satisfying association in which they are able to apply counselling skills and initiate follow-up programmes to help them to adjust to their illness and care. Their knowledge and skill will also ascertain that patients obtain full evidence-based nursing care. They understand and identify the impact of terminal disease when dealing with clinical or home situation, so that they can be able to assess the outcome of care and give appropriate intervention. Competence also includes the ability of the nurses to use the e11 function health patterns to assess the patient. Gordon Morgan, according to Doenges and Moorhouse, devised 11 functional health patterns to be used by nurses in nursing process to provide more comprehensive nursing assessment of the patient. This will help the nurses to give holistic care to patients [18].

The model of palliative care put together by the Canadian Hospice and Palliative Care Association (CHPCA) [19] is the model that is used to guide this chapter. This model is effective because it was developed to plan, evaluate and develop educational programmes [19]. In adopting this model, the paper considered the prominent position of the hospital management, without which it would be impossible to develop a programme for home care. The key role played by nurses as members of the palliative care team begins as soon as diagnosis is confirmed by the physician. Based on gaps identified after confirmation of diagnosis, the model provides guidance in tracking and tracing each patient, and planning home care. Communicating the true position of diagnoses at this stage is very important as it will help to reduce anxiety—after which, follow-up and home care measures will then be put in place.

Two fundamental elements in the framework as utilised are the 'square of care' and the 'square of organization'. As set out in the model [19], the 'square of care' has six components and the 'square of organization' has six stages that are relevant to palliative care integration. The composition of the conceptual framework is shown in **Figure 2** covers all phases of a palliative care programme, service or group. The patient and family are at the middle of the joint square, and their needs decide the concerns to be covered, the care necessary and the purposes and means to deliver care [20].

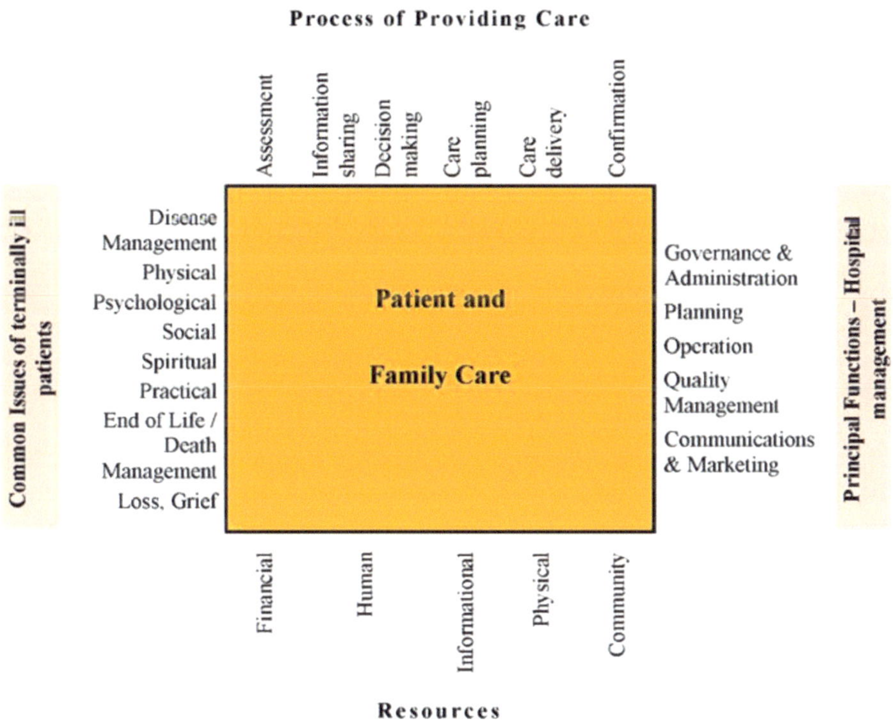

Figure 2.
Square of care and organisation (Source: adopted from CHPCA).

The Square of Care refers to the six important phases during the process of rendering care to patients and family. The phases of square of care include:

- assessment
- information sharing
- decision-making
- care planning
- care delivery and
- confirmation, and demonstration that they relate to the concerns (or areas) that patients and families usually encounter.

Square of organisation also has six stages, which comprise:

- governance and administration
- planning
- operation
- quality improvement communication/marketing
- collection and use of data.

The main concepts of the model are the standards and regulatory beliefs that were established and decided upon through a national consensus-based practice [20].

There should be plans for both the health care professional and patients/families to manage physical and psychosocial suffering and to get ready for the likelihood of advanced disease. This aspect of palliative care involves ways to provide physical and emotional care that will help patients to get through treatments. It enhances patients' compliance with disease management, helps them accept changes in care and prepares patients and their families for the tasks ahead if the disease eventually does not lead to a cure.

3.1 Application of the model

Based on the model of palliative care as developed by CHPCA, the model takes into consideration the prominent position of the hospital management without which it will be impossible to develop any programme of such magnitude [19, 20]. This is because, a lot of things will be considered, especially, developing human resources example training of palliative care nurses, setting up palliative care team, providing other means of integrating palliative care into daily care of patients. Again, patients and families should also be seen at the centre of developing this programme as compliance is the key to success of any programme.

A nurse as an important member of palliative care team has an important role to play as soon as a patient is indicated for home care. Based on the gaps identified, after confirmation of diagnosis, tools that are going to be adapted will be used to track each patient; communication of the true position of diagnoses at this level is very important as this will help to reduce anxiety and follow-up measures will then be put in place. Studies conducted by Temel et al. indicate that patients who had palliative care integrated into normal treatment had a better outcome even when they were diagnosed at the advanced stage of the disease than patients who managed with only normal treatments [21].

4. The relevance of spirituality in health care

Spirituality is a part of holistic care for clients and families. Patients getting palliative care benefit much from the special care that is devoted to physical, personal and social needs [22]. Spiritual care is seen as very significant for a lot of terminally ill patients, but professionals have trouble determining what such care they could embrace. From the viewpoints of the patients/clients at the end of life, their family caregivers and health care workers, the main aims are: to search the notion of spirituality and the meaning of this term; to discover beliefs, understandings and prospects with respect to spirituality, spiritual needs, pain or distress and spiritual care and, eventually, to see how spiritual care can best be provided for patients at home in a depressed economy.

Spirituality and health is an increasing new area of health care; the first textbook on spirituality and health was published by Oxford University Press [23]. Puchalski et al. established that patients would like their spirituality to be addressed in their health care. As the trends and research developed, ethical queries began to come up as to the definition of spirituality within medical care, its role in patient care and the implementation of spiritual care in the clinical setting.

Rosser and Walsh are of the opinion that spirituality takes account of an individual's beliefs, values, identity, a sense of meaning and purpose [5]. Some people see religion as being a component of spirituality. Wright and Neuberger designate spirituality to be pertained to how we see ourselves in the pattern of things, how we relate to other human beings and the wider world and how we ascertain meaning, purpose and association in life [24]. By its very nature, spirituality is often subjective, absolute and personal. In addition to the suggested principles for health care professionals to take care of the whole person, together with the patient's spirituality, studies have established that patients appreciate a more whole-person emphasis on care and value health care professional's probe into their spiritual beliefs [25].

Spirituality according to some schools of thought covers the confidence in self and others and this may include a belief in a divine being or higher authority [26]. The RCN also describes the following as factors of spirituality:

- hope
- strength
- trust
- forgiveness
- love
- relationships
- creativity
- self-expression [26].

If patients' needs could be recognised early and their care adequately planned to include (but not limiting to) follow-up of all patients diagnosed with terminal illness through telephone calls, home visiting, advanced care planning, assessment and treatment of physical, psychosocial and spiritual aspect of patient's needs, etc., there will be better outcome when the condition reaches advanced stage. Some may reason that because spirituality is so personal, it has no relationship in health care but when the perception of total pain is looked into, it is obvious that spiritual care is a vital element of care [5].

5. The impact of economic depression on health

Economic depression is a period of time of economic slowdown presenting low output, not having enough funds and unemployment. It is considered by its length, abnormal upsurges in unemployment, falls in the obtainability of adequate health services, shrinking output and investment, etc.

5.1 General causes of economic depression

The major causes of economic depression in any given economy (lessons from great depressions, 1981, 1991, 2008 economic recession) may include:

- High inflation, a general rise in price of goods and services—leading to low purchasing power.
- Accumulation of debt servicing especially foreign debt.

- High-interest rate—discouraging investors.
- Fall in aggregate demand; fall in wages, income etc.
- Mass unemployment and general loss of confidence in the government [27]

Health is an essential part of man's existence even in the midst of economic depression. Before the current economic crisis, most present-day societies especially in the developing countries were still suffering disease epidemics while other nations incessantly experienced the endemic diseases affecting millions of lives. The global economic crisis persists to worsen the structure and purpose of the health sector. The economic depression has affected several segments of the economy including the health sector, contributing to low output, poor service delivery and poor health outcome. This has led so many people to resort to home care where so much will not be required from them.

The health sector is still struggling to provide rudimentary health care services with the collaborative efforts of government and individuals but determinations to realise this seem unfeasible due to the current state of the economy especially in the developing countries. The current economic position has affected health care funding and the level of support of the public and private health care services particularly among the rural poor is reduced due to increased proportion of poverty [28]. The economic predicament has contributed essentially to poor health outcome; it offers the occasion for careful government health modifications to improve the health system operation [28]. Health is directly or indirectly connected to other sectors such as food security and nutrition, family income generation, housing, education, employment status and other social security services.

Following initial treatment for terminal diseases or elderly patients, they are usually given dates for followed-up appointment in hospital outpatient departments at steady intervals for routine checking in order to assess the patient and timely discovery of recurring of the ailment [29]. This method of follow-up places anxiety on the patient and their family members and most of them defaulted due to religious and cultural beliefs. Secondly, they may complain of inability to travel to the hospital, especially patients living in the rural communities. Most of these patients present late in the hospital either because of poor knowledge, cultural/spiritual beliefs and non-availability of resources for prevention, diagnosis and treatment [28]. Patients and families are not well prepared after diagnosis about the diseases or palliation; this has led to most of the patients not responding to check-up appointments because they are not well informed and no form of follow-up programmes are put in place to track these patients [29].

Based on the above premise, several countries have been able to put in place measures for providing home care services to a lot of their citizenry so as to alleviate the suffering of the poor masses. Most of the developing countries are still struggling as a result of poor economic position of these nations. Home care cannot be instituted without adequate resources.

6. The home care situation in a depressed economy

From a nursing viewpoint, it is imperative to have information about the type of care needed, the explanations of care needed and quality of life among the elderly people and those diagnosed with terminal illnesses living in their own homes, in order to sustain their independence and make best use of their quality of life.

DOI: http://dx.doi.org/10.5772/intechopen.92736

At several stages during our lives, we are each dependent on the care of others [30]. For many, that need comes with old age, chronic illness or ill health. In some occasions, the care is provided by a family member or a friend; in other cases, it comes from a paid care worker such as a registered nurse, a registered practical nurse or a personal support worker. Sometimes, the care is given by a combination of both [30].

This chapter describes the involvements of these three care beneficiaries, their family caregivers and their paid care workers in our survey of the direction of the substantial practices of care associations in home care. Current reorganisation of health and social care services means the home is gradually the site of long-term care and is a place where implications of both home and care must be discussed [31]. The focus on the familiar care points up the diverse forces at work of care through which caregivers, care recipients and home space are established.

Most nurses have their own individual principles and morals, and there are certain professional standards on which all nurses are anticipated to establish their care. Nurses have a duty to make the care of patients their major concern and to practise care giving without harm and efficiently. They must be ethical and truthful [1]. Patients trust their nurses because they believe that, in addition to being experienced, their nurses will not take advantage of them and will demonstrate character traits such as honesty, straightforwardness, reliability and empathy. Good professional decision and behaviour in clinical practice should be patient-centred. It involves nurses understanding that each patient at the end stage of his or her disorder is exceptional, and working in partnership with their patients to discourse the needs and realistic prospects of each patient. The moral pronouncement as proposed by Plato and Aristotle highlighted the part of purpose both in observing what is fair and in permitting us to act reasonably rather than give in to conflicting desires and feelings [32].

Hellström and Hallberg examined people aged 75 years and older dependent on care from professionals and/or a next of kin, their functional health, diseases and complaints in relation to quality of life as perceived by themselves [32]. The study revealed that the number of elderly persons in need of support ranged from 18.5 to 79.1% in the different age groups, and that aid came mostly from informal caregivers [32]. The authors also discovered that assistance from formal caregivers was given in combination with that from a next of kin in 38.8% of the cases. Furthermore, next of kin function more than formal carers; they assisted in all Contributory Activities of Daily Living (CADL) and Personal Activities of Daily Living (PADL) chores, with the exclusion of house cleaning and rendering a bath/shower. Although the respondents had supported themselves, they were also of assistance to another person in 6.5% of circumstances [1].

From the above study, it is seen that care giving at home is mostly carried out by informal caregivers, than the professionals. Patients, therefore, would see care at home more acceptable during this critical period of their lives. Most patients resolved to care at home because their financial status cannot cope with hospital bills, transportation, waiting time in the health care facilities among other reasons that promote home care.

7. The integration of palliative/holistic care in clinical and home-based care in terminally ill patients and the elderly

Nurses are the most valuable member of the palliative care team who are in the best position to look into the physical, purposeful, social and spiritual needs of the patients, but in most situations, they (nurses) are not well-prepared to give the adequate care, especially to elderly and terminally ill patients. The main focus of nursing care as observed is curative approach without taking into consideration effective communication between them and patients/families the truth about diagnosis/prognosis of the disease, lack of patient and family readiness as a result of inadequate training/discharge planning and lack of follow-up [33].

Specifically, since there are no functional palliative care programmes in most health care facilities, the phases being addressed are:

A. Outpatient clinics

B. Hospital service

C. Home care service

D. Approach to care

A. Outpatient clinics:

1. Staff: Palliative care physician and nurse to be identified
2. Terminally ill patients identified after diagnosis is confirmed
3. Visit: To plan routine visit as necessary
4. Symptom assessment in clinic: Routine assessment during every visit by the nurse and physician
5. Psychosocial assessment in clinic: Routine assessment and discussion of goal with patient and family, support system, psychosocial distress and discussion on advance care planning according to their willingness
6. Telephone follow-up: Routine by the nurse after each visit
7. On-call service: 24 hours on-call service to be clarify during first visit after diagnosis has been established.

B. Hospital service:

1. In-patient care: access to palliative care for symptom management
2. In-patient staff training for nurses: identification of nurses, physician and family caregivers for continued education and training in palliative and home care
3. Palliative care in-patient follow-up: follow-up by palliative care team when the patient is admitted to other unit of the hospital.

C. Home care:

1. Community care contact health centre service: health centre closer to the patient will be identified for care continuation and this would be reassessed at each visit.
2. Communication with the family and community health centre: this should be done routinely.

D. Approach to care:

All care providers: Multidisciplinary, this is hope to address physical, psychological, social and spiritual needs of both the patient and the family identifying other specialist. The approach to care takes cognizance of the fact that the economic depression affects the type of care the less privileged members of the population attained. This may affect proper access to good health care services and as such provision of home care will be beneficial to them where they will be taken care of in their familiar environment.

8. Summary/conclusion

Nurses should strive to always make the most of the short time they have with each patient. As nurses, we need to promote a patient's psychological and emotional well-being in order to facilitate physical healing, especially in a poor economic situation. When we do this, our relationship with the patient alters and develops into something more encouraging than it was before. This contributes to better patient outcomes and can heighten the happiness and perseverance in our work as nurses. By doing this, informal caregivers would emulate and continue home care.

There are many easy ways to develop relationships with patients and encourage a sound psychological, emotional and spiritual environment.

- Learn the patient's name and use it
- Make good, strong eye contact
- Ask how a patient is feeling and honestly care
- Smile and laugh when suitable
- Use relaxing touch
- Assist the patient to see themselves as someone who merits self-esteem
- Maintain their self-worth
- Educate patients on the significance of self-care
- Ask the patient how you can decrease their anxiety or pain

Holistic nursing is the concept of caring for a person as a whole. The purpose is to return the patient as a whole to as close to normal as possible even when receiving care at home. Holistic nursing highlights on the nurses considering the link between minds, body, emotion, spirit, social, cultural, environmental and past relationships in order to return the patient to a whole. This however has not always been likely to attain. The idea of caring for the whole person, not just their physical body, is one that dates back to Florence Nightingale. Florence Nightingale devotedness was to care for those who could not care for themselves. Florence Nightingale herself advocated holistic care by recognising the importance of environment touch, light, scents, music and silent reflection in treatment process.

There is a direct relationship between economy and health and by implication of nursing profession. The present economic depression places an enormous threat as its end is not sure. This chapter therefore tried to bridge the gap between holistic care, palliative care, which embodied all the components of spirituality, and the terminally ill patients needing home care. This has a lot to do with economic situation of the populace, especially in the low- and middle-class countries of the world. Since the elderly and the terminally ill patients preferred home care, it is pertinent that all the components of care be provided to take care of the total man.

Acknowledgements

The authors are grateful to all the authors whose work were cited in this chapter without which it could have been impossible to support the original ideas conceived by the authors.

Conflicts of interest

The authors declare no conflict of interest.

Author contributions

AN, EO and BN designed the study, compiled and wrote the manuscript. All the authors reviewed the manuscript and provided critical comments, read and approved the final version of the manuscript.

Author details

Akon Emmanuel Ndiok[1,2]*, Emilia Oyira[1] and Busisiwe Ncama[2]

1 Department of Nursing Science, University of Calabar, Calabar, Nigeria

2 School of Nursing and Public Health, University of KwaZulu-Natal, Durban, South Africa

*Address all correspondence to: ndioka@unical.edu.ng

References

[1] Chukwuneke FN. Ethics of palliative care in late-stage cancer management and end-of-life issues in a depressed economy. Nigerian Journal of Clinical Practice. 2015;**18**(7):15

[2] Eko JE. Implication of economic recession on the health care delivery system in Nigeria. Social Science. 2017;**6**(1):14-18

[3] Agrafiotis PC. In: Christensen B, Kockrow E, editors. Evolution of Nursing in Foundation of Nursing. Philadelphia: Mosby; 1991

[4] Alligood M, Marriner-Tomey A. Nursing Theorists and Their Work. Maryland Heights, Mo: Mosby/Elsevier; 2010

[5] Rosser M, Walsh HC. Fundamentals of Palliative Care for Student Nurses. Oxford: Wiley Blackwell; 2014. pp. 16-27

[6] Mariano C. An Overview of Holistic Nursing National Student Nurses' Association Imprint February/March 2005. pp. 48-51

[7] de Florence Nightingale TA, Crítica UA. The Florence Nightingale's environmental theory: A critical analysis. Escola Anna Nery Revista de Enfermagem. 2015;**19**:3

[8] Zamanzadeh V, Jasemi M, Valizadeh L, Keogh B, Taleghani F. Effective factors in providing holistic care: A qualitative study. Indian Journal of Palliative Care. Iran. 2015;**21**(2):214

[9] Nightingale F. Notes of Nursing: What It Is and What It Is Not. New York: Dover Publications, Inc. p. 133; 1969. pp. 117-125

[10] Erickson HL. Philosophy and theory of holism. The Nursing Clinics of North America. 2007;**42**(2):139-163

[11] WHO. Strengthening of Palliative Care as a Component of Comprehensive Care Throughout the Life Course. Sixty-Seventh World Health Assembly. 2014 Available from: http://apps.who.int/gb/ebwha/pdf_files/WHA67/A67_R19-en.pdf. [Accessed: 22 January 2020]

[12] WHO. WHO Definition of palliative care. 2014 Available from: http//www.who.int/cancer/palliative/definition/en [Accessed: 22 January 2020]

[13] Boltz K. Integration of palliative care into standard oncology care. Oncology Nurse Advisor. 2012. Available from: http://www.oncologynurseadvisor.com/integration-of-palliative-care [Accessed: 22 January 2020]

[14] National Consensus Project for Quality Palliative Care Consortium Organizations. Clinical Practice Guidelines for Quality Palliative Care. Pittsburgh, PA: National Consensus Project; 2004. Available from: http://www.netce.com/coursecontent.php?courseid=845

[15] Callahan MF, Breakwell S, Suhayda R. Knowledge of palliative and end-of-life care by student registered nurse Anaesthetists. AANA Journal. 2011;**79**:S15-S20

[16] Becker R. Palliative care using: Palliative care nursing skills in clinical practice. Nursing Times. 2009;**105**(5):18-21

[17] Royal College of Nursing. A Competency Framework for Nurses Working in Specialist Care Competencies. 2008. Available from: project.www.ncnm.ic/files/events/08/RCN-events [Accessed: 22 November 2018]

[18] Doenges ME, Moorhouse MF. Application of Nursing Process and Nursing Diagnosis: An Interactive text

for Diagnostic Reasoning. FA Davis; 2012

[19] Canadian Hospice Palliative Care Association (CHPCA). A Model to Guide Hospice Palliative Care: Based on National Principles and Norms of Practice. Revised and Condensed edition. 2013. Available from: http://www.chpca.net/media/319547/norms-of-practice-eng-web.pdf [Accessed: 25 February 2020]

[20] Canadian Hospice Palliative Care Association (CHPCA). 2005. Applying a Model to Guide Hospice Palliative Care. An Essential Companion Toolkit for Planners, Policy Makers, Caregivers, Educators, Managers, Administrators and Researchers. Available from: http://www.chpca.net/media/7458/Applying_a-Model-to-Guide-Hospice-Palliative-Care-.Toolkit.pd [Accessed: 25 February 2020]

[21] Temel JS, Greer JA, Muzikansky A, Gallagher ER, Admane S, Jackson VA, et al. Early palliative care for patients with metastatic non–small-cell lung cancer. The New England Journal of Medicine. 2010;**363**(8):733-742

[22] Edwards A, Pang N, Shiu V, Chan C. The understanding of spirituality and the potential role of spiritual care in end-of-life and palliative care: A meta-study of qualitative research. Palliative Medicine. 2010;**24**(8):753-770

[23] Puchalski CM, Cobb M, Rumbold B, editors. Oxford Textbook of Spirituality and Healthcare. New York: Oxford University Press; 2012. p. 2012

[24] Wright S, Neuberger J. Why spirituality is essential for nurses. Nursing Standard (through 2013). 2012;**26**(40):19

[25] Puchalski CM. Integrating spirituality into patient care: An essential element of person-centered care. Polskie Archiwum Medycyny Wewnętrznej. 2013;**123**(9):491-497

[26] Royal College of Nursing. Spirituality in Nursing Care: A Pocket Guide. London: Royal College of Nursing; 2011

[27] Ishiekwere T. Worst Economic Crisis in 25 Years: What Nigeria Can Do To Get Out of Recession? Sahara Reporters 15th November 2016. Available from: http://saharareporters.com/2016/10/05/worst-economic-crisis-25-yearswhat-nigeria-can-do-get-out-recessiontonyishiekwere [Accessed: 15 November 2018]

[28] Nolan A, Barry S, Burke S, Thomas S. The Impact of the Financial Crisis on the Health System and Health in Ireland. Ireland: Economic and Social Research Institute; 2014

[29] Yang B, Prescott N, Bae E. The impact of economic crisis on health care consumption in Korea. Health Policy and Planning. 2001;**16**(4):372-385

[30] Nwogu CE, Ezeome ER, Mahoney M, Okoye I, Michalek AM. Regional cancer control in south-eastern Nigeria: a proposal emanating from a UICC-sponsored workshop. West African Journal of Medicine. 2010;**29**(6):408-411

[31] England K, Dyck I. Managing the body work of home care. Sociology of Health & Illness. 2011;**33**(2):206-219

[32] Hellström Y, Hallberg IR. Perspectives of elderly people receiving home help on health, care and quality of life. Health & Social Care in the Community. 2001;**9**(2):61-71

[33] Bacon J. Integrating Palliative Care Approach into the Management of Chronic, Life, Threatening Disease [Online]. 2013. Ottawa. Available from: www.hpcintegration.ca [Accessed: 25 March 2019]

Chapter 16

The Need for XR-Measurement of Decision-Making Decline and Conscious-State Transition Impairment before Nonvoluntary Euthanization of Dementia Patients

Farida Hanna Campbell

Abstract

Non-voluntary euthanization of dementia patients, the majority of whom are severely conscious-state transition-impaired because of both high levels of anti-somnogenic cytokine levels and circadian disruption, indicates the lack of measurement of decision-making decline and conscious-state transition in palliative care settings. This chapter explains why and how to setup medically-meaningful tests to collect these measurements based on environmental-interactive parameters of nonconscious testing in circadian calibrated XR or virtual reality platforms. It also mentions worthy opportunities in relationship to the Human Connectome Project, including the Alzheimer's Disease Connectome Project.

Keywords: dementia, euthanization, virtual reality, XR, human connectome project, Alzheimer's Disease, conscious-state transition, decision-making incompetence

1. Introduction

Dementia is a prominent symptom of various diseases and not just a disease in and of itself. It is part of brain disease transition such as following virus-infected inflammation through increased neurodegeneration and brain network dysfunctioning.

It renders difficulty in recognition and response to daily environmental information which are needed in short-term learning and recall and decision-making [1, 2]. In general, one of the most disturbing characteristics of neuroinflammatory diseases is loss of conscious-state transition [3]. This is a type of disability or impairment that results in the presence of persistently high levels of anti-somnogenic cytokines [4, 5], and common to Alzheimer's Disease patients [6]. It is alsoo associated with disruption of circadian synchronization between neuronal networks of the brain [7, 8].

A dementia patient's care-giving team is presumed to include certified doctors and nurses qualified in early diagnosis and strategies for dementia-symptom management. The targets of such caregiving include optimizing physical health, cognition, activity and well-being identifying and treating accompanying physical illness detecting and treating challenging behavioral and psychological symptoms providing information and long-term support to carers (WHO).

Section 4.1 of the Dutch euthanization law [9] declares that euthanasia may be given to a patient who is no longer mentally competent as a result of advanced dementia, and that the doctor does not need to agree with the patient regarding the time or manner of euthanatic execution based on a physician declaration of patient inability to comprehend the subject.

Euthanization is delivered via anesthetics without acknowledging the surge of neurophysiological coherence and connectivity in the forced-dying brain [10] or on the basis of any measured disability of a patient to change from one conscious-state to any other. The degree that sensory information processing and conscious memory, awareness, learning and recall are supposed to be fully disabled [11] by the simple observation of delirium seems to possibly have led to an unchecked medical assumption that an overdosage of anesthetic-euthanatic neurotoxins is sufficient to overcome the disability and trigger instant brain death. However, the research shows that this is invalid and that memory formation- and indeed, brain survival mechanisms - are evolved to be much smarter, enabling survival-related learning related neuronal synaptic plasticity changes to occur even under deep anesthesia [12, 13].

In 2019, 146 dementia patients were euthanized in the Netherlands, 14% less frequently than the previous year [14].

The English version Regional Euthanization Review Committees- The Netherlands, report (2018) [9] states that.

> Dementia
>
> *Two notifications in 2018 involved patients in an advanced or very advanced stage of dementia who were no longer able to communicate regarding their request and in whose cases the advance directive was decisive in establishing whether the request was voluntary and well considered.* See case 2018-41, described in Chapter II, and case 2018-21, published on www.euthanasiecommissie.nl.
>
> *In 144 cases the patient's suffering was caused by early-stage dementia. These patients still had insight into their condition and its symptoms, such as loss of bearings and personality changes. They were deemed decisionally competent with regard to their request because they could still grasp its implications. Case 2018-123, described in Chapter II, is an example.*

But, the section titled Advanced Directive Points to Consider (Section 4.1, f, (see Annual Reports, Dutch Euthanasia Committee [15]) requires physicians to answer: *Are there any contraindications that are inconsistent with the advance directive and preclude the performance of euthanasia?*

If so, this statement represents one opportunity to provide an argument that all dementia patients deserve medically-meaningful conscious-state transition monitoring and decision-competence evidence before non-voluntary euthanization can be legally authorized.

Such monitoring technology would enable demonstration of key factors of non-eligibility when a patient is unable to transition into unconsciousness or brain death instantaneously or for up to 36 hours - even following severe anesthesia and cardiac arrest [16] simply because of the nature of the disease's impact on the brain (see **Figure 1** below).

The euthanization method which is intended as a pain-free killing is error-prone with patient re-awakening rather than instant dying [17, 18] on record. Anesthetic drugs targeted to ion channels affect neuronal activity in the Central Nervous System (including the brain), the peripheral nervous system (PNS) and all connected organs, and the cardiovascular system [19]. Barbiturates such as pentobarbital suppress the central nervous system (CNS) by binding to gamma-aminobutyric acid (GABA) A subtype receptors, alters inhibitory postsynaptic CL- currents while simultaneously inhibiting excitatory presynaptic nerve terminal signal event transmission. This is supposed to sustain the opening of chloride channels and results in the suppressed neuronal activation of oscillations throughout the brain and sensory management throughout the entire system [20–23]. The GABAergic thalamic neurons would also therefore inhibit retinally-driven activity, and likewise disable input to the geniculo-hypothalamic pathway which is activated by crossed retinal inputs leading to the suprachiasmatic nucleus (SCN). In this way, brainwave activities related to conscious-state transition and measured by Bispectral Index (BIS) monitors [24] or Guedel's classification system [25] are logistically absent, thereby theoretically preventing patient awakening and patient awareness or memory.

However, the research shows that brain death and cardiac death are not simultaneously correlated [26–29]). In research review by Robijn (2020) as part of an academic thesis submission, Robijn reports correlation between BIS and the Richmond Agitation-Sedation Scale (RASS) ($p < 0.0004$) including reporting patients 'awake' during euthanization despite observational physician [30] decisions that the patients were dead [31, 32]. Also, memory formation also continues under anaesthesia [12, 33, 34]. On closer inspection of the events, one finds that the high dosage anesthetics such as 9 mg/L pentobarbital intravenous injection used in euthanization in the Netherlands has explicit pharmacological warnings that the neurotoxic compound cannot reach the brain in one minute intravenous application and that that the accelerated injection causes gangrene, body-wide joint pain and tissue irritation for any intravenous-administered dosages above 0.5 mg/l. Furthermore, it reduces IL-1beta cytokine release by only 30–40%, while endogenous tumor necrosis factor (TNF-α) transport becomes elevated in a process that remains

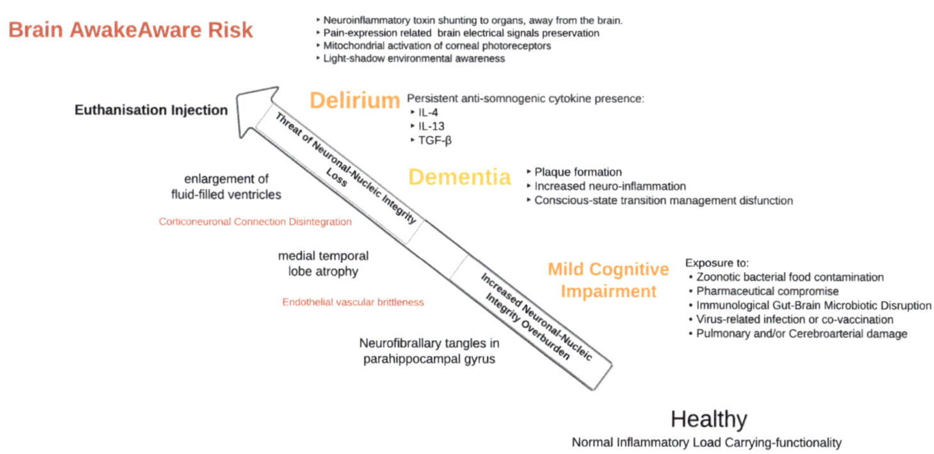

Figure 1.
A list of features in the progression of amnesiac-related brain inflammation from disease or neurological disorders leading to risks that may compromise euthanization patient safety.

persistent on behalf of neurotoxin breakdown and elimination that can last for as many hours as the 36-hour half life of the anesthetic itself [30]. This process is part of inherent mechanisms of survival, regardless the neurotoxic, and it is automatically geared to protect the brain with interleukin-1β (IL-1β), and interleukin-6 (IL-6) pleiotropic mechanisms [6, 35–37].

This is significant considering the fact that, in the Netherlands alone, more than 32,000 killed patients have reportedly also died in conditions of unconsciousness with profound dehydration; and where, at least one pro-euthanization physician promoted the killing of a schizophrenic mentally ill patient to a general public readership with significant reference to the patient's ethnicity and immigrant socioeconomic demeaning reference to drug-addiction [38]. In this chapter, it is particularly relevant to disclose the fact that dementia patients can be proven to be inappropriate for euthanization treatment, both on the basis of their majority high-level of anti-somnogenic cytokine levels and on the basis of brain survival mechanisms that are successful enough to preserve the brain in the oldest dementia-symptomatic victims.

Generally speaking, anesthetics bind to gamma-aminobutyric acid (GABA) A subtype receptors of the central nervous system, the post-synaptic NMDA receptors of hippocampal pathways for memory, and the two-pore-domain K+ channels of the central nervous system, depressing signal transmission associated with conscious awareness for a surgical period. Extreme intravenous euthanatic administration does not reach the brain, according to manufacturer related research and instead produces risk of organ-wide tissue damage plius gangrene [30]. This is because the higher dosages trigger instant release of the pro-inflammatory cytokines tumor necrosis factor α (TNFα), interleukin-1β (IL-1β), and interleukin-6 (IL-6) which are powerful repair and survival brain protective cytokines [39, 40].

These cytokines modulate centers of wakefulness regulation located in the hypothalamus, the basal forebrain and the brain stem by influencing substances involved in sleep–wake-behavior such as adenosine, nitric oxide (NO), nuclear factor-κB (NF-κB), prostaglandin D2 (PGD2), the neurotransmitters γ-aminobutyric acid (GABA), glutamate and norepinephrine, as well as hormones such as growth hormone-releasing hormone (GHRH) and corticotropin-releasing hormone (CRH). However, several key cytokines including IL-4, IL-13 and TGF-β are anti-somnogenic (wakefulness triggering) [41]. If so, queries against forced euthanization of Alzheimer's disease should include high-risk of patient awakening susceptibility during the process, resulting in opportunity for greater error and patient suffering (see **Figure 1** below).

At the time of researching, Dutch physicians reportedly still seem to choose to administer pentobarbital at 9 g/L as the primary euthanatic, which is well above the 0.5 mg/L safe maximum (see online pharmaceutical manufacturing warnings [42, 43]. 71% of patients, dementia and non-dementia, are euthanised at home [30]. Methods of testing brain death and pain detection still include the Bispectral Index monitor (BIS), NeuroSense monitor and Analgesia Nociception Index monitor. There are evidence of pain and suffering, awakening, and discomfort during the euthanization, despite that it is promoted as a dignified pain-free method of termination from irreversible disease conditions [44].

And yet, the law refers to the patient's advance request to receive euthanization on behalf of preserving self-dignity which is separated from medical decisionmaking in itself. If so, there is an unchecked expression that could be interpreted as a mandate to destroy dementia-patients who visibly fail to prevent their symptoms from violating rules of local social dignity. If so, then this contradicts the claim of compassionate reasons for euthanization in the law-making.

In this chapter, a description is given of both. It includes:

I. Measurement of decisionmaking decline in brain-disease related dementia; and,

II. Measurement of conscious-state transition impairment, and capacity to accommodate euthanatic administration.

2. Measurement of decision-making decline in brain-disease related dementia

Decision-making decline in dementia patients [45] can be measured by using tests for autonomic non-conscious learning and recall expression [46]. The rates of learning and recall are measured from responses to an unconditioned stimulus (US) that is associated with a subsequent aversive conditioned stimulus (CS) [47]. Tests are described abundantly throughout the literature as the basis of cognitive *decisionmaking* [48–50] *evaluation.* The results are matched with the arrival of short-term neurosynaptic plasticity changes in corresponding neocortical amygdaloid-hippocampal-prefrontal cortical networks [51], as demonstrated by fMRI images offered in the Human Connectome Project (HCP) database [52, 53], relative to the disease etiology. XR-investigations are appropriate before stages of profound delirium in advanced dementia [54]. Delirium is defined by the Diagnostic and Statistical Manual of Mental Disorders, 5th edition (DSM-5) to include acute disturbance in attention, awareness, and cognition. The European Delirium Association and American Delirium Society (2014) describe its increased mortality rate [55]. Delirious patients suffer from severe disturbances of the circadian system [56]. And so, XR sessions as described in this chapter offer a diurnal monitoring method to predict the arrival of impaired day-night rhythm in patient dementia-related disease progression, long before stages of delirium have arrived.

Portable virtual reality devices that can simulate 360-degrees of 3D- immersive environments in videogame processing have been used in cognitive decision-making diagnostics and therapeutics. They can be scripted with internally-animated virtual cameras and objects, known as *assets* to trigger patient sensorimotor interaction and focus. The engagement parlays into recognition behaviors which can be recorded as data with simultaneous autonomic cardiologic variation measurements as frequently as needed in devices that stream the videogame up to 60 or more frames a second. Also known as serious games or medical virtual reality behavioral tests [54, 57], these videogames require a minimum set of calibration so that the collection of data from the patient (also referred to as the *player*) is medical-meaningful in investigations of decision-making decline and more.

For example, these include psychiatric considerations for:

1. Duration of each session which is minimized to avoid optogenetic influence on the patient bioreceptive retinal cells;

2. Diurnal (circadian) times of day that can report challenges due to brain inflammation transition stages, i.e. from inflammatory repair periods during the night to inflammatory protection during the day;

3. Patient locomotor stabilization and non-navigational requirements against disorientation and injury;

4. Bioperceptive capacity versus retinal limitations that reduce visual motion-detection and circadian synchronization;

5. Headturning rates, restrictions and sensorimotor ease;

6. Heart-rate variation monitoring that is reliable throughout each XR-test session;

7. Saccadic "blink" synchronization with behavioral sampling;

8. Real-world time of day consistency of the XR-session for both scotopic and photopic illumination intensity calibrations;

9. Statistical evenness in game scenes without the use of biased cultural asset-objects in the environment;

10. Geotimestamped coordinates of player position and any testing-related assets and events;

11. Alignment of player data with existing patient psyhiatric evaluations and clinical epidemiological research; plus,

12. Appropriate asset-labeling, tagging, data-reporting standards and patient privacy integrations.

The reader is encouraged to review a detailed description of how these features may be presented in a Supplementary Materials section titled, *Example XR-setup for Decision-making Decline Monitoring of Dementia Patients.*

3. Measurement of conscious-state transition capacity under euthanatic administration

The thalamocortical pathway is central to cortical network information processing during conscious-state transition behavior [58] including auditory and visual sensory information response with emotion-based learning and recall networks. It is influenced by bioperception related retinal vibrations received via the suprachiasmatic nucleus and retinohyptothalamic tract, along with influence from genetic signaling (e.g., CLOCK, BMAL1 and others) governing overall homeostasis [59–61]. The networks include the primary and secondary association area networks of the brain neocortex, as well as networks involving the orbitomedial prefrontal cortex (OMPC, areas 11 & 12) as part of the region described by the limbic cortex and septal nuclei (including the amygdala) on behalf of patient mood regulation monitoring, the hippocampus, the thalamus and basal ganglia which are directly involved in sleep/wake environmental awareness-states [62]. The disruption of these networks occurs from circadian desynchronization and the persistence of neuroinflammation [63]. Images of such disruption and the resulting network changes from neurodegeneration can be seen in detail from fMRI image repositories provided by the Human Connectome Project [52], the Alzheimer's Disease Connectome [64], and similar collections. In fact, a future generation Connectome project might include the complementary circadian-calibrated XR-based data collected from dementia patients across multiple demographics, for key times of day, pre-dawn, mid-day and pre-dusk to dusk. A schematic for a potential model of selected networks with the Human Connectome is shown in **Figure 2**, below.

Currently, no tool exists to measure consciousness or self-consciousness objectively by any machine [65]. In non-communicative patients, its estimation requires the interpretation of motor responsiveness [66]. This response represents active brain processing events in the Primary Motor Cortex (MI, area 4) in the precentral gyrus and the corticospinal tract which has its own relationship to somatotopic organization for specific movement coordination, in general with other sensory processing information via a major thalamic motor nucleus, including its ventral

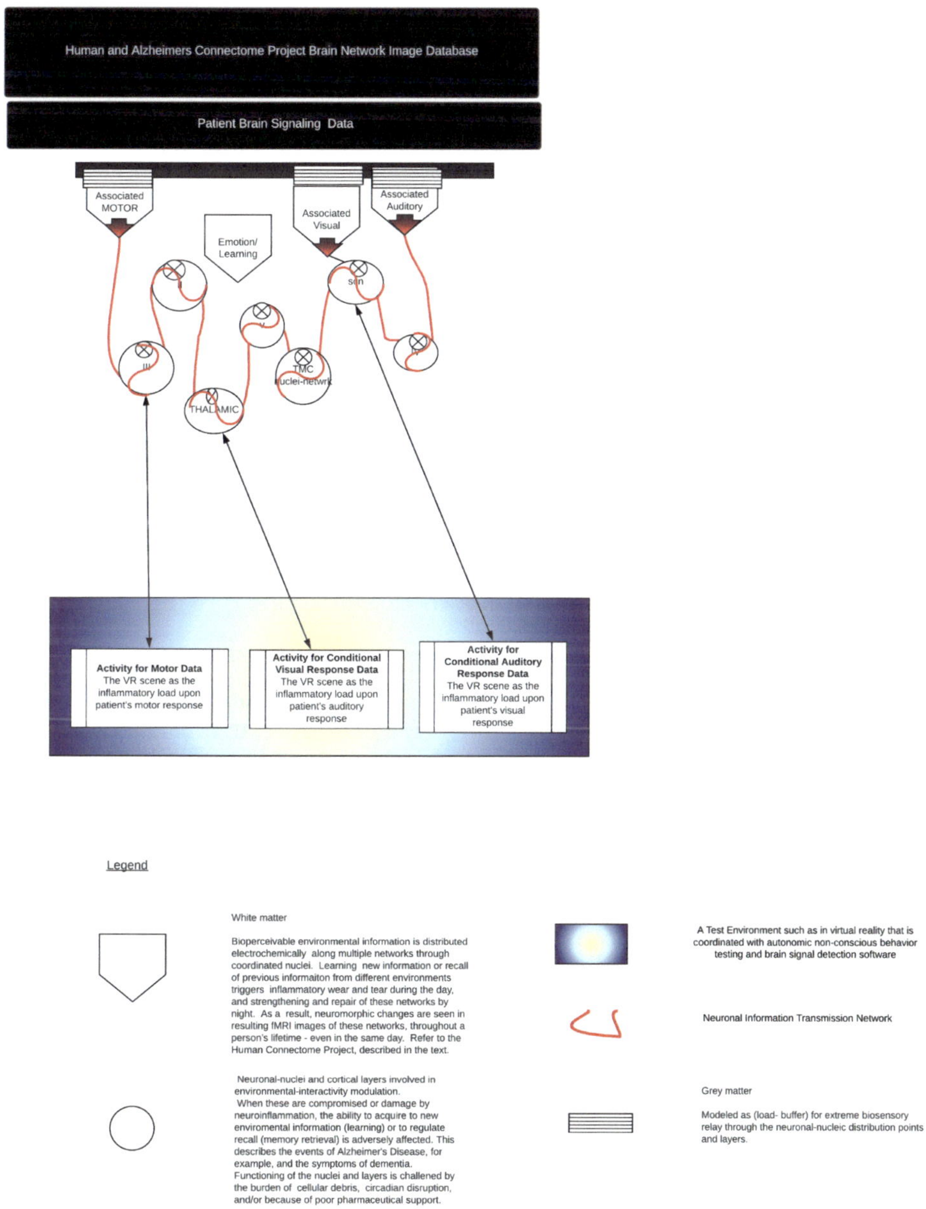

Figure 2.
Schematic example of a selected nucleic-network XR model using the human connectome project (HCP). HCP hosts detailed neuromorphological fMRI datasets combining networks from dementia and related human and animal pathology treatment records. An assembly of virtual reality (XR) monitoring programmes can be organized to support integration with HCP data collections for dementia patients, focusing on any range of selected neuronal-nucleic networks.

lateral nucleus (VL) and Ventral anterior nucleus (VA), and in the presence of dementia-related inflammation [67, 68].

In the Supplementary Materials, a list of some of the parameters are explained so that optogenetic waveform signals are consistent within the virtual reality scene as they are in the natural environment that activates synaptic relays between the intralaminar nucleus of the thalamus and the sensory-information processing cortical networks. These are the same brain regions associated with awareness of self, in relationship to the environment.

Testing in XR can be used to evaluate the degree of this circadian desynchronization in dementia patients, as long as phototopic and scotopic illumination settings are maintained for real-world time-of-day concurrently. γ-Amino-Butyric-Acid (GABA) is necessary for refinement of the circadian firing rhythm that maintains healthy conscious-state transition processes throughout every brain region via the suprachiasmatic nucleus [69] and connecting intergeniculate leaflet (IGL) and retinohypothalamic tract to thalamocortical and related nuclei (**Figure 3**) is responsible for healthy circadian integration of environmental-information throughout multiple cellular oscillations [13] in observable brainwaves.

Circadian daylight regulation [70] via the suprachiasmatic nucleus is also crucial to the production of anti-inflammatory melatonin and so, it would be questionable to find XR-circadian related prosthetics lacking in palliative care for dementia patients.

Melatonin, secreted by the pineal gland, protects neuronal cells with its antioxidant and anti-amyloid properties, and helps to limit or reduce formation of amyloid fibrils involved in Alzheimer-like tau hyperphosphorylation [71, 72]. In neuroinflammatory dementia patients, phase shifts of daylight into dusk trigger agitation, aggression, and delirium during the late afternoon and early evening hours [73], a behavioral regulatory challenge known as *sundowning* [74]. Medically, it is vital to incorporate this condition as a risk of additional suffering during euthanization administration, particularly where euthanatic neurotoxic delivery does not reach the brain and the patient is already conscious-state transition severely impaired (see **Figure 4**).

The XR-tests in conscious-state transition offer an opportunity to evaluate retinal-support as part of psychiatric comfort targets [75] or, to evaluate potential pharmaceutical risk of overdosing a dementia patients.

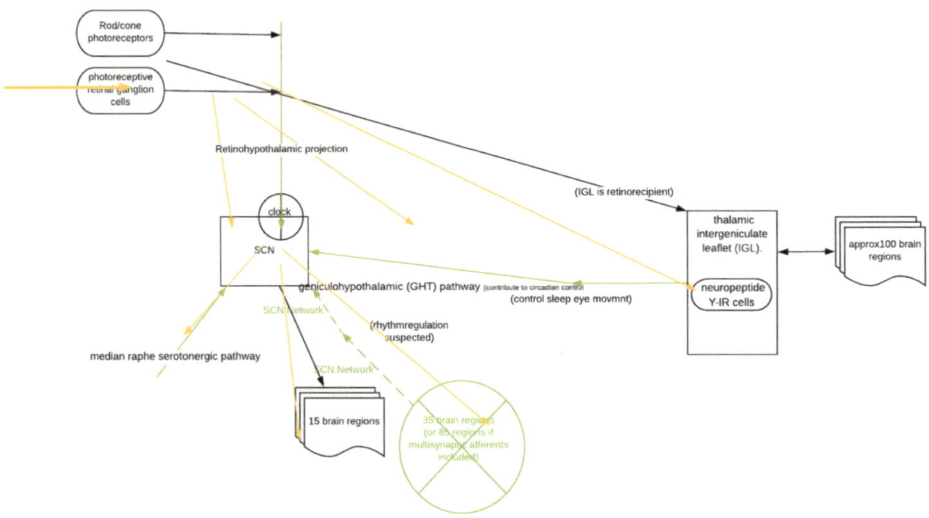

Figure 3.
A simplistic schematic of the bioperception circadian excitatory (yellow) and inhibitory (green) response neuronal-nucleic network relationships, for XR-calibration development purposes.

DOI: http://dx.doi.org/10.5772/intechopen.97384

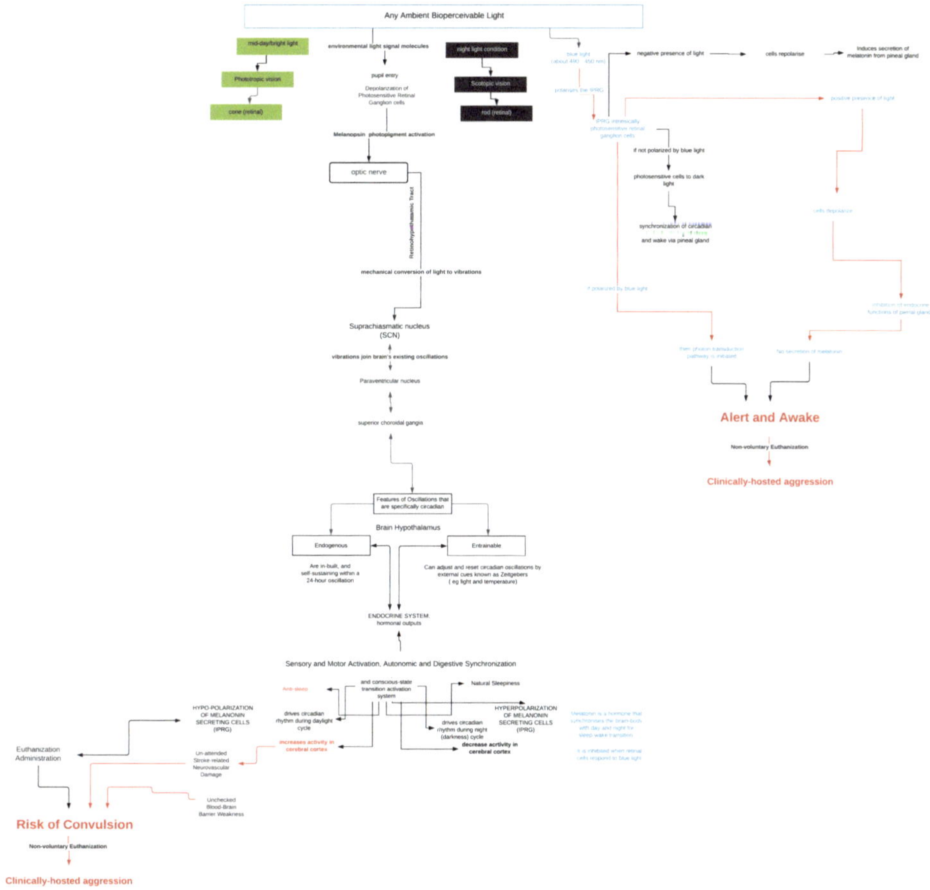

Figure 4.
Relationship of melatonin absence and elevated risk of dementia alert/awake or risk of convulsion.

4. Summary

In this chapter, an XR-based method for evaluating decision-making competence is presented. in reaction to a recent dutch law that suggests decisionmaking incompetence is sufficient grounds for non-voluntary euthanization of dementia patients. Instead, this chapter proposes that decision-making needs to be measured precisely along with conscious-state transition using XR. This is because majority of dementia patients cannot transition from alert or rest state to death state instantly, and that this predisposes them to high risk of brain aware and awake state, including for the duration of the euthanatic product half-life, and despite cardiac arrest. And so, the dutch law which currently only describes patient-disease irreversibility and social dignity loss, appears to overlook the need to evaluate disease conditions and patient conditions for which euthanization is not medically safe and non-voluntary euthanization of such patients is cruelty.

XR-based tests are described as short-instance virtual environmentally-interactive tests, provided in diurnal sessions that have been calibrated to the circadian optogenetic settings of neuronal-nucleic brain thalamocortical networks. The tests provide opportunity to demonstrate neuroinflammation progression and the impact of high expression of anti-somnogenic cytokines, the loss of anti-inflammatory neuroprotective melatonin and circadian desynchronization to the patient. This makes XR-based monitoring in palliative patient caregiving generally valuable as well as key to evaluation of euthanization-readiness.

Acknowledgements

Data collection and sharing for this project was provided by the MGH-USC Human Connectome Project (HCP; Principal Investigators: Bruce Rosen, M.D., Ph. D., Arthur W. Toga, Ph.D., Van J. Weeden, MD). HCP funding was provided by the National Institute of Dental and Craniofacial Research (NIDCR), the National Institute of Mental Health (NIMH), and the National Institute of Neurological Disorders and Stroke (NINDS). HCP data are disseminated by the Laboratory of Neuro Imaging at the University of Southern California.

A. Appendix

A.1 Example XR-setup for decision-making decline monitoring of dementia patients

A.1.1 XR-scene development technology

Any state-of-the-art software can be used for dementia-related testing, such as Unity3D ®, Unreal ®, which are designed for maximum accessibility and ease-of-development for diverse developers. They lack psychiatric calibration and features suited to patient cognitive behavioral environmental-interactive capture and heartrate AI, as well as geographic solar-shadow and weather calibration for both illumination intensity draws and audio. Last but certainly not least, the player analytics do not accommodate sampling frequencies and these will need to be hand-built, which leads to significant reduction in frame rates at the time of this chapter's writing. For this reason data needs to be stored on the device for post-session upload and integration into an appropriate repository. In general, leading palliative care institutions should try to achieve approximately 600 longitudinal sessions per patient for at least 1200 patients56 to generate a suitable diagnostic game AI algorithm [57]. These totals represent average numbers of records submitted to the previously-mentioned Human Connectome Project, for example.

Ethical consideration: Large commercial database hosting sellers are eager to acquire patient data for free. And yet, healthcare costs of the producer, the dementia patient, and the time and technology costs are abandoned or ignored. A fee per interaction should be required from the sellers per frame, and reimbursed towards the patient's full needs, particularly those patients and teams who seek rehabilitation strategies and research for immediate potential curative-care opportunities with XR-related prosthetics.

The simplest platform or device that is VR-enabled and lightweight for hosting a real-time XR-scene for a stationary player is suitable. This can include a basic phone such as a Samsung(R) 10 or 10+ in a Gear VR headset, or an Oculus Rift product, and similar. The ideal software will include AI-calibrated illumination intensity and unbiased wavelength delivery, from a light-emitting diode (such as an AMOLED strip) plus brightness settings that can be adjusted manually by the team. It will also collect geographic coordinates of the player, plus time-of-day and ambient light, pollution and player Fowler's position, heartrate plus saccadic blinking and eye-tracking. The data collected may need to be temporarily stored on the device and so it should also have sufficient hardware capacity both to allow non-occluding GPU rendering and device storage for a 3-minute game processing and behavioral sampling every 30 seconds, minimum at a framerate no less than 32 to 45 frames per second. In a headset, ensure that audio settings conform to any hearing aid or other

DOI: http://dx.doi.org/10.5772/intechopen.97384

prescription settings. The same is true for visual aid adjustments in the VR-headset. Handheld peripherals should not be used or required for dementia autonomic cognitive decision-making and conscious-state transition settings. The patient should not be required to navigate at any time and a member of the diagnostic patient caregiving team is responsible for the condition, use and removal of the XR-assembly from the patient in all sessions.

A.1.2 Significant parameters

Waveform calibration parameters describe phototopic and scotopic settings.

A.1.3 Scene environments

Testing environments for adult-onset dementia-related patients should not be designed to evaluate decisions based on visible timer scoring, navigation decisions through civil-type architecture or semantic response requirements. These do not represent measure states of neuroinflammation-affected decision-making, based on short-term learning and recall.

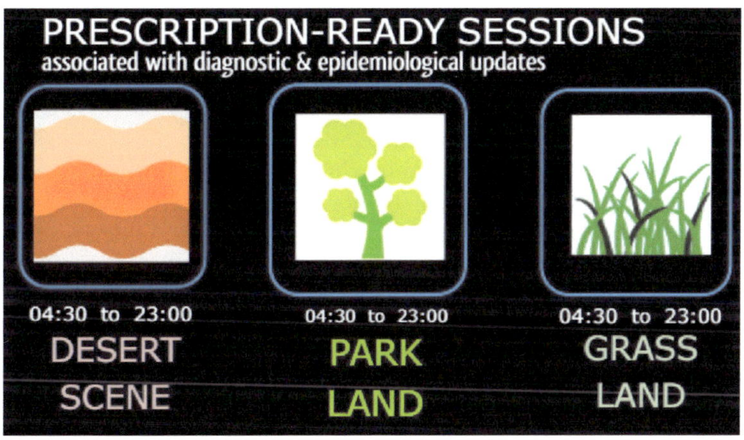

Sky and ground assets above the horizon should be reported in the asset-inventory as either left and right orientable.

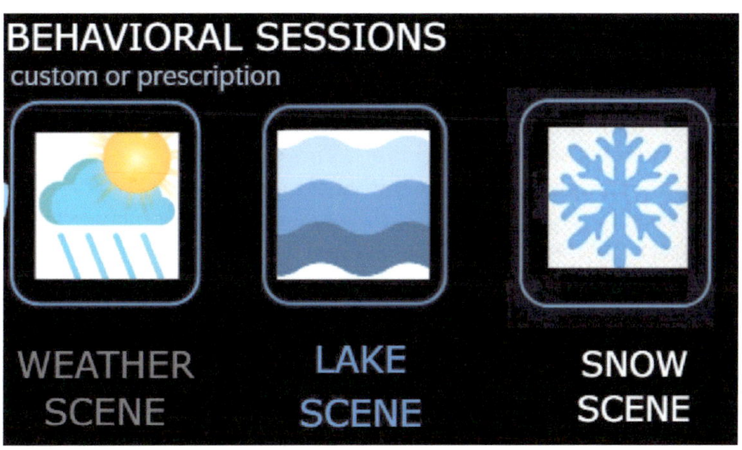

Parameters that describe the maximum spread of the wavelength field such as fulcrum depth and width can also be used to evaluate conscious-state transition where there are compounding or ageing related deficits in one or both hemispheres. These parameters describe the geometric projection of the user's virtual camera-space and orientation of the player's head rotation and line of direction in the virtual scene.

The raycast direction is the parameter used in scripts of assets to report the player's line of direction. The raycast direction describes direction of focus , and is key to describing a change in patient conscious-state. The rate of change of raycast direction is used in behavioral response measurements in recognition and recall of an asset during a nonconscious test.

A.1.4 Light wavelength calibration

Wavelength intensity can be given for assets in parameters from all assets, including sky and ground, vegetation, weather and wildlife. The parameters can be described as0-1 transparency alpha, depth projection, non-spectral shading component size, reflective source component size, rate of single-asset motion (blur), landscape contrast intensity (sharpness), and scene illumination intensity, whichever is appropriate and convenient to describing striking behavioral response differences.

The most critical wavelengths are blue:450–485 nm 620–680 THz 2.64–2.75 eV and red: 625–740 nm 405–480 THz 1.65–2.00 eV on behalf of impact to hippocampal neuronal, and genetic signaling targets involved in transcription/translation feedback loop of CLOCK and BMAL1, and the nucleus basalis magnocellularis projections to the suprachiasmatic nucleus (SCN) mentioned in the main chapter text and shown in **Figure 3**. Cone and melanopsin signaling determines brightness perception. There are references available which suggest that melanopsin excitation takes place at brightness equal to 1 $cd \cdot m^2$ for an equal-energy-spectrum light at 1 $cd \cdot m^2$. The maximum range should lie within 380- 780 nm, which represents the range of skylight visible to human bioperception from pre-dawn to post-dusk.

A.1.5 Retinal luminance

Luminance is in the research to have a defined photon catch of around 480 nm of opsin.

For this reason, maximum error in the device rendering of luminance should be no more than 10% from this value based on maintaining exactly 480 nm spectrally per session.

Mobile device platform manufacturers have responded to health-risk concerns in reported from excess levels of LED blue-light exposure [76]. On the other hand, the research suggests improvements to these same conditions [77, 78]. For these reasons, timing and duration of a virtual reality monitoring session should be coordinated to start at the first eye-blink, and no longer than three (3) minutes. In fact, the first sampling of sensori-motor response and heart rate should be at the instance of the first patient saccadic (blink). This ensures coordination of the data collection with the timing of innate cognitive recognition such as orientation or focus and dorsomedial prefrontal cortex response signaling. It includes the arrival of a new spatial learning event in the hippocampal brain region.

A.1.6 Event rendering

For sky this can also include stimulatory parameters that increase the decision-making integrity challenge, including parameters such as: sky-to-grand relative volume and types of event, such as fog-cloud-rain particle settings. Similarly, parameters for ground can include: ground illumination intensity, ground volume and vegetation-variation, vegetation-windspeed events and so on. Keep in mind that virtual reality involving scores and changing scenes can trigger psychological discomfort, dizziness, eye-strain and even addiction [79–81]. For this reason, there should be only one scene with nature-related motion such as wind in grass or tree branch swaying, and water ripples rather than ground buoyancy.

A.1.7 3D-Audio

Audio settings are vital to immersive realism but, may be varied on left and right, such as for early dementia-related auditory-thalamocortical peri-operative risk evaluation or for patient prescription purposes. Manufacturer settings usually offer sufficient audio control parameters.

A.1.8 Scene bias

No civil society structures, roads, signs whether semantic or drawings, volume-measurement, clock-measurement or human relationship and non-nature type cue references should be included in neurobehavioral XR-testing that is intended to predict the condition of neuronal-nucleic cellular health or tissue functioning.

A.1.9 Behavioral sampling

Thirty second sampling intervals to collect the sensorimotor response and heartrate variation represents successive periods for potential long-term synaptic potentiation in the patient, such as would belong to a learning or decision event based and with matching cerebroarterial blood flow occurring in potential simultaneous XR-fMRI BOLD patient observation. Since daylight variations is composed of wavelengths of light whose frequency and phase change with the position of the sun, it is important to sample for all significant periods of the day in which daylight variation is significant, i.e. the behavioral response from pre-dawn all the way to post-dusk in 3 minute intervals for minimum of 5 or 6 XR-testing sessions, as shown in the sampling tables, below. During an XR-session, wavelight phase information stimulates the retinal cells depending on the device illumination levels (sometimes referred to as *Troland* units, representing retinal illumination from $1mm^2$ pupil area exposed to $1cd/m^2$ (candelas/m^2) of scene light). Light information is translated vibromechanically by the photosensitive retinal ganglion cells onto the suprachiasmatic nuclei cells which directly stimulate the hippocampal neural bed for short-term neuronal growth. The process relies on intracellular transport via light-sensitive heterodimerization which recruits specific proteins in hippocampal neurons, involving recycling endosomes on behalf of neuron axon outgrowth [82]. If XR is used as a circadian prosthetic, this information can be helpful to measuring the amount or volume of full daylight needed for restoring circadian synchronization, using known optogenetic principles of cellular mitochondrial activation and targets in the retinohypothalamic and limbic region circuitry [83].

During a single test event an unconditional stimuli (US) is followed by an unknown conditional stimulus (CS) to the patient, as described in the chapter. This can be for example, a sudden thunder event in a random location that follows the appearance of a bird. The response to the stimuli should be reasonable but significant enough to trigger a cognitive autonomic learning process in healthy controls so that the response behavior is repeated at the next appearance of the same bird, even if the thunder does not occur. In this process, nonconscious autonomic decisionmaking behaviour can be recorded by any XR-scripts that report the raycast change of direction associated with the patient's change of focus and change of heartrate. In Alzheimer's Disease related dementia, for example, there would a noticeable delay in heartrate variation at the time of change of raycast direction. In mid-day testing, learning and recall decisionmaking might appear to be significantly greater than in dusk-based sessions for a wide variety of dementia related diseases. This is because the pathway between the photosensitive retinoganglion cells to the thalamocortical nuclei may be compromised by the disease, such that the hippocampal cells via the retinohypothalamic tract do not receive sufficient daylight phase management information. The loss of daylight wavelength variation from pre-dawn to post-dusk impairs conscious-state transition and increases patient confusion and risk of sleep disruption and hallucination.

A.2 Examples of XR-data-collection setup

Session: Control Mid-day (photopic scene):
Patient device optimization check
Heart rate streaming check.
This requires checking the asset acoustic and animation visibility for distant, near, left and right positions, plus in sky and on ground)
Note: Patient is standing or seated and stationary at all times.
Distant: <20,000m virtual radius
Near: <1000m virtual radius

Nonconscious-asset Type: None Animation Type: None	Start										End
Sampling interval:	00:00:00	00:00:30	00:00:60	00:01:05	00:01:10	00:01:30	00:02:00	00:02:05	00:02:00	02:30	03:00
Heart rate variation											
Sensorimotor response rate-left											
Sensorimotor response rate-right											
Sky Contrast ratio-left	0.1	0.1	0.1	0.1	0.1	0.1	0.1	0.1	0.1	0.1	0.1
Sky Contrast ratio-right	0.1	0.1	0.1	0.1	0.1	0.1	0.1	0.1	0.1	0.1	0.1
Contrast Sky-Ground	0.5	0.5	0.5	0.5	0.5	0.5	0.5	0.5	0.5	0.5	0.5
Rate of conscious-state transition response											
Total Cognitive Responsiveness											
Total Decision-variation											

Session: Pre-dawn (photopic scene):
Nonconscious asset is animated on the ground level, in a distant, near, left or right start position
Note: Patient is standing or seated and stationary at all times.
Note: Patient is standing or seated and stationary at all times.
Distant: <20,000m virtual radius
Near: <1000m virtual radius

Nonconscious-asset Type: Visual and Auditory Animation Type: Approaching	Start (blink)			US left	CS left				US left		End

Sampling times	00:00:00	00:00:30	00:00:60	00:01:05	00:01:10	00:01:30	00:02:00	00:02:30	00:02:32	02:34	03:00
Heart rate											
Sensorimotor response rate-left											
Sensorimotor response rate-right											
Sky Contrast ratio-left	0.1	0.1	0.1	0.1	0.1	0.1	0.1	0.1	0.1	0.1	0.1
Sky Contrast ratio-right	0.1	0.1	0.1	0.1	0.1	0.1	0.1	0.1	0.1	0.1	0.1
Contrast Sky-to-Ground	0.3	0.3	0.3	0.8	0.8	0.3	0.3	0.8	0.3	0.3	0.3
Rate of conscious-state transition response											
Total Cognitive Responsiveness											
Total Decision-variation											

Example Pre- to Post-Dawn Interval: 20-50 minute

Session: Post-dawn (photopic scene)
Ground-level asset-test
Nonconscious asset is animated on the ground level, in a distant, near, left or right start position.
Note: Patient is standing or seated and stationary at all times.
Distant: <20,000m virtual radius
Near: <1000m virtual radius

Nonconscious-asset Type: Visual and Auditory Animation Type: Approaching	Start (blink)			US left	CS right				US left		End
Sampling times	00:00:00	00:00:30	00:00:60	00:01:05	00:01:10	00:01:30	00:02:00	00:02:30	00:02:32	02:34	03:00
Heart rate											
Sensorimotor response rate-left											
Sensorimotor response rate-right											
Sky Contrast ratio-left	0.1	0.1	0.1	0.1	0.1	0.1	0.1	0.1	0.1	0.1	0.1
Sky Contrast ratio-right	0.1	0.1	0.1	0.1	0.1	0.1	0.1	0.1	0.1	0.1	0.1
Contrast Sky-to-Ground	0.3	0.3	0.3	0.8	0.8	0.3	0.4	0.8	0.4	0.4	0.4
Rate of conscious-state transition response											
Total Cognitive Responsiveness											
Total Decision-variation											

Example Post-Dawn to Mid-day Interval: 4 hours

Session: Mid-day (no shadow) (photopic scene)
Nonconscious asset is animated on the sky level, in a distant, near, left or right start position
Note: Patient is standing or seated and stationary at all times.
Distant: <20,000m virtual radius
Near: <1000m virtual radius
Luminance (log cd/m2): 4 to 6
Pupil diameter (mm): 6 to 8
Retinal illuminance (log Trolands): Photopic > 4.5 /Scotopic 0
Active photoreceptors: cones
Color perception/acuity: Good color vision, high acuity

Nonconscious-asset Type: Visual and Auditory Animation Type: Approaching	Start (blink)			US left	CS left or right				US left		End
Sampling times	00:00:00	00:00:30	00:00:60	00:01:05	00:01:10	00:01:30	00:02:00	00:02:30	00:02:32	02:34	03:00
Heart rate											
Sensorimotor response rate-left											
Sensorimotor response rate-right											
Sky Contrast ratio-left	0.5	0.5	0.5	0.8	0.8	0.5	0.5	0.5	0.8	0.5	0.5
Sky Contrast ratio-right	0.5	0.5	0.5	0.5	0.5	0.5	0.5	0.5	0.5	0.5	0.5
Contrast Sky-to-Ground	0.4	0.4	0.4	0.4	0.4	0.5	0.5	0.5	0.5	0.5	0.5
Rate of conscious-state transition response											
Total Cognitive Responsiveness											
Total Decision-variation											

Example Mid-day to Pre-dusk Interval: 6 - 8 hours

Session: Pre-dusk (photopic scene)
Nonconscious asset is animated on the sky or ground level, in a near left or right start position
Note: Patient is standing or seated and stationary at all times.
Near: <1000m virtual radius

Nonconscious-asset Type: Visual and Auditory Animation Type: Approaching	Start (blink)			US left	CS left				US left		End
Sampling times	00:00:00	00:00:30	00:00:60	00:01:05	00:01:10	00:01:30	00:02:00	00:02:30	00:02:32	02:34	03:00
Heart rate											
Sensorimotor response rate-left											
Sensorimotor response rate-right											

DOI: http://dx.doi.org/10.5772/intechopen.97384

Sky Contrast ratio-left	0.5	0.5	0.5	0.5	0.5	0.5	0.5	0.5	0.5	0.5	0.5
Sky Contrast ratio-right	0.5	0.5	0.5	0.8	0.5	0.5	0.5	0.5	0.8	0.5	0.5
Contrast Sky-Ground	0.3	0.3	0.3	0.3	0.8	0.3	0.3	0.3	0.3	0.3	0.3
Rate of conscious-state transition response											
Total Cognitive Responsiveness											
Total Decision-variation											

Example Pre-Dusk to Post-Dusk Interval: 20-50 minutes

Session: Post-dusk (photopic scene)
Nonconscious asset is animated on the ground level, in a near left or right start position
Note: Patient is standing or seated and stationary at all times.
Near: <1000m virtual radius

Nonconscious-asset Type: Visual and Auditory Animation Type: Approaching	Start (blink)			US random	CS left				US random		End
Sampling times	00:00:00	00:00:30	00:00:60	00:01:05	00:01:10	00:01:30	00:02:00	00:02:30	00:02:32	02:34	03:00
Heart rate											
Sensorimotor response rate-left											
Sensorimotor response rate-right											
Sky Contrast ratio-left	0.5	0.5	0.5	0.5	0.5	0.5	0.5	0.5	0.5	0.5	0.5
Sky Contrast ratio-right	0.5	0.5	0.5	0.5	0.5	0.5	0.5	0.5	0.5	0.5	0.5
Contrast Sky-to-Ground	0.2	0.2	0.2	0.8	0.8	0.2	0.2	0.2	0.8	0.2	0.2
Rate of conscious-state transition response											
Total Cognitive Responsiveness											
Total Decision-variation											

Session: Post-dusk (photopic scene)
Nonconscious asset is animated on the ground level in a near, left or right start position
Note: Patient is standing or seated and stationary at all times.
Near: <1000m virtual radius

Nonconscious-asset Type Visual and Auditory Animation Type: approaching	Start (blink)			US random	CS right				US random		End
Sampling times	00:00:00	00:00:30	00:00:60	00:01:05	00:01:10	00:01:30	00:02:00	00:02:30	00:02:32	02:34	03:00
Heart rate											

Sensorimotor response rate-left											
Sensorimotor response rate-right											
Sky Contrast ratio-left	0.5	0.5	0.5	0.5	0.5	0.5	0.5	0.5	0.5	0.5	0.5
Sky Contrast ratio-right	0.5	0.5	0.5	0.5	0.5	0.5	0.5	0.5	0.5	0.5	0.5
Contrast Sky-to-Ground	0.2	0.2	0.2	0.8	0.8	0.2	0.2	0.2	0.8	0.2	0.2
Rate of conscious-state transition response											
Total Cognitive Responsiveness											
Total Decision-variation											

Session: Post-dusk (starry-night scatter) (photopic scene)
Nonconscious asset is auditory in the sky or ground level, in a distant, near, left or right start position
Note: Patient is standing or seated and stationary at all times.
Distant: <20,000m virtual radius
Near: <1000m virtual radius
Luminance (log cd/m2): -6 to -4
Pupil diameter (mm): 7.1 to 6.6
Retinal illuminance (log Trolands): Photopic < -0.62 /Scotopic -4.0 to 0.70
Active photoreceptors: rods
Color perception/acuity: No color vision, poor acuity

Nonconscious-asset Type: Auditory Animation Type:None	Start (blink)			US random				UC random			End
Sampling times	00:00:00	00:00:30	00:00:60	00:01:05	00:01:10	00:01:30	00:02:00	00:02:05	00:02:00	02:30	03:00
Heart rate											
Sensorimotor response rate-left											
Sensorimotor response rate-right											
Sky Contrast ratio-left	0	0	0	0	0	0	0	0	0	0	0
Sky Contrast ratio-right	0	0	0	0	0	0	0	0	0	0	0
Contrast Sky-to-Ground	0.1	0.1	0.1	0.1	0.1	0.1	0.1	0.1	0.1	0.1	0.1
Rate of conscious-state transition response											
Total Cognitive Responsiveness											
Total Decision-variation											

Repeat the above, for Scotopic settings and report.
Compare and analyse daily mid-day decision-variation longitudinal data.
Refer to rate of loss of conscious-state transition as:
Behavioral range > 0

Heartrate variation (time of US event recognition) = Heartrate variation (recall of CS event)

And

Headturn rate or focus > 0 and raycast-direction collides with the CS event location of asset

```
function Update () {
  var hit : RaycastHit;
  if(Physics.Raycast(transform.position, transform.up, hit, 10))
        {
             contact = true;
         }
         else
         {
             contact = false;
         }
```

change to a US-trigger (based on change of raycast direction and speed) relative to patient heartrate variation, for dusk versus mid-day and dawn versus mid-day behavioral responses.

In general, this could verily indicate a medically-prohibitive gradient for euthanatic administration.

A.3 Additional evidence-seeking requirements recommended prior to non-voluntary patient killing including physician account investigation

Behavioural Impairment	• Virtual Reality-fMRI/PET Models • Focus on models of the prefrontal-amygdala circuits and Amygdalo-Prefronto-Dorsostriatal Network reaction times • Include autonomic pavlovian fear-conditioning variations : differences in cerebrovascular response times versus and cardiovascular.
Pain and Suffering	• Include stress-related wipe-out (losses) of immunity-providing gut, blood and genital microbiota (e.g., Lactobacillis, in conversion of tryptophan to kynurenine for neurotransmitter synthesis and neuroinflammation regulation). • Look for increased GI tract permeability and alterations to the neurohumoral communication along the vagus nerve and enteric nervous system, and HPA axis activation • Measure the patient inflammation leading to infection and psychological impairments
Infection and Organ Damage	• Look for records of Increased GI tract permeability and inflammation leading to infection and psychological impairments • Include pharmaceutical induced evidence of Circadian disruption, sleep-interruption • Use medical diagnosis (or absense thereof) to report potential psychiatric neglect of loss of neuronal - and inflammatory repair rates, leading to cognitive disruption, and suicidal drive.
Physical Weakness & Exhaustion	• Compare patient decline with models of post-traumatic stress disorder patients • Target the increased sympathetic tone and decreased parasympathetic activity activation of the stress response and central and peripheral immune cells • Request patient records where physicians failed to examine cardiovascular reactivity and to monitor early signs of onset cardiovascular disease (CVD)

These represent brain neurotoxic inflammatory evidence that are treatable and curable.
When these features are collectively neglected, the patient becomes more dependent on support and may be at higher risk of a non-voluntary commitment to his/her death by physicians or psychiatrists who have not conducted a proper full assessment for a minimum of three months.

A.4 Nervous system relationships for autonomic and conscious behavioral response regulation

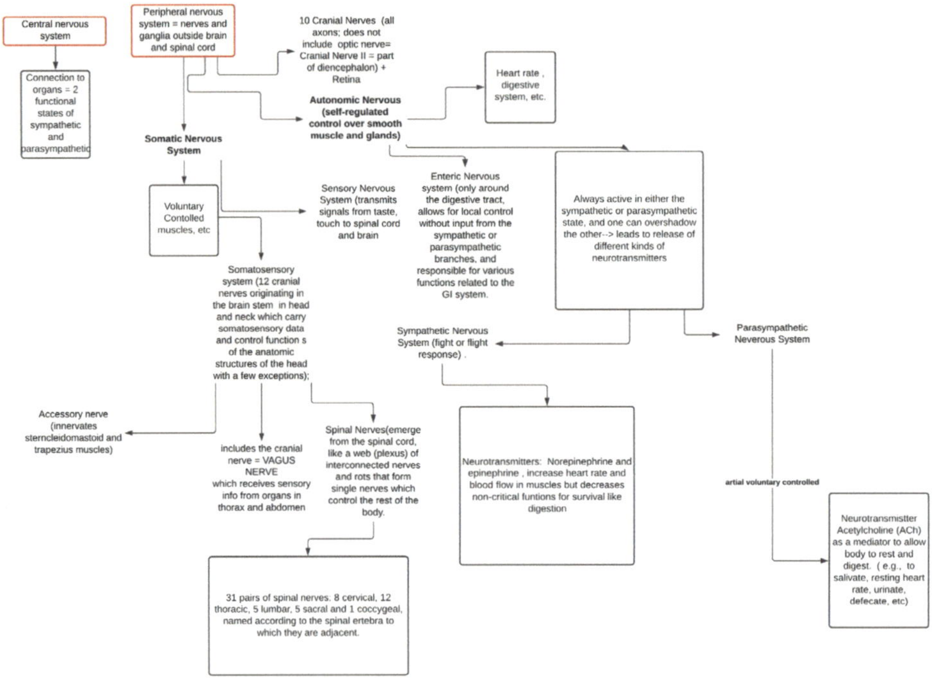

Author details

Farida Hanna Campbell
Epidaurus Telemedical, Leiden, The Netherlands

*Address all correspondence to: hanna.campbell@neuronalregrowth.com

References

[1] Zhang L-Q, Yao J, Gao J, Sun L, Wang L-T, Sui J-F. Modulation of eyeblink conditioning through sensory processing of conditioned stimulus by cortical and subcortical regions. *Behavioural Brain Research*. 2019;359: 149-155. doi:10.1016/j.bbr.2018.10.035

[2] Hocking J, McMahon K. Environmental sound processing: Distinct cortical regions for knowledge about furry, noisy Australian animals. *NeuroImage*. 2009;47:S75. doi:10.1016/ s1053-8119(09)70486-0

[3] Yin L, Bao F, Wu J, Li K. NLRP3 inflammasome-dependent pyroptosis is proposed to be involved in the mechanism of age-dependent isoflurane-induced cognitive impairment. *Journal of Neuroinflammation*. 2018;15(1). doi: 10.1186/s12974-018-1299-x

[4] Mills PJ, Dimsdale JE. Sleep apnea: a model for studying cytokines, sleep, and sleep disruption. *Brain Behav Immun*. 2004;18(4):298-303.

[5] Krueger JM. The role of cytokines in sleep regulation. *Curr Pharm Des*. 2008; 14(32):3408-3416.

[6] Weschenfelder J, Sander C, Kluge M, Kirkby KC, Himmerich H. The influence of cytokines on wakefulness regulation: clinical relevance, mechanisms and methodological problems. *Psychiatr Danub*. 2012;24(2): 112-126.

[7] Kent BA, Mistlberger RE. Sleep and hippocampal neurogenesis: Implications for Alzheimer's disease. *Front Neuroendocrinol*. 2017;45:35-52.

[8] Tranah GJ, Blackwell T, Stone KL, et al. Circadian activity rhythms and risk of incident dementia and mild cognitive impairment in older women. *Ann Neurol*. 2011;70(5):722-732.

[9] Regional Euthanization Review Committees-The Netherlands. RTEjv2018_DEF (1) (2019_11_19 19_28_ 23 UTC).pdf. Published online 2018. https://www.euthanasiecommissie.nl/ binaries/euthanasiecommissie/ documenten/jaarverslagen/2018/april/11/ jaarverslag-2018/RTE_jv2018_English.pdf

[10] Borjigin J, Lee U, Liu T, et al. Surge of neurophysiological coherence and connectivity in the dying brain. *Proc Natl Acad Sci U S A*. 2013;110(35): 14432-14437.

[11] ten Have H, Welie J. *Death And Medical Power: An Ethical Analysis Of Dutch Euthanasia Practice: An Ethical Analysis of Dutch Euthanasia Practice*. McGraw-Hill Education (UK); 2005.

[12] Hadzidiakos D, Horn N, Degener R, Buchner A, Rehberg B. Analysis of Memory Formation during General Anesthesia (Propofol/Remifentanil) for Elective Surgery Using the Process-dissociation Procedure. *Anesthesiology*. 2009;111(2):293-301.

[13] Timofeev I, Bonjean ME, Bazhenov M. Cellular Mechanisms of Thalamocortical Oscillations in the Sleeping Brain. In: Dang-Vu TT, Courtemanche R, eds. *Neuronal Oscillations of Wakefulness and Sleep: Windows on Spontaneous Activity of the Brain*. Springer New York; 2020: 119-170.

[14] van de Wier M. Jacob Kohnstamm-Euthanasie is geen recht.pdf. *Trouw*. https://www.trouw.nl/nieuws/jacob-kohnstamm-euthanasie-is-geen-recht~bf4a9d1a/?referrer=https%3A% 2F%2Fwww.google.com%2F.Published April 12, 2019.

[15] Ministerie van Volksgezondheid W en S. Annual reports. Published December 27, 2016. Accessed March 16, 2021. https://english.

euthanasiecommissie.nl/the-committees/annual-reports

[16] Tiainen M, Poutiainen E, Kovala T, Takkunen O, Häppölä O, Roine RO. Cognitive and neurophysiological outcome of cardiac arrest survivors treated with therapeutic hypothermia. *Stroke*. 2007;38(8):2303-2308.

[17] Friberg H, Westhall E, Rosén I, Rundgren M, Nielsen N, Cronberg T. Clinical review: Continuous and simplified electroencephalography to monitor brain recovery after cardiac arrest. *Crit Care*. 2013;17(4):233.

[18] Rudolph SS, Barnung S. Survival after Drowning with Cardiac Arrest and Mild Hypothermia. *ISRN Cardiology*. 2011;2011:1-2. doi:10.5402/2011/895625

[19] Waszkielewicz AM, Gunia A, Szkaradek N, Słoczyńska K, Krupińska S, Marona H. Ion channels as drug targets in central nervous system disorders. *Curr Med Chem*. 2013;20(10): 1241-1285.

[20] Morgan KG, Bryant SH. Pentobarbital: Presynaptic effect in the squid giant synapse. *Experientia*. 1977;33 (4):487-488. doi:10.1007/bf01922226

[21] Leslie SW, Friedman MB, Wilcox RE, Elrod SV. Acute and chronic effects of barbituartes on depolarization-induced calcium influx into rat synaptosomes. *Brain Res*. 1980;185(2):409-417.

[22] Baudoux S, Empson RM, Richards CD. Pentobarbitone modulates calcium transients in axons and synaptic boutons of hippocampal CA1 neurons. *Br J Pharmacol*. 2003;140(5):971-979.

[23] Schober A, Sokolova E, Gingrich KJ. Pentobarbital inhibition of human recombinant α1A P/Q-type voltage-gated calcium channels involves slow, open channel block. *British Journal of Pharmacology*. 2010;161(2):365-383. doi: 10.1111/j.1476-5381.2010.00886.x

[24] Willingham MD, Karren E, Shanks AM, et al. Concurrence of Intraoperative Hypotension, Low Minimum Alveolar Concentration, and Low Bispectral Index Is Associated with Postoperative Death. *Anesthesiology*. 2015;123(4):775-785.

[25] Drew BA. Arthur Guedel and the Ascendance of Anesthesia: A Teacher, Tinkerer, and Transformer. *J Anesth Hist*. 2019;5(3):85-92.

[26] Lutz PL. Mechanisms for anoxic survival in the vertebrate brain. *Annu Rev Physiol*. 1992;54:601-618.

[27] Shewmon DA. Brainstem death, brain death and death: A critical re-evaluation of the purported equivalence. *Issues Law Med*. 1998;14:125.

[28] Sanders L. Body & brain: "Wave of death" not a last gasp: Rat brain activity seen nearly a minute after decapitation. *Science News*. 2011;180(5):8-8. doi: 10.1002/scin.5591800504

[29] Wijdicks EF. The diagnosis of brain death. *N Engl J Med*. 2001;344(16): 1215-1221.

[30] Campbell FH. Title: Neuroinflammatory Pain in Dutch Methods of Euthanasia. Published online July 1, 2019. doi:10.13140/ RG.2.2.15139.81440

[31] Robijn L. Towards the improvement of continuous sedation until death in nursing homes. Published online 2020. Accessed February 28, 2021. https:// biblio.ugent.be/publication/8676651

[32] Rys S, Mortier F, Deliens L, Bilsen J. The Practice of Continuous Sedation Until Death in Nursing Homes in Flanders, Belgium: A Nationwide Study. *Journal of the American Geriatrics Society*. 2014;62 (10):1869-1876. doi:10.1111/jgs.13073

[33] Kerssens C, Gaither JR, Sebel PS. Preserved memory function during

bispectral index–guided anesthesia with sevoflurane for major orthopedic surgery. *The Journal of the American Society of Anesthesiologists*. 2009;111(3):518-524.

[34] Kerssens C, Lubke GH, Klein J, van der Woerd A, Bonke B. Memory function during propofol and alfentanil anesthesia: predictive value of individual differences. *Anesthesiology*. 2002;97(2):382-389.

[35] Cai Z, Pang Y, Lin S, Rhodes PG. Differential roles of tumor necrosis factor-alpha and interleukin-1 beta in lipopolysaccharide-induced brain injury in the neonatal rat. *Brain Res*. 2003;975 (1-2):37-47.

[36] Sappington RM, Chan M, Calkins DJ. Interleukin-6 protects retinal ganglion cells from pressure-induced death. *Invest Ophthalmol Vis Sci*. 2006;47(7):2932-2942.

[37] Calderón-Garcidueñas L, Cross JV, Franco-Lira M, et al. Brain immune interactions and air pollution: macrophage inhibitory factor (MIF), prion cellular protein (PrPC), Interleukin-6 (IL-6), interleukin 1 receptor antagonist (IL-1Ra), and interleukin-2 (IL-2) in cerebrospinal fluid and MIF in serum differentiate urban children exposed to severe vs. low air pollution. *Front Neurosci*. 2013;7:183.

[38] de Visser E. "Zijn doodswens stond niet op papier. Ik zei_ jullie hebben zijn lichaam, maar ik heb zijn ziel" _ De Volkskrant.pdf.https://www.volkskrant.nl/mensen/zijn-doodswens-stond-niet-op-papier-ik-zei-jullie-hebben-zijn-lichaam-maar-ik-heb-zijn-ziel~bc861190/?fbclid=IwAR3J8z5dDIAo1uq-hzJBqfbe0UDboTfOmUKbIWlW-aOgjCts-bdRwGt5Mkc&referrer=https%3A%2F%2Fwww.linkedin.com%2F. Published August 16, 2019.

[39] Kennedy RH, Silver R. Neuroimmune Signaling: Cytokines and the CNS. *Neuroscience in the 21st Century*. Published online 2015:1-41. doi:10.1007/978-1-4614-6434-1_174-1

[40] Kennedy RH, Silver R. Neuroimmune Signaling: Cytokines and the Central Nervous System. *Neuroscience in the 21st Century*. Published online 2016:1-41. doi:10.1007/978-1-4614-6434-1_174-2

[41] Alt JA, Sautter NB, Mace JC, Detwiller KY, Smith TL. Antisomnogenic cytokines, quality of life, and chronic rhinosinusitis: a pilot study. *Laryngoscope*. 2014;124(4):E107-E114.

[42] Nembutal (Pentobarbital)_ Uses, Dosage, Side Effects, Interactions, Warning.pdf.

[43] Pentobarbital Monograph for Professionals - Drugs.com.pdf.

[44] Torjesen I. Assisted dying methods can lead to "inhumane" deaths. *BMJ*. 2019;364:l797.

[45] Dimech J, Agius E, Hughes JC, Bartolo P. Challenges faced by patients, relatives and clinicians in end-stage dementia decision-making: a qualitative study of swallowing problems. *J Med Ethics*. Published online August 3, 2020. doi:10.1136/medethics-2020-106222

[46] Williams LM, Liddell BJ, Rathjen J, et al. Mapping the time course of nonconscious and conscious perception of fear: an integration of central and peripheral measures. *Hum Brain Mapp*. 2004;21(2):64-74.

[47] Tallot L, Graupner M, Diaz-Mataix L, Doyère V. Beyond Freezing: Temporal Expectancy of an Aversive Event Engages the Amygdalo–Prefronto–Dorsostriatal Network. *Cereb Cortex*. 2020;30(10):5257-5269.

[48] Rolls ET. The cingulate cortex and limbic systems for emotion, action, and

memory. *Brain Struct Funct*. 2019;224 (9):3001-3018.

[49] Paulsen JS, Heaton RK, Sadek JR, et al. The nature of learning and memory impairments in schizophrenia. *J Int Neuropsychol Soc*. 1995;1(1):88-99.

[50] Suarez-Jimenez B, Albajes-Eizagirre A, Lazarov A, et al. Neural signatures of conditioning, extinction learning, and extinction recall in posttraumatic stress disorder: a meta-analysis of functional magnetic resonance imaging studies. *Psychol Med*. 2020;50(9):1442-1451.

[51] Dallérac G, Graupner M, Knippenberg J, et al. Updating temporal expectancy of an aversive event engages striatal plasticity under amygdala control. *Nat Commun*. 2017;8:13920.

[52] Elam JS, Van Essen D. Human Connectome Project. *Encyclopedia of Computational Neuroscience*. Published online 2015:1408-1411. doi:10.1007/978-1-4614-6675-8_592

[53] Haak KV, Beckmann CF. Plasticity versus stability across the human cortical visual connectome. doi:10.1101/520395

[54] Tong T, Chan JH, Chignell M. Serious Games for Dementia. In: *Proceedings of the 26th International Conference on World Wide Web Companion*. WWW '17 Companion. International World Wide Web Conferences Steering Committee; 2017:1111-1115.

[55] Ely EW, Shintani A, Truman B, et al. Delirium as a predictor of mortality in mechanically ventilated patients in the intensive care unit. *JAMA*. 2004;291 (14):1753-1762.

[56] Figueroa-Ramos MI, Arroyo-Novoa CM, Lee KA, Padilla G, Puntillo KA. Sleep and delirium in ICU patients: a review of mechanisms and manifestations. *Intensive Care Med*. 2009;35(5):781-795.

[57] Lau HM, Smit JH, Fleming TM, Riper H. Serious Games for Mental Health: Are They Accessible, Feasible, and Effective? A Systematic Review and Meta-analysis. *Front Psychiatry*. 2016;7:209.

[58] Castro-Alamancos MA, Connors BW. Short-term plasticity of a thalamocortical pathway dynamically modulated by behavioral state. *Science*. 1996;272(5259):274-277.

[59] Cardoso-Cruz H. Dynamics of circadian thalamocortical flow of information during a peripheral neuropathic pain condition. *Frontiers in Integrative Neuroscience*. 2011;5. doi: 10.3389/fnint.2011.00043

[60] Blatter K, Cajochen C. Circadian rhythms in cognitive performance: methodological constraints, protocols, theoretical underpinnings. *Physiol Behav*. 2007;90(2-3):196-208.

[61] Mistlberger RE, Buijs RM, Challet E, et al. Standards of evidence in chronobiology: critical review of a report that restoration of Bmal1 expression in the dorsomedial hypothalamus is sufficient to restore circadian food anticipatory rhythms in Bmal1-/- mice. *Journal of Circadian Rhythms*. 2009;7(0):3. doi:10.1186/1740-3391-7-3

[62] Bodien YG, Chatelle C, Edlow BL. Functional networks in disorders of consciousness. In: *Seminars in Neurology*. Vol 37. NIH Public Access; 2017:485.

[63] Araújo SES, Mendonça HR, Wheeler NA, et al. Inflammatory demyelination alters subcortical visual circuits. *J Neuroinflammation*. 2017;14 (1):162.

[64] Jahanshad N, Rajagopalan P, Hua X, et al. Genome-wide scan of healthy human connectome discovers SPON1 gene variant influencing dementia severity. *Proc Natl Acad Sci U S A*. 2013; 110(12):4768-4773.

[65] Laureys, Steven, Fabien Perrin, and Serge Brédart. "Self-consciousness in non-communicative patients." *Consciousness and cognition* 16.3 (2007): 722-741.

[66] Malagurski, Brigitta, et al. "Topological disintegration of resting state functional connectomes in coma." *NeuroImage* 195 (2019): 354-361.

[67] Harding A, Halliday G, Caine D, Kril J. Degeneration of anterior thalamic nuclei differentiates alcoholics with amnesia. *Brain*. 2000;123 (Pt 1):141-154.

[68] Aggleton JP, Sahgal A. The contribution of the anterior thalamic nuclei to anterograde amnesia. *Neuropsychologia*. 1993;31(10): 1001-1019.

[69] Ono D, Honma K-I, Yanagawa Y, Yamanaka A, Honma S. GABA in the suprachiasmatic nucleus refines circadian output rhythms in mice. *Commun Biol*. 2019;2:232.

[70] Tjebbe vanderLeest H, Rohling JHT, Michel S, Meijer JH. Phase shifting capacity of the circadian pacemaker determined by the SCN neuronal network organization. *PLoS One*. 2009;4(3):e4976.

[71] Wang J-Z, Wang Z-F. Role of melatonin in Alzheimer-like neurodegeneration. *Acta Pharmacol Sin*. 2006;27(1):41-49.

[72] Campbell FH. Calibration of Virtual Reality to bridge the Circadian Genetic Expression Data Gap in Computational Psychiatry for Alzheimer's Disease and Aging-related dementia. Published online January 1, 2019. Accessed July 30, 2019. https://www.researchgate.net/publication/334769295_Calibration_of_Virtual_Reality_to_bridge_the_Circadian_Genetic_Expression_Data_Gap_in_Computational_Psychiatry_for_Alzheimer's_Disease_and_Aging-related_dementia

[73] Todd WD. Potential Pathways for Circadian Dysfunction and Sundowning-Related Behavioral Aggression in Alzheimer's Disease and Related Dementias. *Front Neurosci*. 2020;14:910.

[74] Volicer L, Harper DG, Manning BC, Goldstein R, Satlin A. Sundowning and circadian rhythms in Alzheimer's disease. *Am J Psychiatry*. 2001;158(5): 704-711.

[75] Soltan A, Barrett JM, Maaskant P, et al. A head mounted device stimulator for optogenetic retinal prosthesis. *J Neural Eng*. 2018;15(6):065002.

[76] Chellappa SL, Steiner R, Oelhafen P, et al. Acute exposure to evening blue-enriched light impacts on human sleep. *J Sleep Res*. 2013;22(5):573-580.

[77] Meldrum D, Herdman S, Moloney R, et al. Effectiveness of conventional versus virtual reality based vestibular rehabilitation in the treatment of dizziness, gait and balance impairment in adults with unilateral peripheral vestibular loss: a randomised controlled trial. *BMC Ear Nose Throat Disord*. 2012;12(1):3.

[78] Peñate W, Pitti CT, Bethencourt JM, de la Fuente J, Gracia R. The effects of a treatment based on the use of virtual reality exposure and cognitive-behavioral therapy applied to patients with agoraphobia. *Int J Clin Health Psychol*. 2008;8(1). https://www.redalyc.org/html/337/33780101/

[79] Regan EC, Price KR. The frequency of occurrence and severity of side-effects of immersion virtual reality. *Aviat Space Environ Med*. 1994;65(6): 527-530.

[80] Passamonti L, Riccelli R, Lacquaniti F, Staab JP, Indovina I. Brain responses to virtual reality visual motion stimulation are affected by neurotic personality traits in patients with persistent postural-perceptual

dizziness. *J Vestib Res*. 2018;28(5-6): 369-378.

[81] Park SY, Kim SM, Roh S, et al. The effects of a virtual reality treatment program for online gaming addiction. *Comput Methods Programs Biomed*. 2016; 129:99-108.

[82] van Bergeijk P, Adrian M, Hoogenraad CC, Kapitein LC. Optogenetic control of organelle transport and positioning. *Nature*. 2015; 518(7537):111-114.

[83] Zhou B, Yu P, Lin M-Y, Sun T, Chen Y, Sheng Z-H. Facilitation of axon regeneration by enhancing mitochondrial transport and rescuing energy deficits. *J Cell Biol*. 2016;214(1): 103-119.

Chapter 17

The Challenges Facing Palliative Care Advocacy: What Is in a Name?

Maria Teresa Garcia-Baquero Merino, María Victoria Roqué Sánchez, Katherine Pettus and Micaela Menarguez Carreño

Abstract

The need for Palliative Care (PC) continues to grow throughout the world, requiring continuous development, true to its "ethos." As awareness grows so does the expectation for timely response and policies to potentiate its delivery. The scientific dimension of its philosophy, underpinned by research and scientific practice, looks to explain its nature, origin and concepts, models and theories within which it is delivered. The concept *palliation* is widely used; yet, it is understudied by academics and clinicians. Interestingly, it is increasingly questioned by society and other specialists, calling for it to "be debated and essentially contested". Our aim is to contribute to society's understanding of palliative care so that they can have a clear and truthful awareness of the complex implications of its mission. We approach the different concepts, scientific theories and structures can be achieved by following different pathways, including defining its "ethos": personality or nature, manifest in the very formulae by which PC places itself before those who need it. What a fascinating topic it is to research and write on!, phenomenological in its base, it shows how different translations of the Anglo-Saxon PC influence its understanding and much needed expansion. Semiotics are at the base of the essence of how palliative care might be assumed and promoted. PC is, for sure, one of the most important, existential spheres to apply our knowledge today and a novel promising methodology to apply the semiotic and phenomenological approaches learning of different aspects of cultural transfer processes.

Keywords: palliative care, scientific conceptualization, linguistics, advocacy, ethos, spirituality

1. Introduction

The extension and transferability of what has come to be known as PC [1, 2] has become stalled in some countries [3]. Many believe it to be a consequence of inadequate funding or even political indifference [4]; others question whether it might be due to lack of conceptual intelligibility and transferability across languages and call for a fresh PC [5, 6] definition that incorporates its philosophy and ethos while being fully transferable across countries and cultures.

But what can be said to constitute, identify and define the *Palliative Care Ethos?* With the patient at its centre, PC looks for direction in their own and their loved ones' narratives:

'You can tell them all that it was all right', was the unpretentious and comforting message Cicely Saunders was asked to pass on to a lady's relatives once she had died. It was important for that patient to let her loved ones know that she had not gone through a strange, dramatic, or just unlucky experience, (...) written up as such without sentimentality or sensationalism, but a common experience ordinary people have always faced, writes D. Clark [7]. A good example of the rich exchanges full of meaning and depth that can take place within the ordinary *delivery* of PC. So beautifully common in many ways; and yet, so elusive to capture in a defining snapshot to apprehend its uniqueness.

'The joy, purpose and meaning of medicine has been codified, sterilized, protocolised, industrialized and regimented' says Dr. Eric Levi [8]: a stark reminder of the reality in ever-advancing health systems which seem to have forgotten the more *artistic* aspects of medicine which allows compassion to highlight our common humanity, a fundamental aspect of PC.

2. The purpose of medicine

Medicine is as old as humankind itself [9]. At first it was mythological, the causes of diseases were attributed to the gods or spirits, subsequently acquiring a more scientific character as it was recognized that diseases had physical or environmental causes.

Hippocrates has been considered the father of scientific medicine. The Hippocratic Corpus [10], with its 53 books, has philosophical and ethical writings such as the Hippocratic Oath and Aphorisms, as well as others of medical order consisting of 7 books on Epidemics, 4 on the Regime, 4 on Diseases, 2 on Predictions, 2 on Women Diseases, Instruments of reduction of Joints and Fractures. Writings used by doctors to learn for centuries. One of these texts, the Hippocratic Oath, remains valid- It concisely points out the duties of doctors, duties that were not imposed on them by the authority of the moment but rather, somewhat self-imposed after assessing the value and importance of their own work. This Oath is a model of professional behavior not only for doctors but for all professions.

Medicine is finite, limited. People will die. Diseases will change, but it always comprises great respect for human weakness. Sometimes we will have patients with acute problems, sometimes chronic conditions, some patients will be conscious and sometimes unconscious, sometimes it will be curable diseases and sometimes incurable, sometimes we will have friendly patients, sometimes we will have patients with diseases that we like to treat and sometimes with pathologies that for the doctor are unpleasant, but they are all our patients, all expect us to treat them with respect, they want to feel taken care of, they want humanitarian treatment.

Our medicalised modern cultures tend to render reason and mystery mutually exclusive, defining "death by disease" as failure, and dying as disgraceful. Providers and policymakers alike marginalize aging and dying individuals, while formulating largely ineffective strategies to prevent deaths from violence or epidemics, terrorism, and famines. Policies to nurture care and support the elderly, those with long terms conditions and children [11–13] born with congenital medical conditions, malformations or different capacities, are too often inadequate and departed from reality. They tend to be declarations of intentions lacking in budgetary provision.

3. Palliative care

3.1 Meaning and fullness of worth within the health and social contexts

It is palliative care mission to demonstrate that each life is morally significant to its natural end, restoring patients' and families' quality of life where possible, and attending meticulously to the dying period when necessary [3, 4].

PC changes the perspective from which the world sees health and social care, since its philosophy gives standing to the multiplicity of beliefs and communication patterns manifest in the collective of suffering patients. This motivates the articulation of a good enough ethic.

Contemporary literature [3] shows researchers' acknowledgement of historically relevant milestones in PC roots from bygone days and subsequent evolution, including Palliative Medicine being recognized in some countries as a specialized field of training and work. There is also explicit acknowledgment of the difficulties affecting uniform implementation of its philosophy and principles. Some projects centre future advances and growth in PC provision with promising results in relation to identifying the founding ethos of PC by reproducing its initial way of showing the depth of society's concern for its more vulnerable members, based on its values when alleviating the suffering experienced while facing aging, disease, life threatening pathologies, dying and death.

Such ventures highlight the importance of setting the scene for possible advances to integrate ethical, legal and social implications in years to come to benefit the many likely to need it. It likens the development of the field to a journey; one that sets off on the knowledge the fullness of meaning and richness of PC can only be approached by taking its long view.

A sound understanding of PC foundational bases [2, 14] facilitates answers to many questions needing an answer, although some voices of those who seek a more bio-physical-psychological palliative care model strongly disagree. It is, for example, motivating to take into account the different creative initiatives born in clinical settings in the context of the COVID-19 pandemic; it confirms how man continues to look for ways to alleviate suffering in the most challenging situations making use of what they have to hand. In our time, the inventiveness brought to the bedside of the dying has been astonishing, giving hope to those of us who want to offer holistic care to those who see their lives threatened, including aging and the natural end of life, by some entity threatened life expectancy.

This chapter will aim to identify what constitutes the enduring ethos of PC as it continues to evolve and grow beyond the walls of St Christopher's Hospice, flagship of Cicely Saunders's endeavor to comfort the dying by letting them know that they matter because they are who they are; and they will matter to us until their last moment of their lives.

3.2 Modern hospice movement evolution

Looking into what is understood by this vocable takes us along surprising trails as a Work of Mercy, with deep ancestral Judeo-Christian roots [2]. It is depicted well in both the Old and the New Testaments, for example, in the Parable of the Good Samaritan and many conceivable and incomprehensible healings. It can be followed in the labour of hospital religious orders over the centuries which persists to this day in initiatives such as the contemporary Pastoral of Health. It is doubtlessly, care that has historically been largely provided by Christian orders that hold to the divine 'Thou shall not kill', and are moved to love and compassion.

In our time, proud of its origins, it is a formalized and widely recognized as a growing medical field which has its foundational modern roots in (Dame) Cecily Saunders's concern and work to remedy the poor medical care being provided to dying hospital patients. Over time, its medicine had shifted [15] the focus away from the needs of those who could no longer benefit from evolving technology and life-saving treatments. But it did not stop there as the medical world continue in its way to ignore those dying in its institutions.

Cicely Saunders, established unambiguous foundations for the Modern Hospice Movement [2], one of which is to be found in the togetherness of Head (mind) and

Heart (compassion and our own vulnerability) when caring for these people. It was not, she explained, an idea that occurred to her, but rather the mandate received from David. David Tasma, a Polish Jew, mortally ill with pancreatic cancer, when, broken by the profound suffering he was experiencing, as he was facing his own mortality so far away from his own country and those he knew and loved well asked her:

"Can you say something to comfort me?" taking Cicely Saunders away from *doing* something to him, or giving him some medication to soothe his distress. A little later, he added "I only want what is in your mind and in your heart."

The Modern Hospice Movement, generally known as *Palliative Care* outside Great Britain, was thus born to use scientific rigor to research and treat symptoms such as pain. Its focus on the holistic needs of patients: physical, emotional, social and spiritual, without forgetting the professional dimension. *Palliative Medicine* is the only medical specialty that recognizes care of the spiritual person as part of its mandate [16]. Its science and care are applicable to any person with an incurable, complex or life-limiting illness; its principles can be applied to that person's care from the time of diagnosis. This means good symptom management plus supportive and holistic care occurring alongside: it may be provided by any health care clinician, using the same principles to provide a 'Palliative Approach' to medical and nursing care.

Palliative is derived from the Latin word '*pallium*' meaning to cloak someone who is ill, sick, lonely or needing protection. Symptoms are eased even if the underlying condition be cured.

Maximizing wellbeing and nurturing the hope to maintain or improve perceived quality of life can be achieved in a variety of ways, however, it is imperative to guide all interventions by a common moral compass which indicate the manner by which teams allows someone to be themselves at what can be an extremely difficult time in their lives. PC strives to acknowledge the person as a whole - addressing snags affecting different aspects of their life. A multi-disciplinary approach supported by the skills of different professionals, pooled and utilized as necessary.

Hospices and Palliative Care Units alike house an ethos of care which should extend beyond their walls to places where symptoms need to be eased, the underlying condition not amenable to be cured [14].

3.3 Limits of action: caring, not killing

PC acknowledges the reality of death and seeks to assist patients and those around them to accept its inevitability accepting dying as a normal part of life, teaching that helping people to die well, i.e. "in peace". Nor should it be confused with actively helping people to die, i.e. to bring their deaths about.

Its distinction with euthanasia is at times obscured by claiming that the outcome (death) is the same for both and that the intention of both is to relieve suffering. These assertions are true, as far as they go, but there is a moral distinction between giving a "lethal injection" and the interventions that constitute palliative care. These interventions include the provision of symptoms relief by titrating medication against the symptoms. The aim being to achieve the best control of symptoms with the least side-effects, for which different medications are available: if one medication does not suit, there are usually others to try. *Giving the right medication for each symptom at the lowest dose necessary to alleviate the symptom.*

Sometimes, there might well be situations where relief of very difficult symptoms, such as pain that does not respond to analgesics and adjuvants or intractable shortness of breath and a number of catastrophic clinical events such as some hemorrhages or pulmonary embolism, can only be achieved by medication doses that result in deep sedation.

The clinical situation might be extremely complex leading to a binary status quo in which the options are either vigil and in unbearable anguish or unconscious and calm. In this scenario, the alternatives are either dying with intolerable suffering while being aware of it or dying comfortably while unconscious. There is no real choice here – the only morally good course is to address the patient's symptoms accepting the side effect of sedation that inevitably accompanies this. The Lex Artis requires that all intervention is proportionate and relief of symptoms and suffering sought at all times by proportionate means, and regular reviews.

A frequently held fear or misapprehension when working to control symptoms is that the therapeutic maneuvers used in the process might be also shortening life and hastening death. Medication used need to be clearly explained regarding its purpose, effects and side effects; morphine is regarded with particular fear and suspicion. However, in most situations its careful titration following best practice guidelines under specialist's advice will alleviate symptoms with no noticeable shortening of life. On the contrary, we should not underestimate the potentially life-shortening effect caused by the stress, and distress, of severe uncontrolled symptoms. This is an area in which good *Palliative Care* is able to help.

PC is certainly able to deliver sound, scientific based care with the vulnerable friendship of the heart. Not many could openly object to these foundations. Yet, many committed practitioners ignore them in their daily practice. Could there be a different reason behind? Or, could it be due to a lack of proper understanding of its place in science, health and social care?

Approaching Palliative Care from the point of view of its conceptual basis opens a fascinating quandary for the studious physician when the need to clarify to others, patients, family, cares, health and social professionals, society in general, what PC is and what is not, presents itself. It takes time and effort to work through it all when helping someone accept our help in a timely fashion. Communicating it in a conceptual nugget what PC is a complex task.

There are definitions put forward by organizations such as WHO and IAHPC. And there are also well defended theses, such as Randall's, to deconstruct and determine how such definitions are rather aspirational "declarations of intention".

WHO's [17, 18] definition includes quality of life in their declaration of intentions. Unquestionably, a very important aspect of the palliative philosophy is its commitment to taking care of well-being by excellent symptom control to help maintain the quality of that life for as long as it such. For many, however, life -in its sanctity- cannot be classified and protected in direct relation to its perceived quality at a given time.

While life itself is an objective good, necessary to enjoy many others, its quality or lack of it, is a subjective good, dependent on many factors. For example, for many, happiness is essential to life and it is the pursuit of that happiness that gives meaning to life. It is particularly suggestive to understand the quality of life perceived by those who have learned to live life through the small, insensitive things that adorn it. While others think that the "core" of life can only make a concrete sense among those who believe in the Transcendent, be it God or not.

Dr. Pettus [19], a political sociologist claims that our modern and medicalized cultures make reason and mystery mutually exclusive, defining death from illness as a failure, and dying as shameful. Suppliers and legislators similarly marginalize older citizens and the dying, while formulating ineffective strategies largely to prevent deaths from violence or epidemics, terrorism or famine. The goal of PC is to support those with an incurable disease so that they can live the rest of their lives as well, and with as much sense as possible, giving them the necessary support when, eventually, they reach the natural end of their lives, and die from their illness.

Painful and distressing deaths without palliative care or relief from physical pain, in remote areas, attract neither political attention nor budgets, says Pettus. A growing effort is being made to establish and advance Palliative Care's contextualized advocacy around the world, based on its own "ethos" and spirituality that ensures its implementation and availability for many.

Those who work advocating PC believe that, to be faithful, the its safeguarding should reflect the "ethos" of the hospice movement. This is a central concern for many, particularly concerned to understand how such ethos could be established and how it could dissipate into loss, disappearing. It is worth knowing the work done by those who care about those intangible aspects of the hospice movement that precisely make it so. A particular apprehension is the one that asks how the "ethos" could be lost by spreading more widely t is marketed while losing its well-founded and carefully established training its approach to transmitting its philosophy and principles.

Cicely Saunders left a great number of written documents. This one is particularly representative of her work:

"The longer I work with the dying and their families, the more I learn about life and the small things that are so important to each one of us. Dying is never easy, it is done differently by each person. Fear of the unknown is what most of us can identify with. Having a terminal illness including diseases of cancer, MND and other neurological illnesses, Dementia will take us all, whether patient or a loved one, to places in our lives we would rather avoid and will often include fear of unknowns. How we often support our patients & families is to get alongside them as best we can and share some of our skills and experience to break down these fears. We don't always get things right because dying is not an exact science. What I think is also true is, yes, we put ourselves forward as a resource for the community, to show leadership in this field, but we can't do this on our own" [16]. She was not a theorist and understood others´ suffering and distress and led the way to alleviate their suffering, advocating for a more comfortable dying process and a more acceptable memory of it to their loved ones who live on.

Nobody should be expected nor forced to consent to all life-prolonging treatment; *Palliative Care* does not preclude receiving life-prolonging treatment and, delivered alongside those treatments and interventions can be really productive. Each person should be able to choose for themselves how much treatment they are willing to tolerate for limited gains in life expectancy, and to refuse treatment they do not wish to receive. There is, however, a responsibility to use this life well in service to the end (and to reach one' full potential).

The challenge is perhaps discerning when is it time to let go of this life, and so it has been since humans inhabit the earth. St. Paul's illustrates this tension well in his letter to the Philippians (1:21–24).

Each individual will expect their remaining life to allow them to be and do what their very own idiosyncrasies such as age, illness or responsibilities to others requires to complete their lives. Often, we meet people who may feel that their life is approaching its natural end and are ready to relinquish this world when their time comes. Nowadays, PC has evolved to offer other services under the name *Supportive Care* [20, 21] based on patient's needs, increasingly used in the acute sector and well accepted by both patients and professionals in the context of potentially curative or life sustain treatments which, nevertheless, can be onerous to receive and follow. To many, the adjective *Supportive* is better accepted and understood than *Palliative.*

It is important to find a common base which help recognize PC under whatever wrapping it might come in. Much confusion has come from the different, often random translations of the vocable *hospitium* [22] which has come to be understood different things in different languages. *Hospices*, as understood from its Anglo-Saxon use, are far more than mere buildings; they house a philosophy of human relationship and hosting which could be considered as direct descendants of the medieval form because behind their assertive philosophy sits a highly personal holistic approach which places the physical, emotional and spiritual welfare of patients and their families at its heart.

Still, many still identify them with places where patients go when there is nothing more to be done, where people go to die. The problem with this, is that much of the suffering that could be alleviated in the right space, is not, because it is left too late, thinking they are places one might go to die.

Much work is nowadays undertaken to facilitate the understanding of terminology in our field, many researchers look and write about palliative care. In Spain where it has been translated as `*Cuidados Paliativos*`, thus stressing its most physically relevant aspects of care. Research groups such as ATLANTES. Instituto Cultura y Sociedad. Universidad de Navarra look for its secret, which they call "The Intangible ".

Our own research to define the ethos of PC moves in the same lines, recalling The Little Prince affirmation "And now here is my secret, a very simple secret: It is only with the heart that one can see rightly; what is essential is invisible to the eye." [23], which links seamlessly with the thoughts of those pioneers whose legacy is now ours to work with and transmit forward "All those intangible values are expressed in concrete actions able to transmit unconditional acceptance and the affirmation of the patient's worth as a person [24].

3.4 Scientific aspects

Having set its humanistic aspects, it is imperative to look for PC scientific bearings.

Much has been written and researched around "the scientific" and the Ethos of Science, which refers to the "toned affective complex of values and norms that is carried out to be binding on the man of science. Rules are expressed in form of instructions, prescriptions, preferences and licences" [25].

It is acknowledged that the end of all science is the extension of agreed knowledge and that it must be able to be explained through its technical methods: "empirically confirmed and logically coherent statements of regularities (these are often predictions)" [26].

PC has a strong humanistic element but it is also science [25, 27]. Predictions are even more important in this field, where informed assumptions are regularly made to underpin decision-making as it is also science and, as such, it must be governed by laws ordering any other science. This issue, together with poor conceptualization, could have contributed to the deficient PC extension [28] and expansion; the fact that some have arrogated themselves the right to choose what aspects of the palliative philosophy and principles to apply, choosing them at convenience, either out of ignorance or neglect might have arrested its expansion.

3.4.1 The science and its philosophy

Cicely Saunders is known to have been a woman of multiple interests which she followed by training to be a nurse, almoner and a doctor. She had other interests such a full understanding of Christianism, Philosophy and is considered to be a humanist. She liked to read and study the different aspects of things in depth, often citing authors and philosophers such as Francis Bacon. Philosophy as science certainly underpins the philosophy of the Hospice Movement. Understanding this, together with the great value she gave to the scientific foundations of palliation brings us to consider the Philosophy of science as necessary.

Science is a limited human activity that has its origin in man's observation of ordinary experiences and his desire to know the truth. In its output, science provides proven knowledge that goes beyond human experience. Its classic ideal seeks to achieve true knowledge based on reason, compatible with that which is provisional and reviewable.

Classical sciences such as philosophy, theology or mathematics share some features with many modern experimental sciences such as physics, biology or neuroscience. However, the notion of science is often applied almost exclusively to experimental sciences.

A broader perspective applies the concept of science in an analogue way. For example, experimental sciences and common philosophy both seek a knowledge that extends beyond ordinary experience; the difference is that the philosophical approach does not willingly exclude anything that can be rationally studied. Experimental sciences self-limit the search for empirical evidence using specific principles of reasoning.

The same reality, for example, the suffering of the human being is the subject of study of different disciplines (biology, sociology, sociology, psychology, medicine, which means that each science has its own objectives, methods and therefore, also, results. A situation which has leads to the fragmentation of knowledge which clouds the understanding of the discipline.

The philosophy of science is a philosophical reflection that seeks to understand the nature and value of science, given that philosophical reflection on scientific activity is carried out from reason. Logic, history, sociology ... but, especially from a meta-scientific perspective, experimental science is a clear test of human ability to transcend what is immediately given to observe by the senses.

Philosophy, as science has evolved in time. Among the current main current currents in the philosophy of science, Thomas S Kuhn's historical 'sociological' approach states that the paradigm shift is not due to logical reasoning but to a process of conversion of scientists.

Science needs to be communicated. Scientific communication demands clear conceptualization. Each concept has a meaning and a reference that does not have to be unique. Thus, terms can refer to many semantic fields (evolution of pain, evolution of human suffering) and encompass in their meaning various mechanisms related to their perception by society at that point in history.

But there is more as concepts, these most elementary scientific constructions can be either qualitative or quantitative.

Quantitative concepts are common in healthcare and have a mathematic expression, (temperature, blood pressure ...) and are called magnitudes. They are associated with methods and measuring instruments, acting as bridges between theory and experimentation, because they make rigorous data processing as possible. These concepts, common to physical aspects of medicine are well used and known: they have extended to less measurable concepts such as physical pain by a number of conceptual models.

Concepts are not static. The understanding of the atom, today is much greater than a few years ago.

Science uses models to simplify reality, idealizing some of its aspects. Some models are schematic representations of what you want to study, while others are much more complex idealizations. PC is defined by many as a phenomenon and as such, for its realization the scientist needs to use informed guess (very common in PC advanced communication) to tease out what properties of phenomena form the appropriate basis for idealization and What features can be ignored.

To achieve which, the role of creativity and interpretation are essential, as is scientific induction, including inference.

For example, about could have been causing the back pain a patent suffers from. Or the reconstruction of a family distress from our knowledge of a patient's disease trajectory. Or extrapolation when a new cluster of symptoms appears in relation to biochemistry analysis results taken a few days before of an election from surveys.

A situation which tries to help complexity using models: The model is a scientific construct between theory and reality. On the one hand, it concretes the theory and on the other it simplifies reality.

Scientific statements, are a very varied type of scientific construction. They range from expressing the data obtained to an experimental measure: "You have cancer causing you pain several times in 24 hours as the analgesic effect wears off". Up until a law is formulated: "Patients with cancer who have continuous pain shouldn't have to earn their analgesia; opiates should be given regularly" stated C Saunders. Like models or concepts, they are not an exact translation of what is going on in nature. The statements and laws that are constructed from them are, by definition, approximate, provisional and contextual, because in the future the concepts can be further specified and the measuring instruments can be improved.

Theoretical Systems arise from statements and laws that articulate and command each other. Well formulated, they become consistent and are susceptible to improvement, at the same time, they remain always open, i.e. they are not closed systems: at least they have initial conditions and contour conditions. They are formulated in a fragmentary way, just as a child acquires greater ease in the management of a language.

Science and scientific proceedings therefore, come supported by complex structures that need understanding and respect. Many work to help others understand these and give us principles to promote respect, setting out the Ethics of Science, worth of a chapter to itself.

Sociologist Robert Merton [29] identifies four institutional imperatives—universalism, collectivism, selflessness, and organized skepticism—such as the ethos of modern science—its "fundamental values." Mertonian laws cover aspects such as: volume of research funds, consistency of the professional network, community collectivism and involvement in non-academic content.

Universalism. Promotes the value of scientific claims for what they bring to society and not by who brings them to the scientific arena or even which personal or scientific background they bring their claims from. Merton recognizes and warns about the power of society at large and a scientific private cosmos which may clash with universalism. "Ethnocentrism is not compatible with universalism," he affirms and requires that "careers be open to talent," because science must be a meritocracy. Therefore, to hinder science ability to nurture knowledge, by excluding capable people from developing their scientific callings on the basis of competence, harms scientific progress at large.

This aspect could be detrimental to PC, where the *friendship of the heart* constitutes one of two foundational cornerstones, without which, extreme over technification and medicalization might overrepresent its science. PC demands more impalpable aspects to achieve its mission and the vast volunteering that support it is testimony of the founder's vision to successfully combine both knowledge and compassionate doing.

Data and theories are valuable assets, continues Merton, which can be cond in models or scientific structures, even named after the scientist behind it when thought to constitute a significant contribution to the field and brings prestige to the so-named person or research group. Such prestige is in itself an honor best respected by those who work in that field, hence the reason why communication of scientific results is prized by science which despises secrecy about them.

He [29] states that *Universalism* is also a democratic principle (laissez-faire), "impersonal criteria of realization and non-fixation of status characterize open democratic society". established scientific knowledge should be accessible to all members of the scientific community to use, explore, etc.

Collectivism, also communism, does not refer to the Marxist-Leninist movement, but to the view that scientific knowledge is a resource to be shared with the entire scientific tribe, regardless of which individual scientists in particular have produced a particular discovery.

One of the things a scientist has to do to meet this standard is to communicate his findings to other scientists. Knowledge that is not made public does not help the scientific community.

Interestingly, Cicely Saunders took good care to encourage collectivism of the scientific ethos [30] of the new field of medicine was set to become. *Palliative Care* was born with no scientific secrets as she sought to tell others what she had found to help the dying from the very beginning when every Saturday morning the met to "work and pray fror Hospice".

Disinterest, maintains that scientific accounts ought not to be personal in their outlook and, rather than empower the individual scientist own plan, they should bring a greater good to a bigger group. Merton [29] argues that disinterest is an institutional obligation, not be disarrayed by individual motives. Individuals should certainly have personal motivators such as scientific awareness, publications, recognition, curiosity, among others. Such desires are licit as far as that will encourage them to work with others to obtain the results that will made the group shine.

"Institutional control of a wide range of these motivations" better characterizes what is fundamental to science and helps avoid science scam. Merton [29] believes this is reinforced by the rigorous monitoring that scientist undergo at the hands of other scientists. Interestingly, he also highlights the connexion researchers establish with their *customers* different from those other professions. Alarmingly, when lay people and scientists establish closer working links, such connection frequently spurs fraud and pseudoscience.

Finally, Organized *skepticism*, encourage omitting one's own judgment and using only empirical and logical criteria. This is frequently the strained connection between and those vital areas inclined to offer judgment.

While difficult, it is comforting to discover that the scientific aspect of Palliative Care, "its head" is up to any other scientific effort, although it is true that there would be much to analyze and work in order to give greater rigor. It is especially relevant to strengthen the learning in countries where *Palliative Care* and Palliative Medicine are not recognized as specialties. This leads to situations in which the expert becomes such by means of an expensive, often online, master degree and short clinical observational stays with experts who are such by the same method, very distant from the structured learning that a four-year specialist training affords the individual.

From its inception *Terminal Care,* as it was our field originally known, it was ambitious in its founder's commitment to practice within scientific frameworks, to research and treat symptoms such as pain [2, 30–32]. The focus being the person as a whole and responding to patients' physical, emotional, social and spiritual needs. Palliative Medicine, is today a consolidated [33] medical specialty which incorporates the care of the spiritual dimension of the individual as part of its decree although, sadly, not in every country.

On the other hand, most cultures and formalized religions [34, 35] have incorporated palliation to their teachings and fullness in some way, having also "come to join the movement" with their own array of richness which, although not known to many until now, has always being present in any human grouping. It is such an interesting and fascinating aspect that deserves another full chapter to really learn how other communities look after their vulnerable members, the ill, the dying and how to support those who are bereaved.

3.5 Patient centred and directed palliation effort: quality of life

It becomes necessary to position ourselves and acknowledge the conceptual mare magnum which too often blurs and disorders the delivery of timely PC, its scientific structures perhaps too vague to work on.

Probably, the best way to understand the undeniable value of PC is to allow others, those who have experienced PC, rather than deliver it, to inform our effort.

Patients´ narrative recounting their experience is full of details; something we become aware of when we introduce someone, visitor or professional from other specialty, to the dynamic of our consultations. We are talking about its other foundation: *"The vulnerable friendship of the heart"*.

As with any vital aspect, and Palliative Care is very much about living life to its natural end, we encounter have a static duality - dynamic, negative - positive, pain-pleasure, darkness-light, night day, death - life experience that makes this field one of very strong contrasts.

How many times have both patients and their families told us that they are "living on a real roller-coaster of emotions, experiences, illusions and losses."?

Hundreds of sick people who tell us about what they experience when the afternoon falls and the day - perhaps their last day - becomes night. Likewise, the desolation of the last sunrise when a new day arrives that they do not know if they will have the strength to face in a dignified way. How much suffering holds the narrative of "I'm afraid of the night in case I die during it. I feel horror at dawn because I am still alive and have to face a new day and I don't know if I can."

As professionals, it is in these moments of very personal, intimate exchange and confidence, when we confirm that something very special imprints character to our work. Yes! something that reaches the other. Just as their desolation reached us. For me, the question is "how could we find what that something is?"

Occasionally, it's rare but extraordinarily motivating, people look us in the eye and ask "And how can you do this every day? Sometimes they tell how they have seen us tend to another patient and have seen the pain in our eyes. They insist "where do you get the strength to come back the next day with a smile? Where does the inspiration come from for your eyes to shine when you approach me, broken my useless body? Me who with my pain caused you pain?" We respond with professionalism, humanism and simplicity. In that therapeutic space, we left something of us. It is very likely that in such a personal exchange, the very spirit of PC is contained.

It would therefore appear that experiencing PC is possible by both: those who need it and those trained to deliver it. As an experience it falls into the phenomenological sphere which incorporate a combination or synthesis of the positive aspects described, experienced in situations of suffering and uncertainty which can be qualified as intensely relational. If these moments pregnant with human intensity are symbolized by a single quality, it would be one very close to life itself and characterized by light, beauty and love gathered in one. A phenomenon that can be experienced but difficult to describe and be identified by the someone else, not actively involved or not adequately trained.

Thus, life to its end can be a wonder in the development of images and s never seen before, thoughts never before thought, realities never dreamed of, constantly emerging, constantly reminding us that the person's individual universe might not yet have reached the limits of its possibilities.

Palliative Care might well be the force able to bring forward the life that remains as such, as an evolving universe, says R. Bruening, an organic chemistry scientist who says his work is that of anti-cancer drug maker and CEO. Practising good Palliative Care can help whoever receives it to reach their own, yet unrealized, potential as a human being.

These profound understandings come from experience; the problem is that trying to quantify subjective experience is like trying to create a metric for a favorite color. Or flavor of ice cream. Or to measure suffering by the volume of tears cried. It is also possible to use Scientific constructs and models to objectivize the experience.

Indeed, WHO's definition of Palliative Care, considered by some authors to be mere statement of intentions, incorporates the concept of quality of life since a very important aspect of palliative philosophy is its commitment to well-being, quality of life, as long as it exists. Many consider happiness to be essential to closing a full life, and their pursuit of what gives meaning to life. It is particularly suggestive to have learned to live life through the small, insensitive things that adorn it. Others say that the "essence" of life comes to its full meaning depending on how transcendent.

From a metaphysical (spiritual) point of view the essence, as in any matter of vital nature, and Palliative Care is very much about life and living it, incorporates static-dynamic, negative–positive, pain-welfare, darkness-light, night - day, death - life, soul-body duality, which make this field one of very strong contrasts.

It might be that experiencing the essence of Palliative Care is possible: combination- synthesis- of the positive aspects described, experienced in situations of suffering, uncertainty and very, very relational. If these moments pregnant with human intensity are symbolized by a single quality, it would be a very close to life, the very life characterized by - light, beauty and love – gathered in one and become like One, that could be identified.

The European Consortium in Healthcare Outcomes and Cost–Benefit Research's extensive study concluded that those theories based on a QALY approach do not give a true account of the manner real populations performance outlines (Quality Adjusted Life Year) is a non-specific measure of disease burden, which tries to encompass value and amount of life lived; used in economic appraisal to weigh the cost of healthcare interventions and their impact on society as a whole. An entirely foreseeable result: we can no more predict what patients will want or need when a given disease takes hold, than guess that their favorite color or the ice cream flavor they disfavor. Such understandings only come when know when we know them and we spend time with them and they tell us themselves. Or we observe their behavior and possessions as well as their loved ones.

Enabling patients to choose what they can has consequently become very relevant and organizations such as "Nothing about me without me" [35] leading the way help bring forward the more humanistic dimension of PC.

Consent laws focus on the ability to understand illness and treatment options, as well as the consequences of treatment selection or refusal. As patients often are not aware of their own goals and values because and they have not specifically paused to think about them or make them explicit, getting to know the patient through asking the right questions and listening carefully to answers which can be new to the person, can help us understand their choices. We learn what is most important to patients in their life right now, and what would their ideal end of life look like. *Active listening* [35] will afford us the knowledge of their wishes relating to spending time or even dying at home, not wanting to be in bed attached surrounded by machines. We often listen saying little while the patient comes to realize what they want and vocalize some outstanding goals of care. After this, the patient -as the director of a well-rehearsed orchestra and the entire palliative team came up with a plan of care to meet those goals to the greatest extent possible.

Patient choice, as an entity, must become part of the medical Curriculum and take its rightful place as a basic starting point of all good medicine.

Bereavement is not to be forgotten. Frequently, the bereaved come with a card, cake or fruit to let the professionals know they are grateful for the great care provided to their loved one. They do not mention a single common research metric, but the team are motivated by their gratitude in remembering their patient. It is a very humbling experience as we are reminded of the uniqueness of each life and the impact of our common humanity.

4. Chapter motivation and scientific interest

After almost 30 years of combining multilingual medical care in three countries with a special interest in *Palliative Care* practiced at all levels of care in the country in which it had its modern origin and at the political-organizational level of the country of origin itself, the pressure to address its expansion from different perspectives: conceptual, semantic and semiotic; anthropological, philosophical, political and welfare, of confronting the intrinsic philosophy seeking what imprints character on a multi -professional attention at the international level at a time when there is great confusion as to what constitutes the delicate spirit of a movement that has its roots in medieval *hospitium*. What remains today in a health system carelessly over-mechanizing its practice within a society that turns its back on the truth of that fluid *charity* of religious orders that knew how to welcome, attend, assist, care for and treat exhausted pilgrims [35] who had undertaken journeys with genuine hardship of those who did not know whether they would be able to return home?

The rigorous search for intangible fundamentals to make them available to all involved, within a strict research framework will result in new knowledge that, made available to all, results in undisputed palliative conceptions and important new paradigms.

The real impact on the defense of life in the context of an announced death is indisputably revealed by the immediate practical applicability of the theories used. These are issues that arouse great interest in acquiring greater knowledge, apprehensible by those who develop their clinical activity in this field.

The Anglo-Saxon *Palliative Care*, known among Spanish speakers as "*Cuidados Paliativos*", changes the perspective from which we see the process of dying and death itself contributing to facilitate vital fullness and that the sick or close individual achieves his or her potential as a person even in the midst of complex multidimensional needs.

Cicely Saunders'original biography [36] relays how she established that one of its the modern Hospice movement underpinning values would be thinking and incorporating "Those who one day will come to join us" referring to professionals from diverse specialties, countries and bringing their own contribution to the field strengthening.

Undoubtedly the urgent demographic need means that many of us allow ourselves to call what is nothing more than a part of the original Palliative Care, a successor of Canadian origin of the previous "Terminal Care" [30, 32]. Contemporary Palliative Care has not made a full conceptual incorporation making, in my opinion, imperative the need to adjust foundational concepts.

International contemporary PC has not always made full conceptual incorporation, making it necessary the effort to adjust current impressions to the foundational ethos of the discipline, maybe contributing to the serious contemporary problem of PC's lack of expansion in some places, even regressing in some countries unable to take roots in different cultures and new times. A phenomenon that could be contributing to a great confusion of what can be legitimately undertaken to facilitate the end of life.

The IAHPC. Global Consensus based palliative care definition [6], found it necessary to incorporate a glossary to define a long list of terms, an indication of the difficulty to agree on them when used in different languages and settings.

An example of this situation has come to worry many during the current pandemic: While in the Anglosaxon countries it is said to have come of age and helped reinforce services and support colleagues and professionals, in other countries, their activity has been reduced.

The growing interest in the political and institutional sphere PC has fostered in the COVID -19 demands increasing determination in its organizational assistance and political levels. Might It be possible that the careful conceptual clarification of terms common in the palliative field eases their extension and promotion? [36].

The depth of PC ethos, wherever it might lay, should be preserved to some level. Its transformation into *Cuidados Paliativos* is work in progress since 1989 [37] and continues to attract interest to clarify evolving conceptions [38]. It has slowly started moving over the years from *Cuidados* to a broader and less physical *atención*, (attention), to be true to its authentic foundational philosophy and inherent principles, their safeguarding of which should reflect the spirit of the modern hospice movement as it was when St Christopher's Hospice first opened its doors. How it adapts and evolves is a central concern for many, characteristically uneasy about understanding how such ethos could be more widely established and how to prevent it from dissipation until lost, disappearing under the increasing technology laden healthcare services. It is worth getting to know the work undertaken by those for whom intangible aspects matter, precisely because they constitute the hospice movement founding heritage. A particular apprehension is that the "ethos" could be lost by spreading more widely if it is "marketed", while losing its well-founded and carefully established approach to convey its philosophy and principles.

Interestingly, it precisely the collaborative effort between PC and other hospital specialties which is contributing significantly to its interdisciplinary progression and consolidation. The support of classic specialties, which once questioned the specific object of Palliative Medicine, a different entity from PC, is key to its advancement and development.

It is worthy of consideration the fact that Palliative Medicine is the only medical specialty that

a. Does not wrap its expertise around an organ, as Cardiology or Gastroenterology do; or group by age, as Geriatrics or Pediatrics do; or even an entity such as Infectious diseases or Virology.
b. Has adjectivized its specialism to qualify the medical expertise offered.
c. Is truly transverse across all other areas of expertise, from Neonatology to Neurosurgery passing through Organ Transplantation and Primary Care.

It is, therefore hardly surprising its practitioners need to explain what they do and who they are many times a day!

A recent piece work reviews some important milestones in PC's history and development from which Palliative Medicine spirals in many countries; analyses its evolution in the world, studying current issues concerning consistency in its implementation and some possible projections for future progress and expansion, seen from the perspective of a central issue:

"What exactly constitutes the ethos of PC faithfully replicating its philosophy and founding principles wherever it is applied or used?" The author concludes that coming to that knowledge would help facilitate possible future advances that integrate ethical, legal and social implications in years to come that truly benefit those with palliative needs.

PC delivery and benefits fall under the Philosophy Phenomenological arena while the conceptualization of the main terms on which research is centered around its practice, as the phenomenon investigated. Conceptual construction. Life to its end is a prodigy in progress. Images and s never seen before, thoughts never before thought, realities never dreamed of, constantly emerging, constantly reminding that individual universe that it has not yet reached the limits of its possibilities. The essence of PC could well be life that remains as such, as an evolving universe. Or perhaps the sick person's journey to his deepest self than the professional is more of a witness than an escort.

To identify themes to be found in the English and Spanish literature a systematic search was conducted (**Table 1**).

From those, the summary, the most important ideas to consider include

Palliative Care comes to change the perspective from which we see the process of dying and death itself contributing to facilitate the vital fullness and that the sick or close individual achieves his potential as a person even in the midst of complex multidimensional needs.

Cicely Saunders, as included in her biography [2], spoke of the PC bases would include "Openness to those who will come" referring to professionals from diverse countries and cultures who, one day, would join the Modern Hospice Movement. They would bring new ways to alleviate and contribute their own culture, ways of doing and even different specialties and specific needs in the final phase of different diseases. Another base was to be the *Freedom of the Spirit.*

Wanting to know what constitutes the essence of PC is a complex task; our search shows the need to do an in-depth analysis of the terminology used and its conceptual adequacy.

A relevant finding was the fact that other concepts such as *essence*, might be used to make reference to what philosophy and ethos bring. "Essence" is a term of alchemy from Latin *essere* (to be), then arguably embodies "meaning", "purpose". From a metaphysical point of view, it could be considered as the possibility of filling the living space of the individual with information gained through experience.

MESH Terms	
"Palliative" (and) "Care" (and) "Ethos"	
32	Other non-randomized, quasi-experimental, descriptive (comparative, correlation), case–control, cohort studies
1	Reports or opinions from expert committees or the clinical experiences of respected authorities
1	Systematic reviews and meta-analysis. Controlled Randomized studies
8	Books and Book Chapters
9	Clinical guides, documents
2	Thesis

Table 1.
Palliative care ethos literature review.

5. Conceptualization

To the scholar mind, a multi-faceted approach is prerequisite to adequately conceive PC from the conceptual, semantic and meaning, anthropological, philosophical and political angles without forgetting that of *actively caring for others´* wellbeing and assisting them. There could be different ways to unveil its intrinsic philosophy by seeking what imprints character to a movement which began well before Medicine itself was considered an entity, from the medieval hospitium [39] (pl hospitia) hɒˈspɪtɪə Greek: ξενία, xenia, προξενία and positions the scholar in front of is the ancient Greco-Roman concept of hospitality as a divine right of the guest and a divine duty of the host. An archaic place of shelter for travelers, especially one kept by a monastic order, that we are trying nowadays to adapt to a very different society with unmet needs.

The encounter with the ancient vocables that give name to this *caring* movement whets the scholar's appetite to learn more about the semantic and semiotic correspondence of the most commonly used words in PC in order to fully understand the impact of language and its own development in its evolution.

A straightforward methodology pathway leads us to study the roots of the discipline key words, analyzing their semantic transformation over time to witnessing their morphological evolution and conceptual spirit of each vocable. Grounded on a careful conceptual description of those words used in the palliative field could facilitate its extension and promotion which should benefit more people.

5.1 Language and conceptualization

Linguistics is a science which object of study is language. Its analysis places language in context, as it takes into consideration social, cultural, historical, and political factors influencing language.

Conceptualization consists of processes observing language production. It takes language-specific perspectives and event understanding.

Such process is still little understood by the experts [40] in the field. At the same time, we find ourselves at a point in the history of the Modern Hospice movement when it seems to be imperious to start a rigorous process around strong, concise and unambiguous definitions. This is due to the expansion of the discipline throughout the different countries with their cultures and languages which need to adapt to a new way of formalized compassion. Within PC, too many words are translated almost literally from the English language, resulting in numerous concepts with multiple scopes or dimensions, often inaccurate. This is confusing and makes it hard to transmit the science to others outside the field as they are incapable of conceiving its objective without further clarification. Existing PC definitions are being currently contested, probably because concepts are neither tangible nor concrete. Characterizations of our field based on abstract concepts make for confusion needing an effort to interpret conceptually by act or process of forming a general notion or idea.

Interest in this matter comes from personal experience of palliation in both the Anglo-Saxon and Iberian cultures and language and observing the inadequate adoption of terminology without the right notions behind. We defend the proposition that it is important to know what notions different authors might use to refer to PC and establish which of those most faithfully represent its most intimate nature.

There are interesting efforts to establish useful, replicable models. Some are orientated to [41] building digital domain ontologies, incredibly interesting and potentially game changing in niche areas used across the world. However, the model chosen to conceptualize is one by Flores Talavera G. [42] for reasons relating to its clarity, teaching dimension and the fact that she writes in Spanish.

Professor Talavera's process guides the investigator to initiate conceptualization by undertaking documentary research on the meaning of the key terms; including a review of the meanings and clarification of semantic confusions, looking at the appropriate dictionaries to contextualize it and learn about the possible conceptual evolution of the term. She then suggests consultation of Thesauruses in which the terms are described in the way they are used by scientists followed by accounting for the definitions of the term from a specific perspective. - In specialized dictionaries (Philosophy, Psychology, Sociology, and Physicians and Education) and conceptual essays, definitions located in sources to broaden the search horizon to find the "sense" of the term.

It is then possible to compare related terms using three processes: defining each one of them, establishing similarities and then establishing differences. This would then facilitate term characterization by establishing its most important characteristics, not of the word but of the complex reality that the term tries to elucidate.

To consider types and uses of the object (term) of study from its conceptual definition and expand the understanding of the meaning and reality intended to be explained, it is useful to identify the key ones.

5.2 Palliative care conceptualization

Conceptual purity of words used in the palliative field could facilitate its extension and promotion by examining its intrinsic philosophy understanding *what* it is that imprints character to a movement that began from the medieval hospitium and has foundational Judeo- Christian roots.

Applying the chosen methodology to the conceptualization and semantics of the original Palliative Care entails an interesting linguistic and geographical *iter* that could decisively contribute to the dissolution of the original *karos* philosophy observed in some situations. There should have been a process of content-rich implementation, in its place this is truncated by a less nuanced implementation marked by external and constant pressure to achieve tangible and quantitatively relevant results.

5.2.1 Representative terms and words used in international palliative care

The number of terms that could be analyzed in order to be conceptualized could might be thought to be huge. This is not the case as there are a handful of terms, key to impulse palliative programs (**Table 2**).

However, there is a number of them that deserve immediate attention as they are used, maybe even abused, too frequently. An appropriate conceptualization of these is urgent due to their weight in planning, policy – making and the delivery of excellent *Palliative Care.*

Although it is a very specialized subject and deserves a full piece of work with more specialist direction, we present a first attempt here.

To begin with, and following the first two process points from guideline, we can start from the top of the organizational and planification pyramid from which all policy flows to inform health and social care, there are two vocables that could be used better to achieve the sought-after results.

	Dates from	Meaning	Original language (s)	Contemporary use	Of note
Hospice noun *Hospitium*	*late 17th century.*1818.	Rest house for travellers	French *hospice* "hospital, almshouse" Old French *ospice* "hospice, shelter," ,"hospitality," 13c. Latin 1. *hospitium* "hospitable reception, entertainment; hospitality, bonds of hospitality, relationship of guest and host 2.*hospes* (genitive *hospitis*) "guest; host," also "a stranger, foreigner"	1879.Sense of "home for the aged and terminally ill " 1978is first attested as *hospice movement*	The term “Hospice” is strongly repudiated in Spanish- Palliative Care Unit is used instead Used in the Netherlands as *Hospitium,* places for those who don’t want euthanasia and go there for protection.
Implement verb *implemere* noun *Implementum*	*Verb.* early 18th century. 1707 *Noun,* in late Middle English. First used circa 1707c. in Scottish English. Legal term meaning "fulfilment,"	Verb: 1.-To put (a decision, plan, agreement, etc.) into effect. 2.- To start using a plan or system 3.- To complete, perform, carry into effect," *Noun* Used to refer to different artifacts: furniture, gear, or dress’.	Late Latin*: implementum*; *implere*: filling up Made of two Latin vocables In (towards the center) Plere (to fill up) (Greek polis, many) Partly from Medieval Latin implementa (plural Partl from late Latin Implementum ‘filling up, fulfilment’, both from Latin implere ‘fill up’ (later ‘employ’), from in- ‘in’ + Latin plere ‘fill’.		From it comes implementation, its use first recorded 1913.
Implant *verb* *Noun*	16th Century 1540c 15th Century	*Verb* I.Transitive 1a: to fix or set securely or deeply 1b: to set permanently in the consciousness or habit patterns: inculcate 2. to insert in living tissue II.Intransitive To undergo implantation *Noun*	Old French *Emplanter* French *“to insert, engraft”* Medieval Latin. *Implantus* In (towards the centre) Plant (see in, to plant, and observe)	*Noun* Modern use From 1886 Meaning "surgically implant (something) in the body", originally of teeth. which is attested by 1981 short for breast implants (1976). 1890, "thing implanted;"	If you implant an idea or attitude in people, you make it become accepted or believed.

		graft "to plant in" abstractly, of ideas, emotions, etc. "to plant", literally "plant in," from assimilated form of in- "into, in, on, upon". –		1941 as "action of implanting," from implant	
IMPLEMENT /IMPLANT	The difference between the notions conceived through these two verbs is very important. Implementing a Palliative Care Program speaks of "working at it" and "being part of the development". While implanting a Palliative Care Program talks about "having something new to deal with or to put up with". Something that needs to be taken into account by politicians, managers, et as it might mean the difference between people being engaged or not.				
PALLIATIVE *ADJ.* *PALLIATIF* *PALLIATUS* *VERB* *NOUN* *PALLIATIVUS* *VERB* LATIN *PALLIARE*	Early 15c., Dates from 1724. As a verb, used since 1779.	"serving to mitigate or alleviate" (a wound, illness, etc.); other meanings "cloak, cover, concealing;" from "under cloak, covert," from Latin *pallium* "a cloak" *'to cloak',* *´to protect´* ´to conceal,"	*Adj.* French *Palliatif,* Late Latin *Palliatus* "cloaked," from past participle of Late Latin *palliare* "cover with a cloak, conceal," *Noun.* Medieval Latin *palliativus* *Verb.* Medieval Latin *palliare*	"serving to extenuate by Excuses or favorable representation". "that which mitigates or extenuates,". Used by politicians and journalists to express strong actions or will.	
CARE *Noun* *Verb*	circa. 1400 Circa 1580. Circa 1520s- 1550s	a. the provision of what is necessary for the health, welfare, maintenance, and protection of someone or something. (safe keeping, supervision, custody, charge, protection,keeping) b. serious attention or consideration applied to doing something correctly or to avoid damage or risk. (caution, carefulness, wariness,awareness, heedfulness,heed) D. Meaning "object or matter of	Old English *caru*, *cearu* "sorrow, anxiety, grief," also "burdens of mind; serious mental attention" Late Old English "concern, anxiety caused by apprehension of evil or the weight of many burdens," Proto-Germanic **karō* "lament; grief, care" Source also of Old Saxon *kara* "sorrow;". The primary sense is that of inward grief, and the word is not connected, either in sense or form, with L. cura, care, of which	C."charge, oversight, attention or heed with a view to safety or protection" is attested from; The sense in *care of* in addressing (used from 1840).	Of all the different meanings of Care, only *Cuidados* & *Cura are* used in Spanish. There is a reluctance to Attend, Assist, have regard for etc..

		concern" is from To take care of "take in hand, do"; take care "be careful" also is from Negative sense 1.Old English "To be anxious or solicitous; grieve; feel concern or interest, 2. "Proto-Germanic "grief, care" 3. Old Saxon *karon* "to lament, to care, to sorrow, complain," 4. Old High German "complain, lament," 4.Gothic *karon* "to be anxious"), said to be from PIE root *gar- "cry out, call, scream" (source also of Irish *gairm* "shout, cry, call;"). 6. Latin "curar". think, consider. Positive sense senses, such as "have an inclination"; "have fondness for" seem to have developed later as mirrors to the earlier negative ones. a. feel concern or interest; attach importance to something. (be concerned,worry (oneself) trouble oneself, bother,mind) b. look after and provide for the needs of. (look after, take care of, tend, attend to,mind, minister to	the primary sense is pains or trouble bestowed upon something. [Century Dictionary] Old High German *chara* "wail, lament;" Gothic *kara* "sorrow, trouble, care". 1.Old English *carian, cearian* 2. "Proto-Germanic **karo-* "lament," 3. Old Saxon *karon* 4. Old High German *charon* 5.Gothic *karon* "to be anxious" said to be from PIE root *gar- "cry out, call, scream" (source also of Irish *gairm* "shout, cry, call;"). 6. Latin *Cogitatus*, *cura*. Co (combined, global) Agitare (to get moving, agitate, think things through) Cogitare – to think with movement. (To be moved to ...)		
ATTEND *Aspect of Care* *Verb*	Late 14c. 12c 14c	a."giving heed," "attention, attentiveness," b. "to direct one's mind or	Both *verb* and *noun* share origen from two Latin vocables a. Latin *attentionem* (nominative	Very little in Spanish Palliative Care	Attention "Mental heeding" This finding is highly relevant as id

Attention *Aspect of Care* *Noun*		energies," "Mental heeding" "give heed to," literally "to stretch toward", "be subject to" (now obsolete), "direct one's mind or energies" (archaic), from (…)	*attentio*) *ad* "to, toward" + *tendere* "stretch," b. Old French *"atendre"*	directed related to Cicely Saunders´s *"Active listening"*
ASSIST *Aspect of Care* *Verb*	early 15c 14c	*assisten* 'take one's stand'. stand by, take a stand near, attend," to set, place, cause to stand," *assister* "to stand by, help, put, place, assist" to help someone, aid, collaborate, cooperate, benefit	Origen from two Latin vocables Ad- to; + iuvare – "to help" from *ad-* 'to, at' + *sistere* Late Middle English, from Old French Latin *assister* "	Related: Assisted; assisting gives way to Medical assisted suicide attested from 1884
INSIST Aspect of Care	1580s 14c.	"take a stand, stand on, stand still; follow, pursue; insist, press vigorously, urge, dwell upon," from in- "upon" "take a stand," from PIE *si-st-, reduplicated form of root *sta- "to stand, make or be firm."	French *insister* Or directly from Latin *insistere* from root *en "in") + *sistere*	Interesting use of *insist* tends to happen when patient´s symptoms or family anguish are present.
ASSISTANCE & ASSIST Aspects of Care Noun*(s)*.	early 15c., 1570s	take one's stand by', 'take one's stand'. "act of helping or aiding; help given, aid," from the respective verbs "to help, aid, give assistance or support to in some undertaking or effort," "stand by, take a stand near, attend," To take a stand; to set, place, cause to stand"an act of assistance," from assist" stand still.	Late Middle English: from Old French *assister*, from Latin *assistere* 'from ad- 'to, at' + sistere from Old French *assistance* and Medieval Latin *assistentia*, Late Latin *adjuva* Latin *assistere* from assimilated form of *ad* "to" + *sistere*	

Table 2.
Palliative care terminology: vocables evolution through time and languages

I. Hospice

Noun.
Dates *from late 17th century*, 1818.

Meaning: 1. Greek: ξενία, xenia, προξενία.
2. "rest house for travellers"

From: Greco-Roman concept of hospitality as a divine right of the guest and a divine duty of the host.

French *hospice* "hospital, almshouse".

Old French *ospice* "hospice, shelter," also "hospitality," 13c.),

From Latin *hospitium* "hospitable reception, entertainment; hospitality, bonds of hospitality, relationship of guest and host.

From *hospes* (genitive *hospitis*) "guest; host," also "a stranger, foreigner". and positions the scholar in front of is the ancient.

II. Implement [43–46]

Verb. /ˈɪmplɪmɛnt/
Dates from the early 18th century.
Meaning: 1. To put (a decision, plan, agreement, etc.) into effect.
2. To start using a plan or system
3. To complete, perform, carry into effect," 1707

From Late Latin: *implementum*; *implere*: filling up.

Made of two Latin vocables

1. In (towards the center)
2. Plere (to fill up) (Greek polis, many)

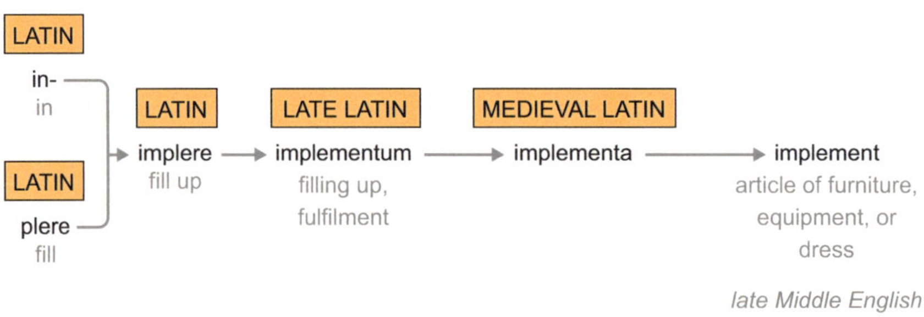

Noun. /ˈɪmplɪmɛnt/
Used in late Middle English to refer to different artifacts: furniture, gear, or dress'. Originates in part from the medieval Latin *implementa* (plural), in part from late Latin *implementum* 'filling up, fulfilment', both from Latin *implere* 'fill up' (later 'employ'), from in- 'in' + Latin plere 'fill'.

First used circa 1707 initially in Scottish English. As a noun it was a legal term meaning "fulfillment," From it comes implementation, its use first recorded 1913.

III. Implant [43–46]

Verb.
Dates from 1540, Old French.

Meaning:

I. Transitive verb
1a: to fix or set securely or deeply
1b: to set permanently in the consciousness or habit patterns: inculcate
2: to insert in living tissue

II. Intransitive verb
To undergo implantation.

If you implant an idea or attitude in people, you make it become accepted or believed.

Medieval latin.

In (towards the center).
Plant- see in, to plant, and observe.
implant (v.)

1540s, "to plant in" (abstractly, of ideas, emotions, etc.), from French *implanter* "to insert, engraft" (alongside Old French emplanter "to plant"), literally "plant in," from assimilated form of in- "into, in, on, upon" (from PIE root *en "in") + planter "to plant" (see plant (n.)). Meaning "surgically implant (something) in the body" is from 1886, originally of teeth. Implanted is attested earlier, from early 15c., probably based on Medieval Latin *implantus*. Related: Implanting.

Noun.
implant (n.)

1890, "thing implanted;" 1941 as "action of implanting," from implant (v.). Related: Implants, which is attested by 1981 as short for breast implants (1976).

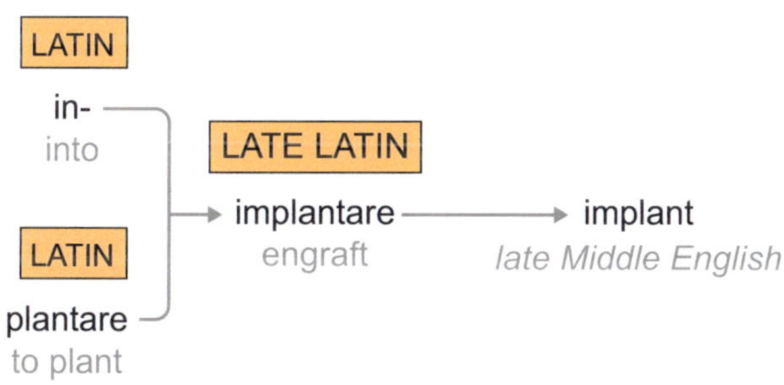

late Middle English: from late Latin implantare 'engraft', from Latin in- 'into' + plantare 'to plant'. (Oxford Languages Definitions)

implant (v.) 1540s, "to plant in" (abstractly, of ideas, emotions, etc.), from French implanter "to insert, engraft" (alongside Old French emplanter "to plant"), literally "plant in," from assimilated form of in- "into, in, on, upon". (Online Etymology dictionary).

Relevance: The difference between the notions conceived through these two verbs is very important. Implementing a Palliative Care Program speaks of "working at it" and "being part of the development". While implanting a Palliative Care Program talks about "having something new to deal with or to put up with" Something that needs to be taken into account by politicians, managers, et as it might mean the difference between people being engaged or not.

IV. Palliative Care

The term "Cuidados Paliativos" (Spanish/Portuguese) seem not to have incorporated the richness of meaning *Palliative Care* has afforded those who request, practice and receive it in the Anglo-Saxon context.

IV.a. Palliative

As a concept, in my experience, requires much explanation to those who encounter it for the first time, both as a patient or carer and as professionals. Explaining its meaning and aims to the general public can be very challenging indeed, although it must be said it has brought about really creative ways of explaining it in a practical way.

It is said that its use in English has seen a significant increase in the last 200 years due to the development of *Palliative Care.* Its Spanish translation is often used in politics such as in "we are going to remedy such a situation without palliatives", as a plural, indicaring with harshnesh.

IV. Palliative [43–46]

Adj.
Early 15c., french Palliatif, "serving to mitigate or alleviate" (a wound, illness, etc.); other meanings "cloak, cover, concealing;" from.

From Late Latin *Palliatus* "cloaked," from past participle of Late Latin palliare "cover with a cloak, conceal,"

Noun. Medieval Latin *palliativus* "under cloak, covert," from Latin *pallium* "a cloak" (see pall (n.)).

Dates from 1724.

Meaning"serving to extenuate by excuses or favorable representation". "that which mitigates or extenuates,"

Verb.
1779c. from the verb palliare 'to cloak','to protect′. (Online Etymology Dictionary)

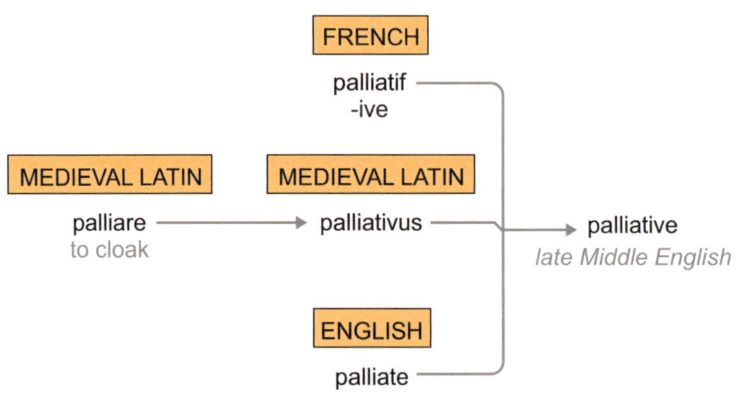

late Middle English (as an adjective) from French palliatif, –ive or medieval Latin palliativus, from the verb palliare 'to cloak'.

IV.b. Care [43–46]

The Spanish and Portuguese vocables "Cuidar" and "Cuidados" fall short of representing its multiple meanings within this context. The question to try to answer is: could this happen because it ignores certain conceptual aspects such as those of "that I care about the other", "care", "pay attention", "assist", "give assistance to", "medically treat." beyond "hacer curas" (wound and dressing management) and "curar" (cure in English) that has been reduced to in the Spanish language (while trying to offer its whole range of attentions)?

1. Noun
Origen
Old English *caru*, *cearu* "sorrow, anxiety, grief," also "burdens of mind; serious mental attention".
Late Old English "concern, anxiety caused by apprehension of evil or the weight of many burdens,"
Proto-Germanic **karō* "lament; grief, care" (source also of Old Saxon *kara* "sorrow;". The primary sense is that of inward grief, and the word is not connected, either in sense or form, with L. cura, care, of which the primary sense is pains or trouble bestowed upon something. [Century Dictionary].
Old High German *chara* "wail, lament;" Gothic *kara* "sorrow, trouble, care".
Dates from c. 1400

Meanings.

a. the provision of what is necessary for the health, welfare, maintenance, and protection of someone or something. (safe keeping, supervision, custody, charge, protection,keeping)
b. serious attention or consideration applied to doing something correctly or to avoid damage or risk. (caution, carefulness, wariness, awareness, heedfulness, heed)
c. "charge, oversight, attention or heed with a view to safety or protection" is attested from;

The sense in *care o*f in addressing (1840).

d. Meaning "objcct or matter of concern" is from 1580.

To take care of "take in hand, do" is from 1580s; take care "be careful" also is from 1580s.

2. Verb
Dates from

a. Old English *carian, cearian.*

Meanings

a. "be anxious or solicitous; grieve; feel concern or interest,
b. "from Proto-Germanic *karo- "lament," hence "grief, care".

Source also of Old Saxon karon.
"to lament, to care, to sorrow, complain," Old High German *charon* "complain, lament,"
Gothic karon "to be anxious"), said to be from PIE root *gar- "cry out, call, scream" (source also of Irish *gairm* "shout, cry, call;").
If so, the prehistoric sense development is from "cry" to "lamentation" to "grief." A different sense evolution is represented in related Dutch *karig*

"scanty, frugal," German *karg* "stingy, scanty." It is not considered to be related to Latin cura. Positive senses, such as "have an inclination" (1550s); "have fondness for" (1520s) seem to have developed later as mirrors to the earlier negative ones.

a. feel concern or interest; attach importance to something. (be concerned, worry (oneself), trouble oneself, bother, mind).
b. look after and provide for the needs of. (look after, take care of, tend, attend to, mind, minister to).

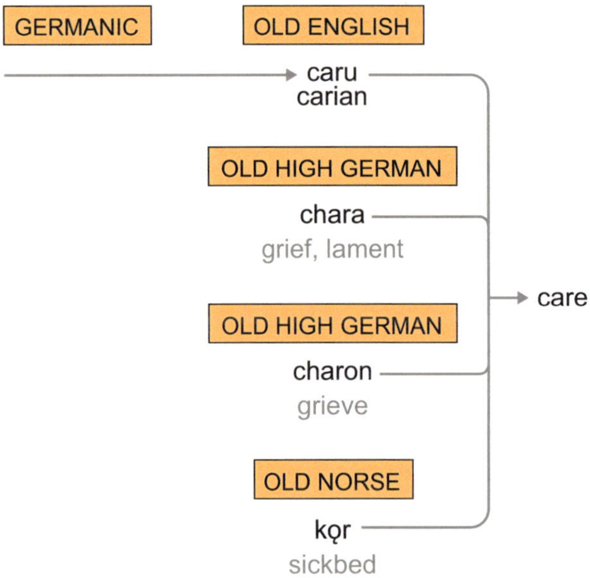

Old English caru (noun), carian (verb), of Germanic origin; related to Old High German chara 'grief, lament', charon 'grieve', and Old Norse kǫr 'sickbed'.
Proto-germanic. Karo. "Lament, grief, Care".
Old Saxon. Chara; wail, lament.
Old high German. Charon To wail.
Old English. Carucearu. "Sorrow, anxiety, grief".
Old English. Carian, cearian. "Be anxious, to grief, to feel concern".

"CARE".
To find the Spanish *Cuidados* translation, we need to look further and find how *care* has other interesting close relations that help work with a more active manner of manifesting one's need of being attended to.

Cogitatus (Latin)

Origin & history
Perfect passive participle of *cōgitō* ("think, consider").

Participle
cōgitātus *(masc.)* (*fem.* Cōgitāta, *neut.* cōgitātum)

1. thought, having been thought.
2. considered, having been pondered.

Descendants

- Asturian: *cuidáu*
- Galician: *coidado*

- Portuguese: *cuidado*
- Spanish: *cuidado*

Latin: cogitatus
Co (combined, global) Agitare (to get moving, agitate, think things through)
Cogitare – to think with movement.
The same studies could be undertaken for all of *Care* meanings and "close friends".

IV.b1 To Attend to [43–46]

1. *Verb*
   Dates from.
   a. Late 14c.

Originates from

a. Latin attentionem (nominative attentio).
b. Old French "atendre"(12c.)

Meaning

a."giving heed," "attention, attentiveness," 1300,
b. "to direct one's mind or energies,"

IV.b2 Attention

ad "to, towards" (see ad-) + tendere "stretch,"
Noun
Ad (to).
Tendere (stretch) one's mind to.
Dates from early 14c, 1300.

Originates from
Old French *atendre* "to expect, wait for, pay attention" (12c., Modern French attendre) and directly from Latin.

Meaning
–Attention "Mental heeding".

Note.
This finding is highly relevant as id directed related to Cicely Saunders's "*Active listening*".
"give heed to," literally "to stretch toward", "be subject to" (now obsolete), "direct one's mind or energies" (archaic), from (...).
(Online Etymology Dictionary)

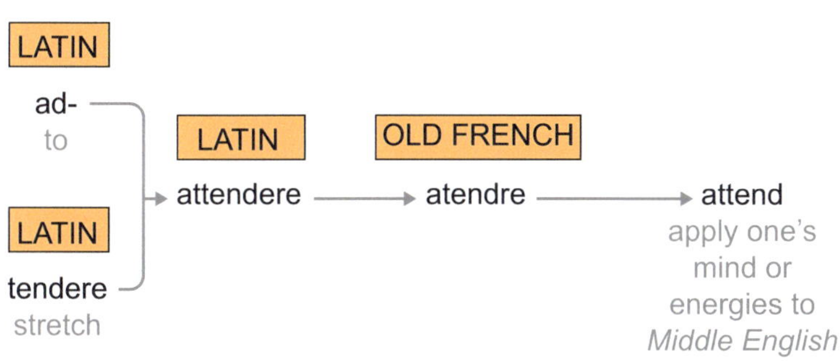

Middle English (in the sense 'apply one's mind or energies to'): from Old French atendre, from Latin attendere, from ad- 'to' + tendere 'stretch'.

IV.b3 To Assist [43–46]

Verb. Ad- to; + iuvare – "to help" from *ad-* 'to, at' + *sistere* 'take one's stand'.
Late Middle English, from.
Old French Latin *assister* "stand by, take a stand near, attend,"
from assimilated form of ad "to" (see ad-) + sistere "stand still, take a stand; to set, place, cause to stand,"
from PIE *si-st-, reduplicated form of root *sta- "to stand, make or be firm."
Latin *assister* Take one's stand by".
Originates

1. early 15c., *assisten*, "to help, aid, give assistance or support to in some undertaking or effort,"
2. 14c old French *assister* "to stand by, help, put, place, assist"

Dates
to help someone, aid, collaborate, cooperate, benefit.

IV.b4 To Insist

Dates 1580s,

Originates
French *insister* (14c.)
Or
directly from Latin *insistere.*
"take a stand, stand on, stand still; follow, pursue; insist, press vigorously, urge, dwell upon," from in- "upon".
(from PIE root *en "in") + sistere "take a stand," from PIE *si-st-, reduplicated form of root *sta- "to stand, make or be firm."
assist (v.) Related: Assisted; assisting. Medical assisted suicide attested from 1884.

IV.b5 Assistance

late Middle English: from Old French *assister*, from Latin *assistere* 'take one's stand by', from *ad-* 'to, at' + *sistere* 'take one's stand'.

Noun.
"act of helping or aiding; help given, aid," from the respective verbs.
Dates
early 15c.,

Originates from
from Old French *assistance* and Medieval Latin *assistentia*, Late latin adjuva

Meaning
"to help, aid, give assistance or support to in some undertaking or effort,"

Originates
Latin *assistere*
"stand by, take a stand near, attend,"
from assimilated form of ad "to" (see ad-) + *sistere* "stand still,

Meaning
To take a stand; to set, place, cause to stand,
"from PIE *si-st-, reduplicated form of root *sta- "to stand, make or be firm."

Related: Assisted; assisting. Medical assisted suicide attested from 1884.
assist (n.) 1570s, "an act of assistance," from assist.

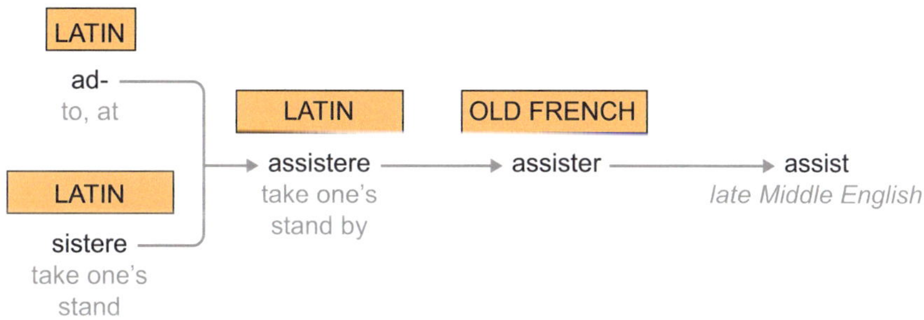

late Middle English: from Old French assister, from Latin assistere 'take one's stand by', from ad- 'to, at' + sistere 'take one's stand'.

6. Conclusion

Can you say something to comfort me? The Polish man Cicely Saunders considered to have been the *Palliative Care* patient to set the bases for the Modern Hospice Movement, asked her. A beautiful research question which proves incredibly difficult to give an answer to in a timely, honest and personalized way [46, 47]. A question that demands words constructed and delivered in a soothing, comforting manner. A question that leaves out action, doing to, as we often want to do: administering medication, offering therapeutic and surgical options less sought than human verbal interaction.

Language in its different forms is very important to transmit knowledge, affection, security ... and so much more too. PC uses not only spoken and written language but also body language. Language requires the support of concepts known, accepted and used by most. We conclude that too often those notions are not crystal clear and can provoke rejection, fear, isolation, doubt and increase the very suffering they should help alleviate.

Standing for and advocating for the promoting and contributing to the expansion and of Palliative Care [48], clear messages are important to avoid creating confusion. These messages should state truths such as "Palliative Care facilitates the process of dying without interfering with its natural course beyond the legitimate and ethical limits". It's a complex phenomenon that recognizes the intrinsic reality of professional work while touching on the most humane and compassionate principles of the art of palliating.

Today there is no doubt that the expansion and scope of Palliative Care is neither the desired nor the necessary [49]. In this the agreement is widespread. Where there is no agreement is in why this situation and therefore how to overcome it.

To appreciate and love something, it is necessary to know it. The better we know it, the easier it becomes to enjoy its bounties. The less we know it, the longer it will take us to accept it while finding what is needed to accept its place in our lives.

How much more difficult it is to accept something new when our life is threatened by a medical condition and we feel forced to face our own mortality. This is the reality found by professionals who try to introduce *Palliative* or *Supportive Care* to reinforce the person's own strengths, both natural and acquired.

It is at that point that the professional needs to give the sick and their family a master class on what they do, what they offer, where and when. Were they going to be seen by the cardiologist, the question might be "is that for the heart?" The number of questions that come up before accepting *Palliative* or *Supportive Care* are many more and are related to many different facets and it takes time to address each one of them appropriately. It has been the linguistic, semantic and its meaning and their impact on the patient's outcome that has fascinated me after many years working in the field and observing the change in the often the angry, frightened and frustrate people I meet when responding to a colleague's call for help and the relaxed, understanding, grateful and collaborative demeanor in the, by then patient under our care, we leave behind. Often part of our goodbye includes the question "will we see you again?" We have managed to establish a connection with the patient by spending time with them and their family and by talking to them about our role in their situation.

At a time when reassurance, otherness and presence can communicate so much, the power of language is immense in relationships that are short at the same time as they are intense.

Our work confirms the power of words and the importance of exerting the *Active Listening* key in the holistic care promoted by Cicely Sanders to alleviate Total Pain [7]. It pioneers in the recognition of scientific linguistics as fundamental to improve delivery of Palliative Care improving quality of translation to new languages. This will need promoting due care is taken by working towards methodologically scientific ways of conceptualization in language production with language-specific perspectives and event construal for different cultures who communicate in different languages.

An exciting topic to research, *Palliative Care Linguistics* will need further work in the future because, just as Cicely Saunders said about *pain* "There is so much to learn about explaining palliative concepts and the models of care!"

This chapter invites the reader to recognize the relationship between the expansion of PC and the appropriate conceptualization of the ideas, terminology and words used by those working in what constitutes its "deepest core", where its true significance is.

Additional information

Figures in this chapter are adapted from Oxford Languages Definitions & Online Etymology Dictionary.

Author details

Maria Teresa Garcia-Baquero Merino[1,2*†], María Victoria Roqué Sánchez[1], Katherine Pettus[3,4,5] and Micaela Menarguez Carreño[1]

1 Universidad Católica San Antonio de Murcia (UCAM), Spain

2 Palliative Care Consultant, UK

3 Palliative Care at International Association Hospice Palliative Care (IAHPC), USA

4 Columbia University, USA

5 Health Law and Policy, University of California San Diego, USA

*Address all correspondence to: mtgarcia@ucam.edu

†Madrid first Regional Palliative Care Coordinator 2008–2016.

References

[1] Saunders C. (2001). The evolution of palliative care. Journal of the royal society of medicine. journals.sagepub.com

[2] DU BOULAY, S., & RANKIN, M. (2007). Cicely Saunders: the founder of the modern hospice movement. London, SPCK.

[3] García-Baquero Merino MT. (October 2018) Palliative Care: Taking the Long View. Frontiers. Pharmacology. 9:1140. doi: 10.3389/fphar.2018. 01140.

[4] Pettus K. 2017. Palliative Care: The Pearl of Great Price. Huffington Post electronic.

[5] Randall F., Downie R S. (2006). The Philosophy of Palliative Care: Critique and Reconstruction. Oxford University Press

[6] IAHPC. Global Consensus based palliative care definition. (2018). Houston, TX: The International Association for Hospice and Palliative Care. Available from https://hospicecare.com/what-we-do/projects/consensus-based-definition-of-palliative-care/definition/ [Accessed February 1 2021]

[7] Clark, D. (1999). Total pain', disciplinary power and the body in the work of Cicely Saunders, 1958–1967. Social science & medicine, 49(6), 727–736.

[8] Levi E. (2016). It's time to reclaim the heart of medicine. Available from https://www.kevinmd.com/blog/post-author/eric-levi [Accessed February 2021]

[9] Longrigg, J. (2013). Greek rational medicine: philosophy and medicine from Alcmaeon to the Alexandrians. Routledge.

[10] Miles, S. H. (2005). The Hippocratic Oath and the ethics of medicine. Oxford University Press.

[11] KR Hexem, CJ Mollen, K Carrol. (2011) How parents of children receiving paediatric palliative care use religion, spirituality, or life philosophy in tough times. Journal of Palliative Medicine. online.liebertpub.com

[12] B McNamara. (2004). How parents of children with life threatening conditions draw upon religion, spirituality, or life philosophy is not empirically well described. Social science & medicine Elsevier

[13] PL Hudson, S Aranda. (2004). Meeting the supportive needs of family caregivers in palliative care: challenges for health professionals Journal of palliative medicine. online.liebertpub.com

[14] Kazanjian A. (2010) Cultural conceptualizations of hospice palliative care: more similarities than differences. Palliative Medicine. 24(5):510–522. DOI: 10.1177/0269216309351380.

[15] Saunders C. (1978). The Philosophy of Terminal Care. First published in The Management of Terminal Disease, 1st ed, ed. C. Saunders, pp. 193–202. London. Edward Arnold.

[16] Saunders C. (November, 1965). 'Watch with me'. Nursing Times. 61 (48):1615–1617.

[17] Stjernswärd J, Colleau SM, Ventafridda V. (1996). The World Health Organization Cancer Pain and Palliative Care Program. Past, present and future. J Pain Symptom Manage;12: 65–72.

[18] Foley, K. (2005). The Past and Future of Palliative Care. The Hastings Center Report, 35(6), S42-S46. Available from http://www.jstor.org/

stable/24290050 [Accessed February 13, 2021]

[19] Pettus K. (2015)"Expert Patients" Moved by Love — Palliative care in a non-denominational ethos. https://globalpalliativecare.wordpress.com/2015/08/

[20] Highet G, Crawford D, Murray SA, et al. (2014). Development and evaluation of the Supportive and Palliative Care Indicators Tool (SPICT): a mixed-methods study. BMJ Supportive & Palliative Care; 4: 285–290.

[21] Hui, D., De La Cruz, M., Mori, M. et al. (2013). Concepts and definitions for "supportive care," "best supportive care," "palliative care," and "hospice care" in the published literature, dictionaries, and textbooks. Support Care Cancer 21, 659–685.

[22] González Luis, José. (1992). "Origen y espíritu de las antiguas peregrinaciones ad loca sancta." Fortunatae número 3.

[23] Twycross R.G . A Time to Die. Christian Medical Fellowship– January 1, 1994. ISBN-10: 0906747287; ISBN-13: 978-0906747285.

[24] Anderson, M. S., Ronning, E. A., Devries, R., & Martinson, B. C. (2010). Extending the Mertonian Norms: Scientists' Subscription to Norms of Research. The Journal of higher education, 81(3), 366–393. https://doi.org/10.1353/jhe.0.0095

[25] Riesch H, Potter C.(2014);. Citizen science as seen by scientists: methodological, epistemological and ethical dimensions, Public Underst Sci. 23:107–120.

[26] Anderson, M. S., Ronning, E. A., Devries, R., & Martinson, B. C. (2010). Extending the Mertonian Norms: Scientists' Subscription to Norms of Research. The Journal of higher education, 81(3), 366–393. https://doi.org/10.1353/jhe.0.0095

[27] Kamal, A. H., Harrison, K. L., Bakitas, M., Dionne-Odom, J. N., Zubkoff, L., Akyar, I., Pantilat, S. Z, O'Riordan, D. L., Bragg, A. R., Bischoff, K. E., & Bull, J. (2015). Improving the Quality of Palliative Care Through National and Regional Collaboration Efforts. Cancer control: journal of the Moffitt Cancer Center, 22(4), 396–402. https://doi.org/10.1177/107327481502200405

[28] Kuhn TS. 1970 (1962). The structure of scientific revolutions. (268-269). 2nd ed., The University of Chicago Press, Chicago;

[29] Merton, R K (1942): "Science and Technology in a Democratic Order" Journal of Legal and Political Sociology: 1, 115-126. [Traducción al español como "La estructura normativa de la ciencia" en el volumen II de "La Sociología de la Ciencia" Alianza Editorial 1977, traducción de The Sociology of Science – Theoretical and Empirical Investigations, 1973]

[30] Hamilton, J. (1995). Dr. Balfour Mount and the cruel irony of our care for the dying. CMAJ. 1;153(3):334–6. PMID: 7542165; PMCID: PMC1487213.

[31] Mount B. https://www.lifenews.com/2013/04/14/founder-of-palliative-care-balfour-mount-opposes-euthanasia/ [Accessed February 2021].

[32] Mount B. M. A Personal Odyssey. Illness, Crisis & Loss, 11(1), 90–103

[33] Selman L, Speck P, Gysels M, Agupio G, Dinat N, Downing J, Gwyther L, Mashao T, Mmoledi K, Moll T, Sebuyira LM, Ikin B, Higginson IJ, Harding R. (2013) 'Peace' and 'life worthwhile' as measures of spiritual well-being in African palliative care: a mixed-methods study. Health Qual Life Outcomes; 11:94.

[34] Selman L, (2012). Spiritual well-being and its assessment among patients receiving palliative care in South Africa and Uganda. Unpublished doctoral dissertation, King's College London.

[35] Delbanco, T., Berwick, D. M., Boufford, J. I., Ollenschläger, G., Plamping, D., & Rockefeller, R. G. (2001). Healthcare in a land called People Power: nothing about me without me. Health expectations, 4(3), 144–150.

[36] Boulay du Shirley & Rankin, M. (2011).Cicely Saunders. Fundadora del movimiento Hospice de Cuidados Paliativos. Edición Española. Palabra hoy, traducido de DU BOULAY, S., & Rankin, M. (2007). Cicely Saunders: the founder of the modern hospice movement. London, SPCK.

[37] Gómez-Batiste, X., Porta-Sales, J., Pascual, A., Nabal, M., Espinosa, J., Paz, S. & Geli, M. (2007). Catalonia WHO palliative care demonstration project at 15 Years (2005). Journal of pain and symptom management, 33(5), 584–590.

[38] Gómez-Batiste, X., Blay, C., Roca, J., & Fontanals, M. D. (2012). Innovaciones conceptuales e iniciativas de mejora en la atención paliativa del siglo XXI. Med Paliat, 19(3), 85–86.

[39] González Luis, José. (1992) "Origen y espíritu de las antiguas peregrinaciones ad loca sancta." Fortunatae número 3.

[40] Von Stutterheim, C., & Nüse, R. (2003). Processes of conceptualization in language production: Language-specific perspectives and event construal. Linguistics, 41(5), 851–881.

[41] Biebow, B., Szulman, S., & Clément, A. J. (1999, May). TERMINAE: A linguistics-based tool for the building of a domain ontology. In International Conference on Knowledge Engineering and Knowledge Management (pp. 49–66). Springer, Berlin, Heidelberg.

[42] Flores Talavera Gabriela ¿Cómo hacer la conceptualización para un marco teórico? Blog Formando Investigadores. Lunes, 14 de febrero de 2011.

[43] Cambridge inglésdictionary.cambridge.org

[44] Merriam-Websterwww.merriam-webster.com

[45] Online Etymology Dictionary. https://www.etymonline.com/. Fuentes: Weekley's "An Etymological Dictionary of Modern English," Klein's "A Comprehensive Etymological Dictionary of the English Language," "Oxford English Dictionary" (second edition), "Barnhart Dictionary of Etymology," Holthausen's "Etymologisches Wörterbuch der Englischen Sprache," Kipfer and Chapman's "Dictionary of American Slang."

[46] Oxford Languages Definitions (online) Academic. www.oed.com

[47] Global Palliative Care. (2017) Reflections from the periphery. https://globalpalliativecare.wordpress.com/2017/02/

[48] Sprangers MA, Sloan JA, Barsevick A, et al. (2010). Scientific imperatives, clinical implications, and theoretical underpinnings for the investigation of the relationship between genetic variables and patient-reported quality-of-life outcomes. Qual Life Res. 19: 1395–1403.

[49] Knights D. et al., (2020). Upside down solutions: palliative care and COVID-19. BMJ Supportive & Palliative Care.

Chapter 18

Perspective Chapter: Who Is Making Decisions? An Open Letter to Healthcare Professionals in the Developing World

Rasheed Ofosu-Poku

Abstract

The educational standard of people living in low- and middle-income countries (LMICs) such as Ghana is relatively low. Thus, most resources of information about health available on electronic and print media remain to a large extent non-beneficial to them. They rely mostly on healthcare professionals to discuss about their health, illnesses, resources available for care, and how and to what extent the available resources can meet their needs and expectations. Some healthcare professionals in these LMICs, instead of taking the opportunity to carry out these educational and empowering discussions with patients and their families, assume a paternalistic role, making decisions unilaterally and involving them only minimally in providing care. This article, instead of being written as a scholarly referenced paper exploring ethical issues of autonomy and informed decision making, has been worded as a letter to healthcare professionals. Although it addresses healthcare professional in LMICs in general, it does not in any way imply that none adheres to these important ethical principles.

Keywords: healthcare professionals, informed decision making, autonomy, paternalistic, patients and family

1. Introduction

The educational standard of people living in low- and middle-income countries is very low, with one-third of its youth dropping-out of school before secondary level of education [1]. The literacy level among graduates of tertiary educational institutions in most low- and middle-income countries is also low [2]. On account of this poor literacy rate, majority of people living in these countries depend on healthcare professionals for information about health and illness [3]. A similar situation exists in Ghana, a lower middle-income country.

The burden of chronic non-communicable diseases in Ghana is rising [4], and the importance of patients and their families understanding the disease they are suffering from, the treatment modalities available, and the objective of each modality is crucial to adherence to therapy [5–7]. However, in the course of caring for patients in the last few months to a year of life, the author has noted a generally poor level of knowledge among patients and families about the disease affecting

IntechOpen

them and the objective of therapy they have sometimes received for several months. They, therefore, present to the palliative care unit with expectations of cure and expressions of feeling of anger at and disappointment with healthcare professionals for not being open to and honest with them from the beginning.

This article has therefore been addressed to colleague health professionals as a letter, to highlight the voices and cries of these patients and their families, and to appeal to healthcare professionals to involve them actively rather than passively in their care.

2. The letter

My dear colleagues,

I would like to congratulate all of you – doctors, nurses, pharmacists, laboratory scientists, health information officers and other healthcare professionals in the world in general and developing countries in particular – for the tremendous work you do every day and the sacrifices you make for your patients.

We, however, do not have to let the feeling and thought of having done or sacrificed a lot cause us to relent on our efforts. We cannot rest until our patients and their families are satisfied with the care we provide. How can we get them satisfied and grateful for the care we render?

How can patients and their families be satisfied and grateful for what we do if they do not understand their illness, our plan of management, and the role they have to play towards care? Thus, our goal – patient and family satisfaction – seems an impossible feat without discussing with them what we think is happening, the services available to meet their healthcare needs, and the possible consequences each course of action chosen may result in.

My dear colleagues, patients and their families are not oblivious of what is happening to and around them. They know the signs and symptoms they present with better than us. Our specialty is in our ability to connect the different issues they present with to make meaning – to arrive at a diagnosis. When they present to us, they seek first to understand what exactly is happening to them; then what we can offer and how what is being offered will help them.

Unfortunately, on both counts, health professionals in low- and middle-income countries such as Ghana generally perform below expectation. How much do we discuss with patients and their families to help them understand what they are experiencing? Most of the time, we say nothing after hearing their issues and asking a number of questions; we just hand over a prescription and/or laboratory request. Few times, especially when the patient has a life-limiting illness and wishes to understand what is happening to them, we tell them half-truths under the guise of 'protecting them' or 'maintaining their hope'. Really? Are we protecting them or protecting ourselves? Do we not fear admitting that we do not have all the answers, and that we cannot offer cure?

Does the course of a life-limiting disease change by keeping information away from the patient and/or family? Does it change the fact that our medical or surgical therapy may not offer cure but reduce the disease burden, if anything at all? If our answers to the above are the obvious 'no', then are we not putting the patient and family at a great disadvantage of not putting right their affairs before the disease causes them to be incapacitated?

For a second, let's turn around the table. Ask yourself, 'if I or my relative is suffering from a life-limiting illness, will I want to be told everything so that I am mentally prepared?' For most of us, our answer will be in the affirmative. That information is so valuable, not only in preparing oneself mentally or emotionally towards the imminence of the inevitable, but is the basis for pulling together all physical, social and spiritual resources one can have to cope with the stresses associated with suffering a life-limiting illness. So why keep from patients such valuable information about themselves?

Consider the case of a mechanic who is called upon to attend to a faulty vehicle. After asking a few questions from the driver and checking a few issues on the vehicle, he scribbles a few things on a sheet of paper, directs that whatever is stated thereon be obtained from a particular shop to get the vehicle fixed, and takes his leave. Who can stand that? That is why the mechanic does not even imagine such a situation. Rather, what he does is to explain to and show the driver what he thinks is wrong, what he can do about it, what is unavailable and has to be purchased, where to purchase it, and the options available to resolve the fault so that the driver will make a choice – an informed choice, an informed decision. So why is this logical principle so challenging for most healthcare professionals?

The argument of 'the patient/family must ask if they have any questions' is feeble. Over the course of time, we (health professionals) have succeeded in creating around us an aura of being 'superhuman' rather 'gods'. We have successfully replaced respect for the profession with fear of the professionals. Thus, our patients and family cannot even ask us what we think about their illness. The result is that they will go to those who will provide them information about the illness to help them make meaning of the situation. As to whether that information is true or false is really a secondary matter to them. One would be surprised to learn how much patients and their families pay for seeking such care that only causes their health to get worse. In the end, they report to the hospital with the patient in a worse state after exhausting all their resources. Interestingly, our reaction as healthcare professionals is to blame them for not reporting to the hospital at the outset. What we fail to recognize is that we are primarily responsible for their course of action. The earlier we as healthcare professionals begin to look within ourselves – our attitudes and actions – to identify our role in improving the image of our professions and the healthcare system, the better it will be for ourselves and the people we have pledged to serve.

Another intriguing related issue is how healthcare decisions are made in a system where patients and family have little information. Do clinicians just make unilateral decisions for patients and their families? If no, on the basis of what information do they contribute to decision making about their care or the care of their loved ones? Only two logical conclusions come to mind, either clinicians really make decisions unilaterally for patients and their families, or they provide some information and impose their decisions. In both cases, such clinicians occupy the role of 'fathers' to the patient and family. That is, they convey to patients and their families through actions the following message: *"we are more knowledgeable and experienced than you in caring for the sick. We want to do 'A' and 'B' for you or your relative. Just do it and ask no questions because you, like a child, have no knowledge and experience in healthcare".*

That is exactly how patients and their families feel. Hence, they ask no questions. When they get fed up with prescriptions and laboratory requests for which they see no direct benefit to the wellbeing and quality of life of the patient, they request discharge. No amount of words can change that decision because they have gone through such an awful experience with healthcare professionals that, they would rather stay home and die in peace. That is their reaction; they are not involved actively in any decision making, but when they make the only decision about their care that has actually come from them, we try to talk them out. That will not work.

O my dear colleagues, where is the ethical principle of autonomy we learnt during our training? Why have we regulated informed decision making to the background and harnessed for ourselves a paternalistic role in rendering care in the 21st century.

O my dear colleagues, let us keep in mind that patients have the right to every information about themselves and their care. They have the right to seek another opinion from any other person they desire even if we disagree with their choice. Our responsibility is to provide them all the information they need to make whatever decision is right to them, and to provide them the best care we can offer in the context of their decision. There should be no coercion or imposition of decision.

If we really desire the best for our patients and their families, we must completely deflate our pride and come down to their level, offer them every information they need to know regarding their illness and the care we are providing, involve them actively in decision making at every step of treatment, and respect their decisions even if we are uncomfortable with it. If this simple but golden principle is kept in view, the public perception about healthcare professionals practicing allopathic medicine will totally transform and we will in no time be their first and only choice in seeking healthcare.

Yours sincerely,

Rasheed Ofosu-Poku.

The author is a nurse specialist in palliative care at the Komfo Anokye Teaching Hospital in Ghana. Palliative care services in Ghana are available in isolated facilities in Kumasi (Komfo Anokye Teaching Hospital), Accra (Korle-Bu Teaching Hospital) and the Eastern Region (Tetteh Quarshie Memorial Hospital). With respect to human resource, the number of trained clinicians providing palliative care services is inadequate to meet the need of the hospitals and the administrative regions within which they are found. Thus, many patients who need palliative care never get the chance to receive it. Furthermore, most patients and families who eventually get referred for palliative care live for a few more weeks to few months, and are thus unable to obtain all the benefits associated with palliative care services. The lack of a national policy on integration of palliative care within Ghana's healthcare system is, perhaps, the greatest contributory to the inadequate availability of palliative care services in the country.

The availability of essential drugs such as opioids is crucial to the practice of palliative care. In Ghana, morphine is increasingly being made available as a prescription-only drug in pharmacies in its major cities. However, other essential opioids such as methadone are completely unavailable for use in palliative care. Thus, pain management is less than optimal in patients with severe renal impairment and those with bone metastases whose pain is difficult to control with other opioids. Fentanyl transdermal patch is available in only few pharmacies in the two major cities of Accra and Kumasi.

Thus, although some effort is being made in Ghana to provide palliative care services, there are many challenges ranging from lack of a national policy on palliative care to poor human resource capacity and poor availability of opioids for pain control.

Acknowledgements

I am grateful to my colleagues (Ms. Gladys Anyane, Ms. Alberta Delali Dzaka, Ms. Mary Owusu Appiah, Dr. Michael Owusu-Ansah, Dr. Anita Eseenam Agbeko and Dr. Kathryn Spangenberg), all members of the Palliative Care Team of the Komfo Anokye Teaching Hospital for their encouragement and review of this article.

Conflict of interest

The author declares no conflict of interest with respect to this article or its publication.

Author details

Rasheed Ofosu-Poku
Directorate of Family Medicine, Komfo Anokye Teaching Hospital, Kumasi, Ghana

*Address all correspondence to: alienph1215@gmail.com

References

[1] T. Khokar, "A crisis in learning: 9 charts from the 2018 World Development Report," *World Bank*, 2017. https://blogs.worldbank.org/opendata/crisis-learning-9-charts-2018-world-development-report (accessed Nov. 30, 2020).

[2] L. Crawfurd, "Literacy of Adults in Developing Countries: New Data from a Skills Survey," *Centre for Global Development*, 2016. https://www.cgdev.org/blog/literacy-adults-developing-countries-new-data-skills-survey (accessed Nov. 30, 2020).

[3] S. Das, M. N. Mia, S. Manzoor, A. Hanifi, S. Hoque, and A. Bhuiya, "Health literacy in a community with low levels of education: findings from Chakaria, a rural area of Bangladesh," *BMC Public Health*, vol. 17, no. 203, pp. 1-10, 2017, doi: 10.1186/s12889-017-4097-y.

[4] Ministry of Health Ghana, *National Policy for the Prevention and Control of Chronic Non-Communicable Diseases in Ghana*, no. August. 2012.

[5] L. R. Martin, S. L. Williams, K. B. Haskard, and M. R. Dimatteo, "The challenge of patient adherence," *Ther. Clin. Risk Manag.*, vol. 1, no. 3, pp. 189-199, 2005.

[6] C. I. Fernandez-lazaro *et al.*, "Adherence to treatment and related factors among patients with chronic conditions in primary care: a cross-sectional study," *BMC Fam. Pract.*, vol. 20, no. 132, pp. 1-12, 2019.

[7] A. Gavrilova *et al.*, "Knowledge about Disease, Medication Therapy, and Related Medication Adherence Levels among Patients with Hypertension," *Medicina (B. Aires).*, vol. 55, no. 715, pp. 1-12, 2019.